AF583554

Slow Cooker

THE ULTIMATE COLLECTION

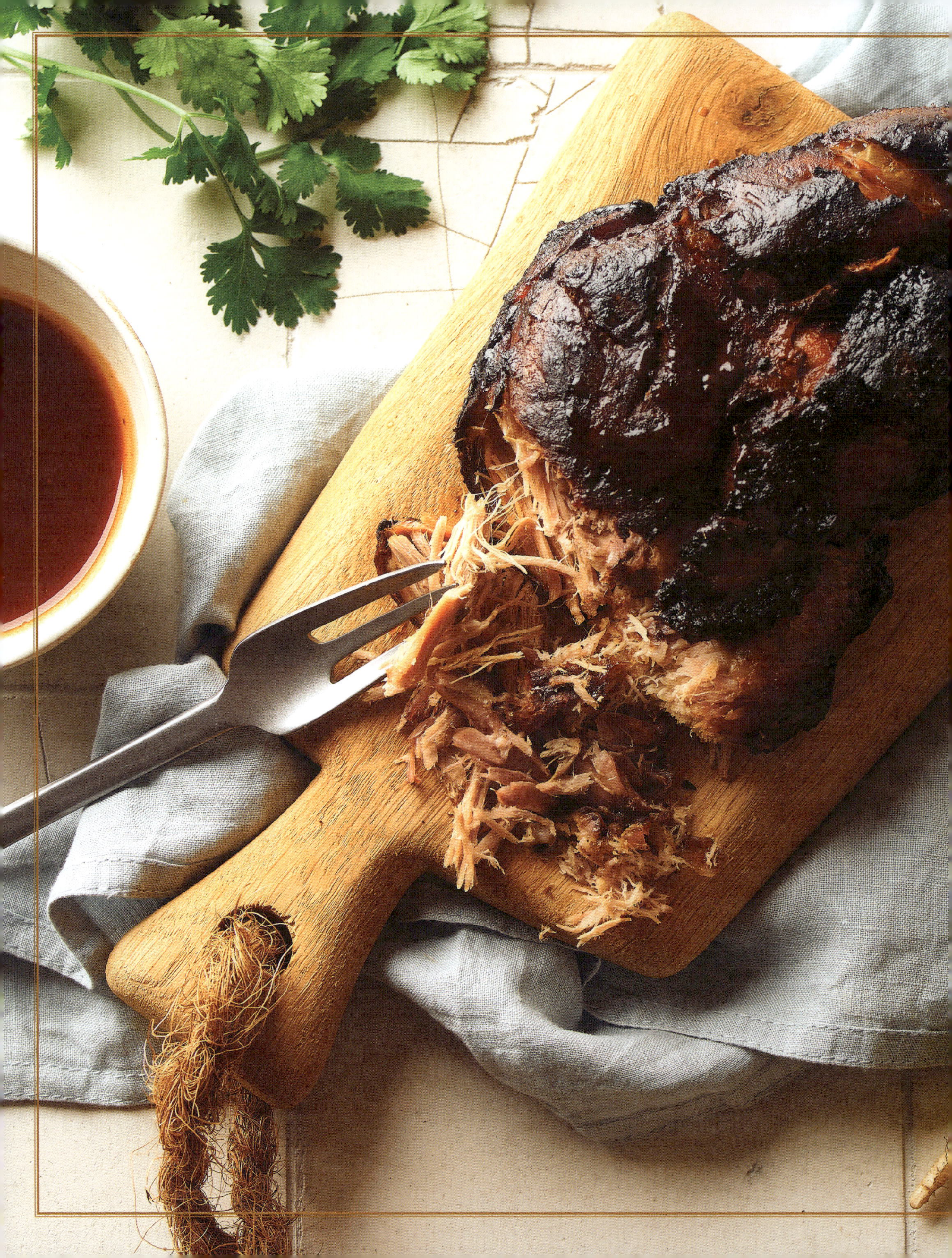

Slow Cooker

THE ULTIMATE COLLECTION

The absolute best recipes, so you can make the most of your appliance.

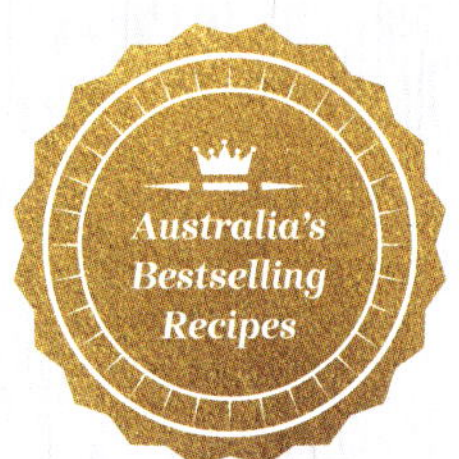

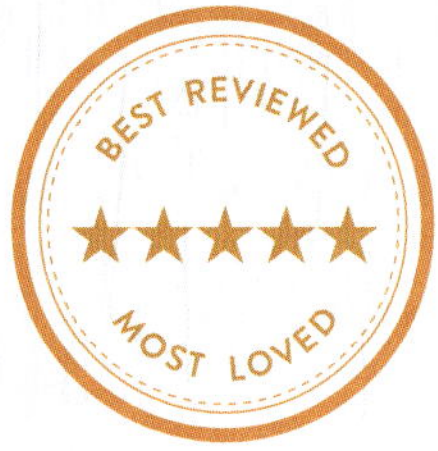

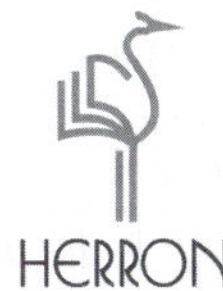

Contents

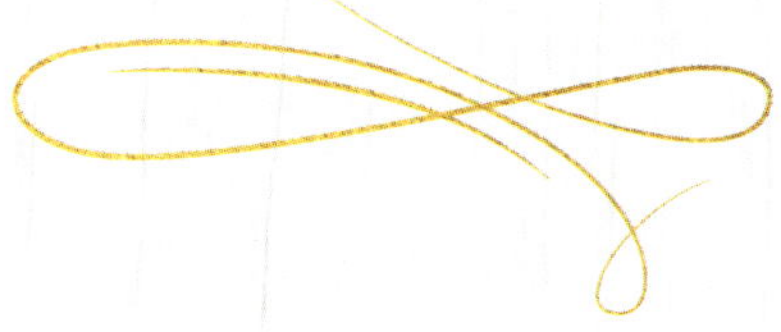

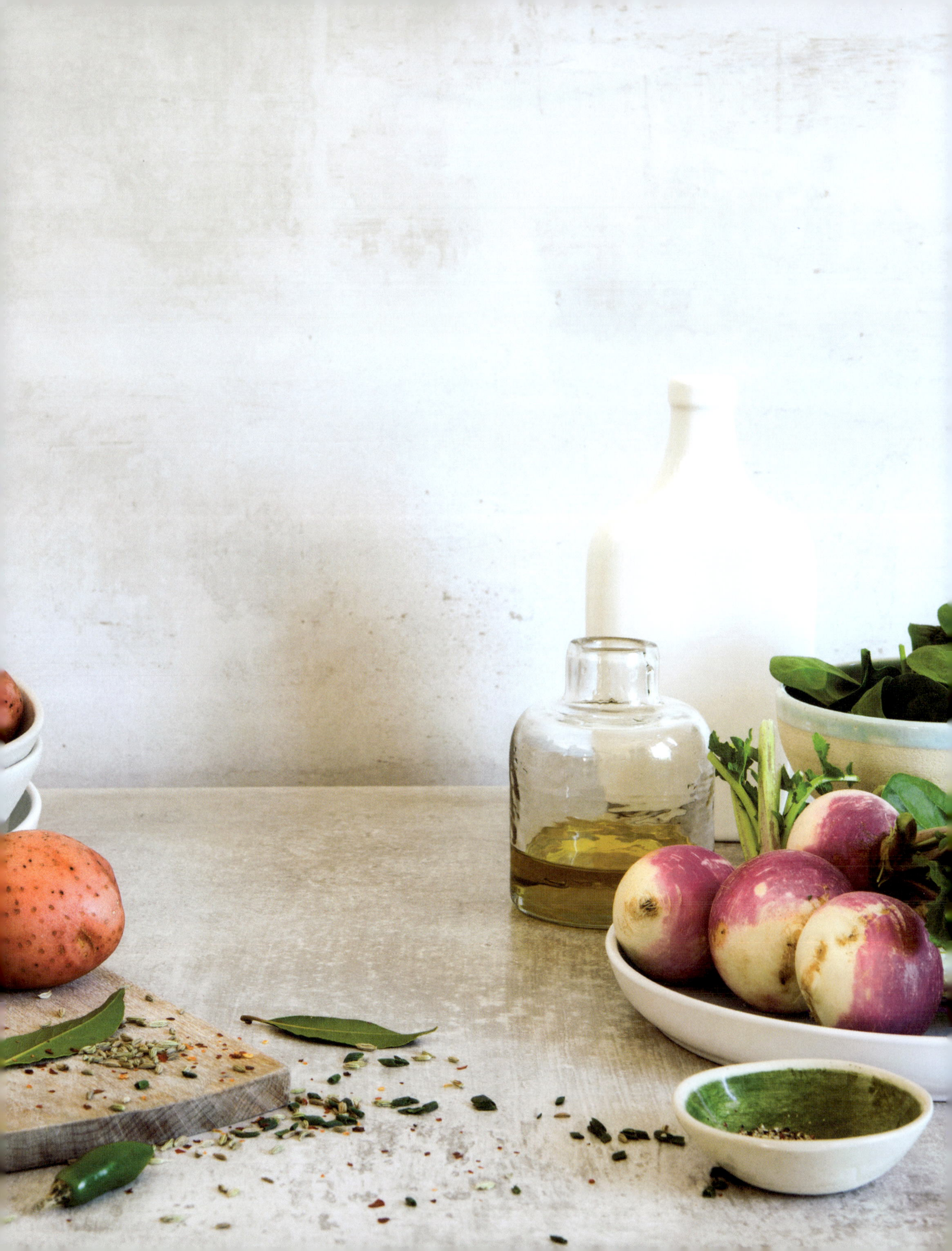

Welcome to the Ultimate Collection of Slow Cooker Recipes.

The recipes in this book are the best of the best. They have been handpicked from a selection of Australia's bestselling slow-cooker cookbooks, so that you have the most useful, versatile and successful collection of recipes in one place. Packed full of inspiration, ideas and practical tips, they will set you on track to slow cooking with ease.

The magical world of slow cooking is here: delicious dinners are ready and waiting at just the flick of a switch. Whether you're a slow-cooking newbie or a dab hand, you'll find everyday go-to recipes in this book, as well as some surprises.

High or low. That's about the only technical instruction your slow cooker requires. Beyond that, you just need to master the basics of how to prepare ingredients, how much liquid to use, and what it is that you want to cook. Slow cooking is the art of the possible and almost anything is possible with this clever device. Whether it's sauces, condiments, curries, soups, Sunday 'roasts' or classic desserts, you can do it in the slow cooker. Dive in with one of the 200+ recipes in this book and you won't be disappointed.

We kick off this cookbook with recipes for red meat: that's the home turf of the slow cooker, which excels in helping you to create tender and flavourful stews and casseroles with almost unbelievable ease. In the next section, chicken and pork get the slow-cooker treatment with an exhaustive range of recipes from barbecue-style to baked, stewed and curried dishes.

Demonstrating the slow cooker's versatility, the next section contains a wide array of interesting recipes for fish and seafood meals, from jambalaya, chowder and fish pie to poached salmon fillets or soused herring.

If you or a family member is vegetarian, you can still make dinner time a breeze thanks to your slow cooker. In the Vegetables section of the book, we provide recipes for classics such as mac and cheese, vegetable ratatouille and vegetarian chilli as well as contemporary dishes such as vegan chickpea balls, quinoa taco mix and sesame tofu.

Finally, delicious and diverse desserts are the slow cooker's secret weapon. It is not just possible, it's incredibly easy to create classic creme brulee, chocolate cake, cheesecake or rice pudding in the slow cooker.

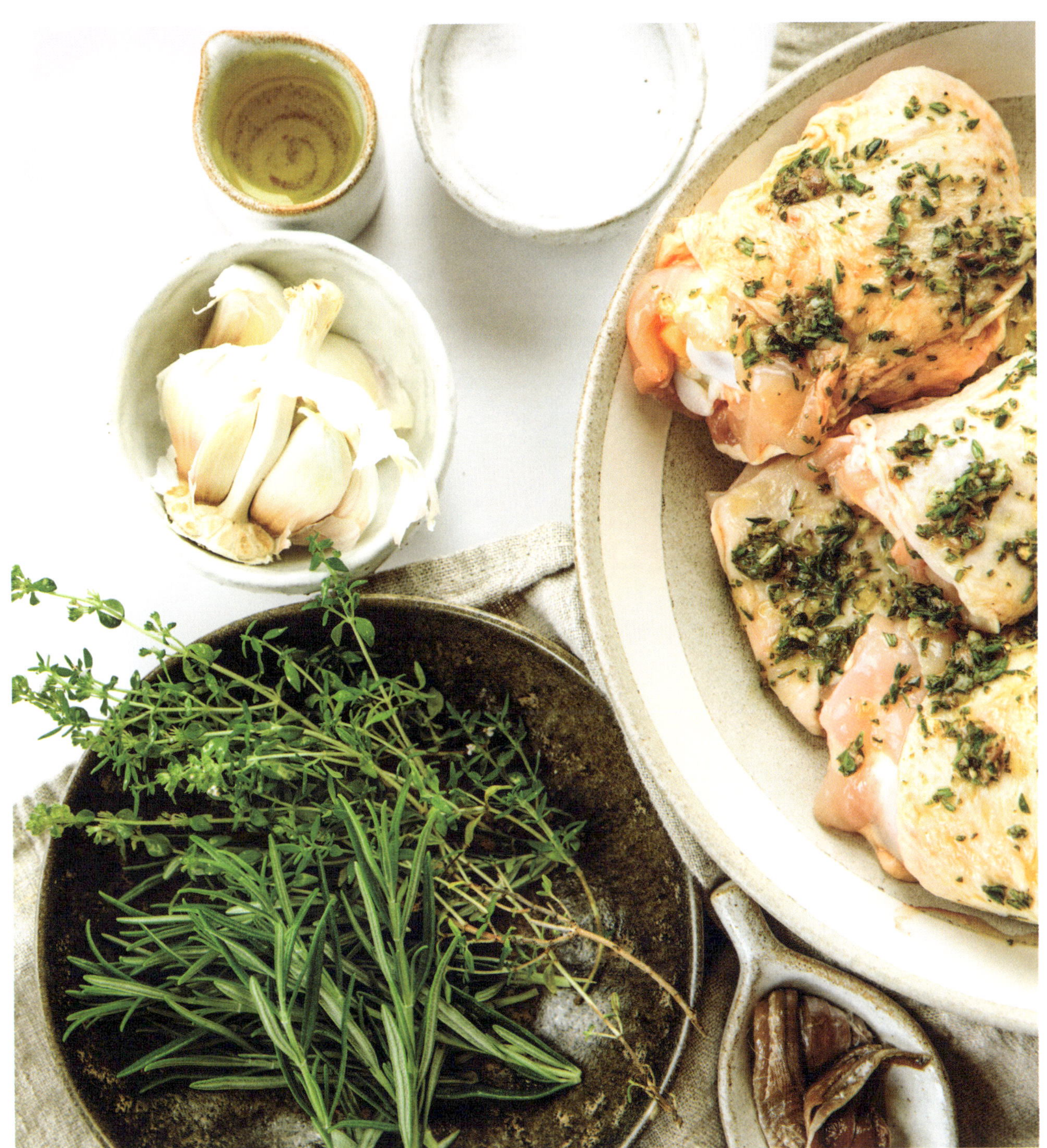

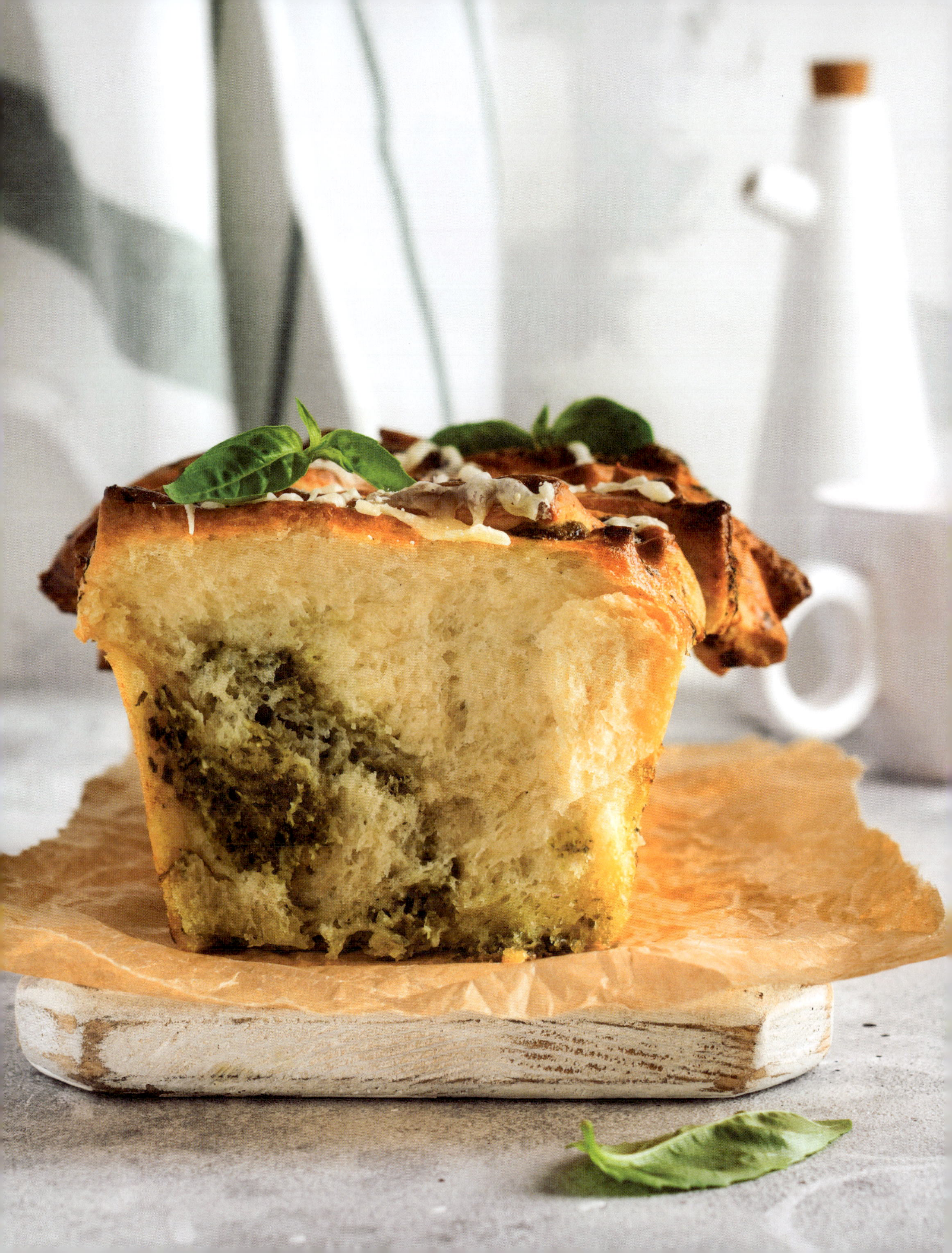

Tips for cooking in a slow cooker

Cooking in the slow cooker is easy, but it's a different method than traditional stovetop or oven cooking, so it's a good idea to follow these simple tips.

KEEP IT CHEAP, SIMPLE AND EASY

While the slow cooker can turn its hand to all kinds of cooking, even baking cakes, it's best suited to stews, casseroles and soups. The beauty of cooking these dishes in the slow cooker is that there is minimal prep required, the meat is generally very tender and cheap cuts of meat can be used. We've provided many recipes like this in this book, so keep an eye out for them and if you are just starting out then focus on these types of recipes first.

You can fry onions or brown meat before placing it in the slow cooker, if you like. Some recipes in this book recommend doing that because it can add extra flavour, but it isn't essential. Experiment and see what suits your tastes and your time frame.

The slow cooker excels with cheap cuts of meat such as pork shoulder, beef brisket or chicken thighs. Even better, you can use less meat than you might conventionally because the slow cooking process extracts a lot of meaty flavours. Bulk up with vegetables or pulses instead.

Preparing food the night before is a good idea. You can place pre-prepared vegetables or meat in the bowl of the slow cooker and leave it in the fridge overnight. In the morning, simply add liquids and turn on the cooker to have a meal ready for lunch or dinner. Likewise, you can cook breakfast items, stock, or anything you like overnight.

Leave your cooker alone after you've switched it on. There's no need to keep checking. Removing the lid releases heat and increases cooking time, so resist the temptation.

ADD LIQUIDS SPARINGLY

The slow cooker does not reduce liquids like conventional cooking does, so don't overdo the liquid that you add in the first place. Use the recipes in this book as your guide and experiment with more or less according to what works for you.

In order to keep food moist, liquids should cover the meat or vegetables in the slow cooker – just.

Never fill to the top of the cooker – depending on the recipe, half full or two-thirds full is enough.

HOW TO THICKEN SAUCES

Just as liquids don't reduce, sauces don't thicken in the slow cooker. But there are some easy ways to create a thicker sauce. Depending on the result you want, consider the following tips for reducing sauces in the slow cooker.

To create a thicker sauce from scratch – toss the meat in flour before placing it in the slow cooker, or if browning the meat in a frying pan add liquids and flour to create a simple sauce, then transfer this to the slow cooker.

To thicken slightly while cooking – remove or place the lid ajar for the final 30 minutes of cooking.

To thicken the sauce significantly while cooking, there are two options – At the end of cooking time transfer the sauce to a saucepan over high heat on the stove, and simmer, stirring, until the desired consistency is reached. Then pour the sauce over the final dish when ready to serve.

Alternatively, combine 1 tablespoon of cornflour with 1 tablespoon of cool tap water and stir to remove any lumps. Pour directly into the slow cooker 20-30 minutes before serving and stir briefly then leave the dish to continue cooking either on high (preferably) or low (if need be).

To thicken dishes that contain potato or root vegetables – add 1-2 raw grated potatoes approximately 30-45 minutes prior to serving.

COOK ON LOW

While the slow cooker offers two temperature settings for the sake of convenience, if the recipe gives the option and if time allows, then cook on the low setting. Most dishes benefit from this longer, slower cooking, which releases extra flavour and tenderises meat even more.

Because of the long cooking time, you can put the slow cooker on in the morning and come home to a cooked dinner.

GLUTEN-FREE ADJUSTMENTS

Many recipes for the slow cooker are naturally gluten-free, while many others can be made so by way of simple adjustments.

Flour is often used to thicken sauces in the stews and casserole dishes that slow cookers are famous for. Plain flour in these recipes can usually be substitued for a gluten-free option such as cornflour or arrowroot.

Some of the recipes in this book call for the addition of pre-made sauces such as teriyaki or Worcestershire sauce. Gluten-free versions of these sauces are generally available to purchase and make for an easy substitution.

Soy sauce appears frequently in the recipes in this book, and when it does, the gluten-free alternative, tamari, is listed in the ingredients list as an alternative.

Some recipes in this book require store-bought tacos, tortillas or breads to accompany them. It is easy to substitute with gluten-free options so that you do not need to miss out on these great recipes.

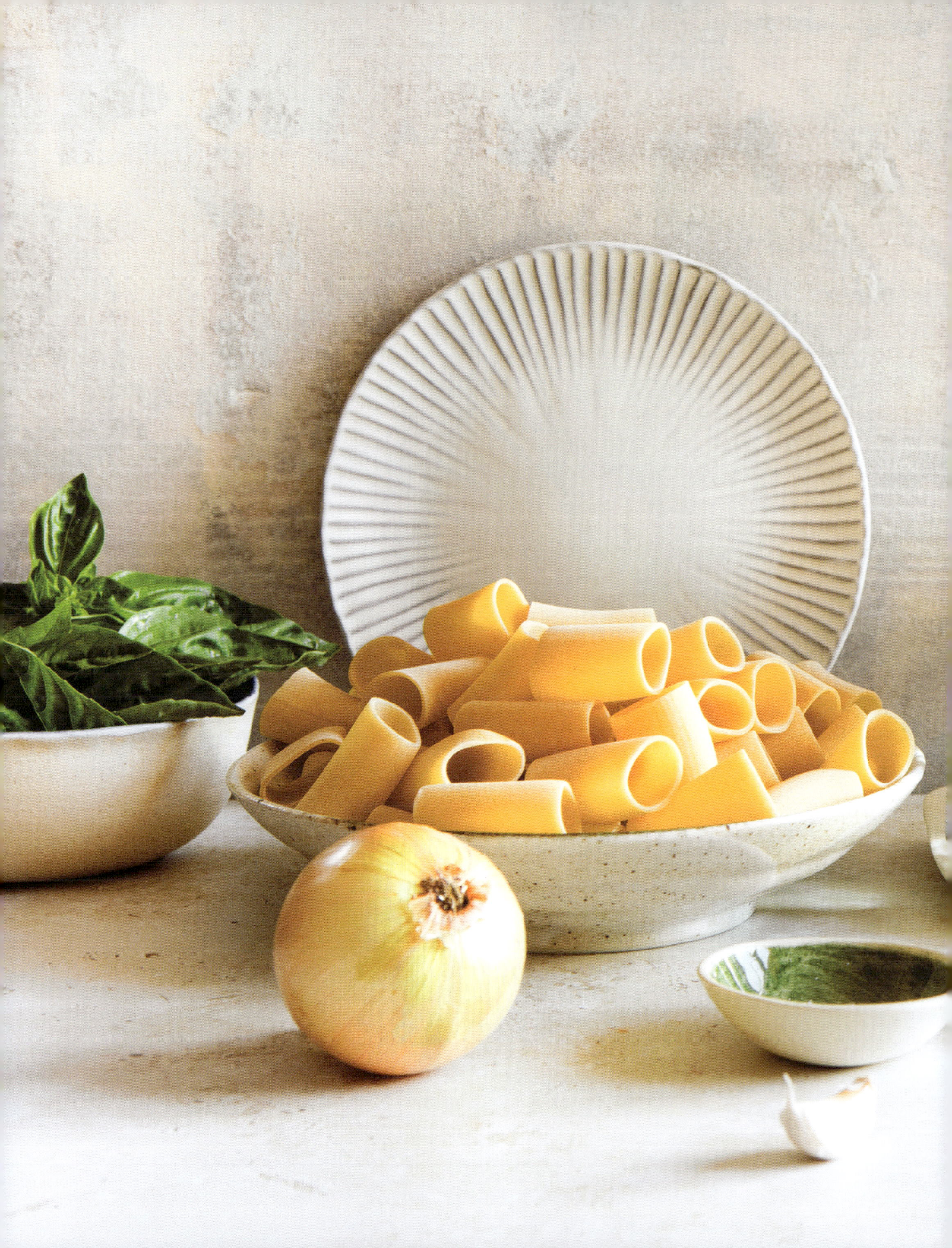

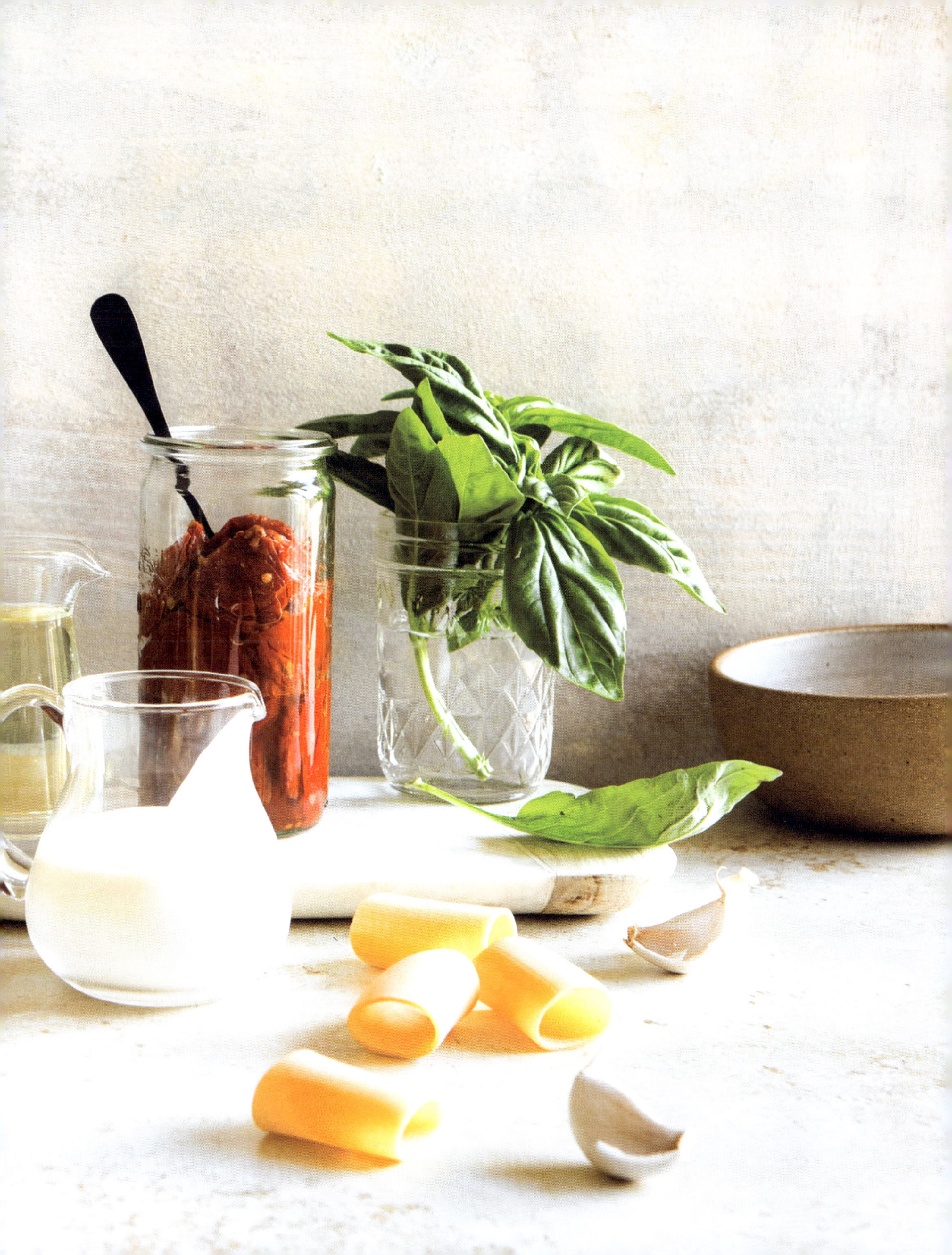

Chapter One

Red Meat

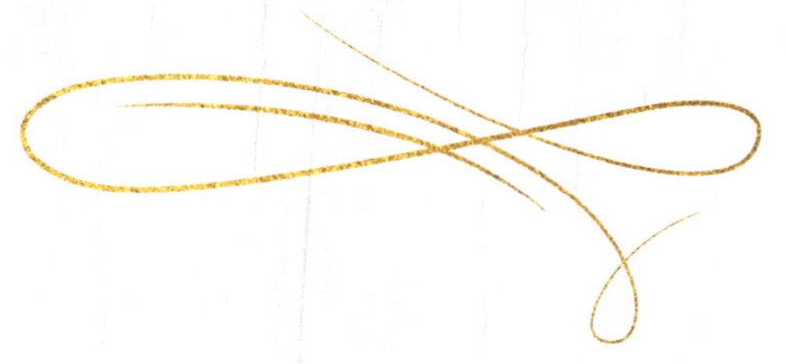

BEEF BOURGUIGNON

4 tbsps plain flour
½ tsp salt
½ tsp pepper
1kg beef chuck steak, cubed
2 tbsps olive oil
1 onion, sliced
2-3 carrots, halved and sliced
225g button mushrooms
6 sprigs thyme, leaves picked
3 cloves garlic, minced
2 bay leaves
1 cup (250ml) red wine
½ cup (125ml) beef stock
1 tbsp tomato paste

Combine the flour, salt and pepper in a large bowl. Add the beef and toss to coat.

Heat the oil in a frying pan over a medium-high heat and add beef. Cook, stirring, for 4-5 minutes until browned all over.

Place the beef along with the remaining ingredients into the slow cooker.

Cover and cook on low for 6 hours or high for 3 hours, until meat is very tender.

Discard bay leaves before serving.

LAMB SHANKS IN GRAVY

½ cup (60g) plain flour
1½ tsps salt
½ tsp pepper
4 lamb shanks
2 tbsps olive oil
2 onions, cut in wedges
3 cloves garlic, finely minced
1½ tbsps chopped fresh rosemary
1 carrot, diced
1½ cups (375ml) beef stock
½ cup (60g) gravy powder

Place flour, salt and pepper in a large bowl. Place each shank in the bowl individually and toss to coat well with the flour. Repeat until all shanks are coated in flour.

Heat the oil in a large frying pan over a medium-high heat. Add the lamb shanks in batches and cook for 2-4 minutes until browned on all sides. Place the browned lamb shanks in the slow cooker with onion, garlic, rosemary and carrot.

Deglaze the pan with beef stock. Use a spatula to scrape up any brown bits. Pour half of the liquid into the slow cooker.

Pour the remaining liquid into a jug with gravy powder. Stir to combine, then pour into slow cooker. Cover and cook on low for 8 hours until lamb is tender.

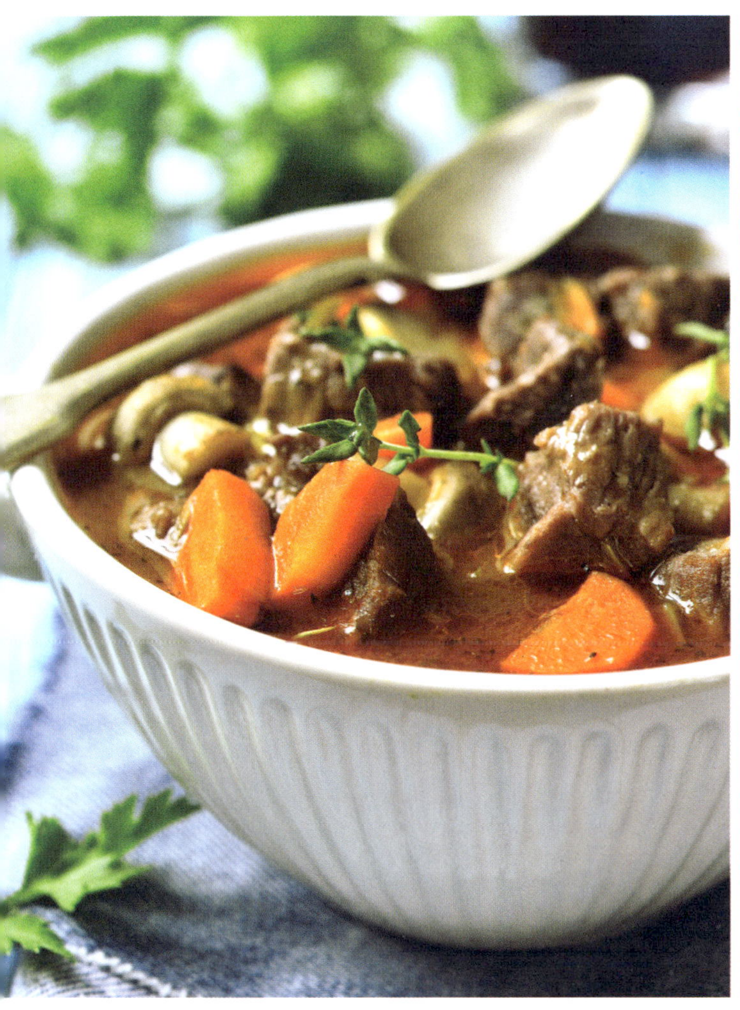

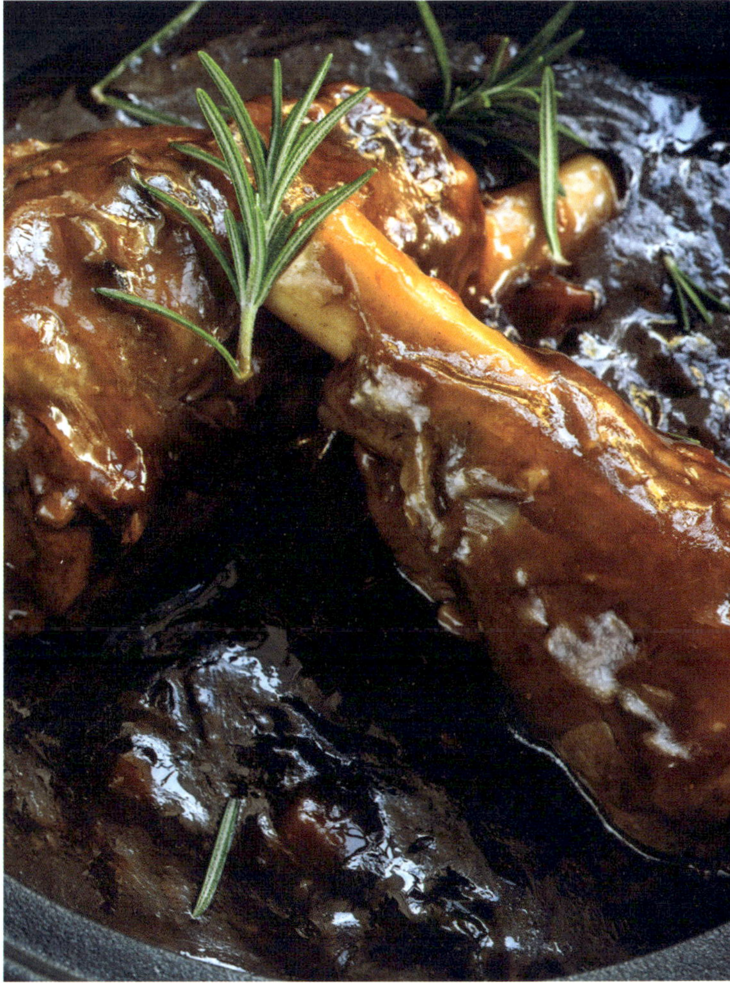

Beef Bourguignon

SERVES 6

COOK TIME: HIGH 3 HRS/LOW 6 HRS

DAIRY FREE

Lamb Shanks in Gravy

SERVES 4

COOK TIME: LOW 8 HRS

DAIRY FREE

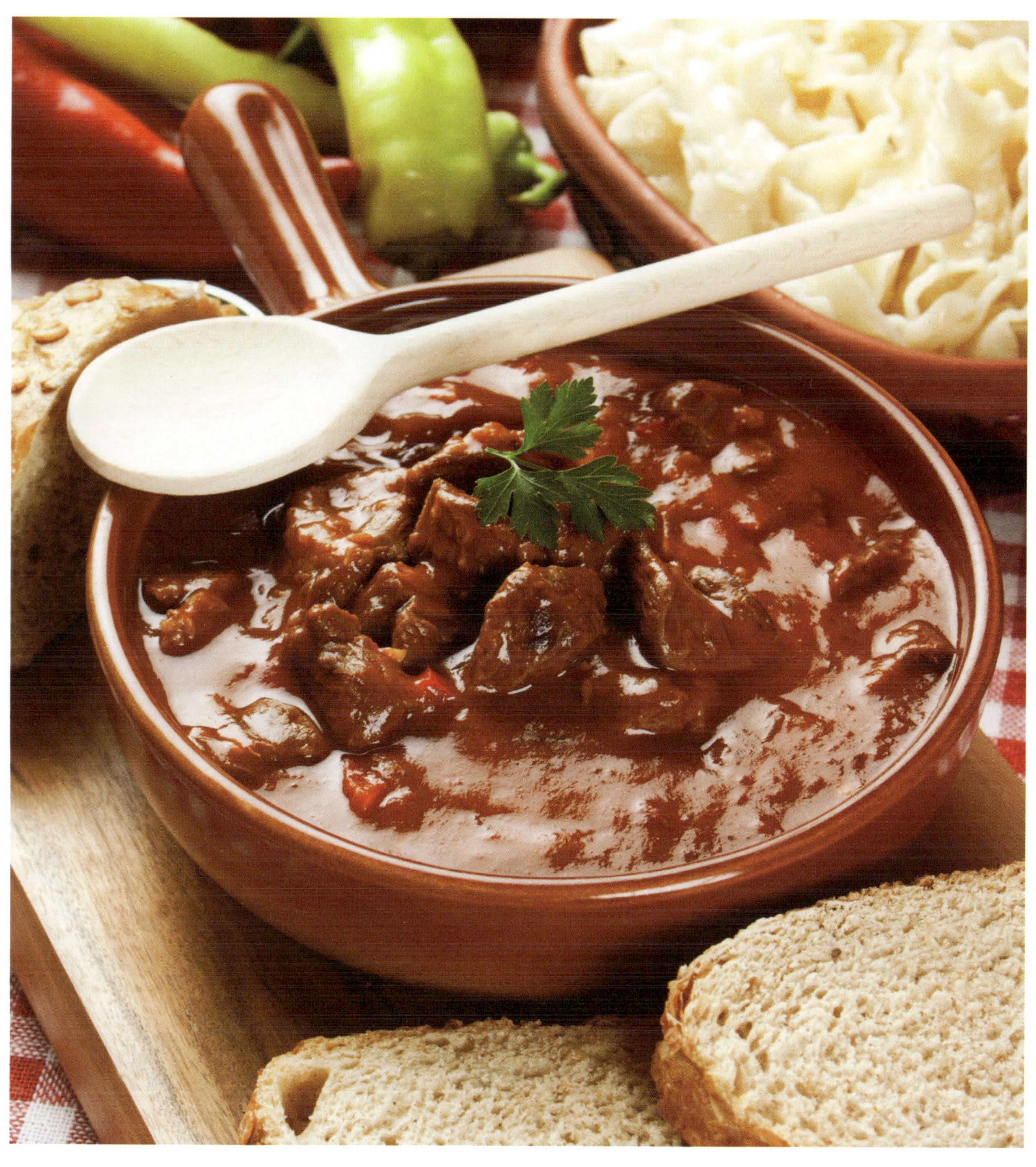

Beef Goulash

SERVES 6

COOK TIME: LOW 8 HRS + HIGH 30 MINS

BEEF GOULASH

1.3kg beef blade steak, cubed
½ cup (60g) + 1 tbsp flour
1 tsp salt
¼ tsp pepper
1 tbsp olive oil
2 tbsps paprika
¼ tsp cayenne pepper
1 onion, diced
1 clove garlic, crushed
1 cup (225g) passata
1 x 400g can diced tomatoes
2 tbsps Worcestershire sauce
6 button mushrooms, sliced
1 tbsp brown sugar
1½ tsps Dijon mustard
2 tbsps lemon juice
1 cup (250ml) beef stock
1 tbsp butter, softened

Place the meat, ½ cup flour, salt and pepper in a plastic bag and shake to coat the meat.

Heat oil in a large frying pan over medium-high heat. Add the meat and cook in batches for 2-3 minutes each until browned. Drain off excess fat.

Place meat in the slow cooker. Sprinkle with paprika and cayenne and stir to ensure evenly coated. Add onion and garlic to slow cooker.

In a mixing bowl, combine passata, diced tomatoes, Worcestershire sauce, mushrooms, brown sugar, mustard, lemon juice and beef stock. Pour over meat.

Cover and cook on low for 8 hours.

Mix the butter and 1 tablespoon flour to make a paste. Add to slow cooker and stir well. Cook on high for 30 minutes or until thickened.

BEEF, BEAN AND SPINACH STEW

3 tbsps olive oil
2 onions, chopped
2 cloves garlic, chopped
1kg stewing beef, cubed
Salt and pepper to taste
1 x 340ml bottle light beer
1 cup (250ml) beef stock
150g fresh baby spinach
2 tbsps finely chopped parsley
2 tbsps finely chopped basil
1 x 400g can cannellini beans, drained and rinsed

Heat half the oil in a large frying pan over medium-high heat. Add onions and garlic and cook for 3-5 minutes until onions are soft. Transfer to the slow cooker.

Season beef with salt and pepper. Heat remaining oil in same pan. Brown the beef cubes on all sides. Transfer to the slow cooker.

Deglaze the pan with beer, scraping up any brown bits with a spatula. Pour beer into slow cooker along with beef stock.

Cover and cook on high for 4 hours or on low for 8 hours.

Add spinach, parsley, basil and beans.

Cook on high for 30 minutes.

Season with salt and pepper before serving.

INDONESIAN BEEF RENDANG

1 tsp lime juice
1 tsp brown sugar
1 large onion, finely chopped
3 cloves garlic, minced
1 tbsp fresh ginger
1 cup (250ml) coconut cream
1 tsp salt
750g beef chuck, diced

Place the lime juice, sugar, onion, garlic, ginger and half the coconut cream in a blender or food processor and blend until smooth.

Pour into a large saucepan and add the rest of the coconut cream. Add the salt, and bring to the boil. Reduce the heat to medium and simmer for a few minutes until the sauce has thickened, stirring occasionally.

Place the meat and sauce in the slow cooker and cook on high for 4 hours or low for 8 hours or until the meat is tender.

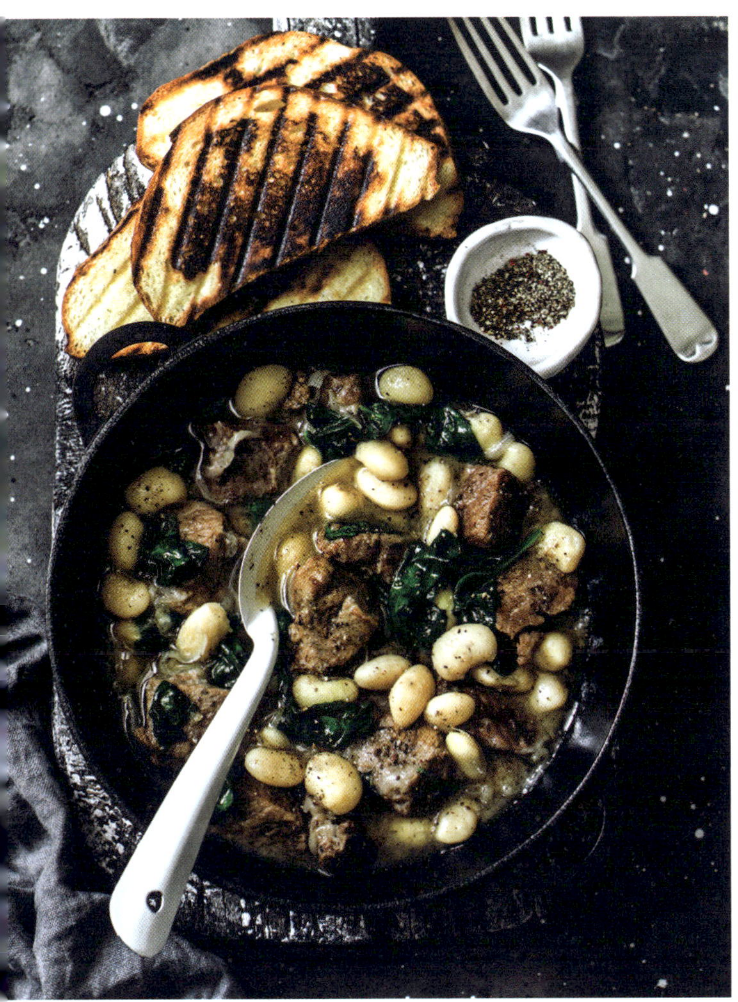

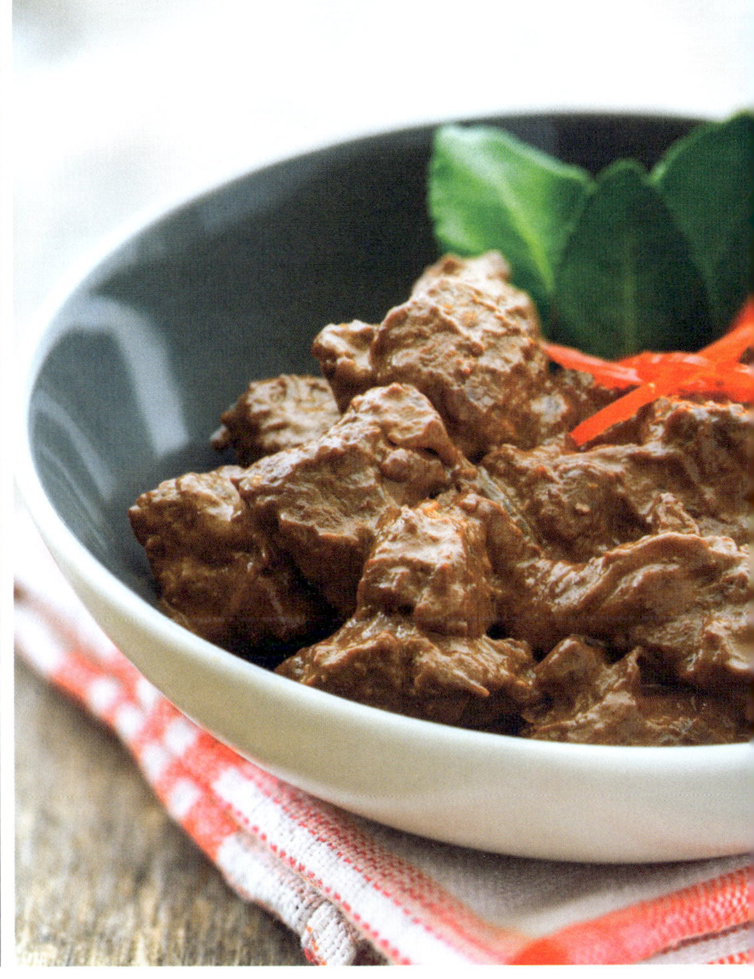

Beef, Bean and Spinach Stew

SERVES 4

COOK TIME: HIGH 4 HRS/LOW 8 HRS

DAIRY FREE

Indonesian Beef Rendang

SERVES 4

COOK TIME: HIGH 4 HRS/LOW 8 HRS

GLUTEN FREE • DAIRY FREE

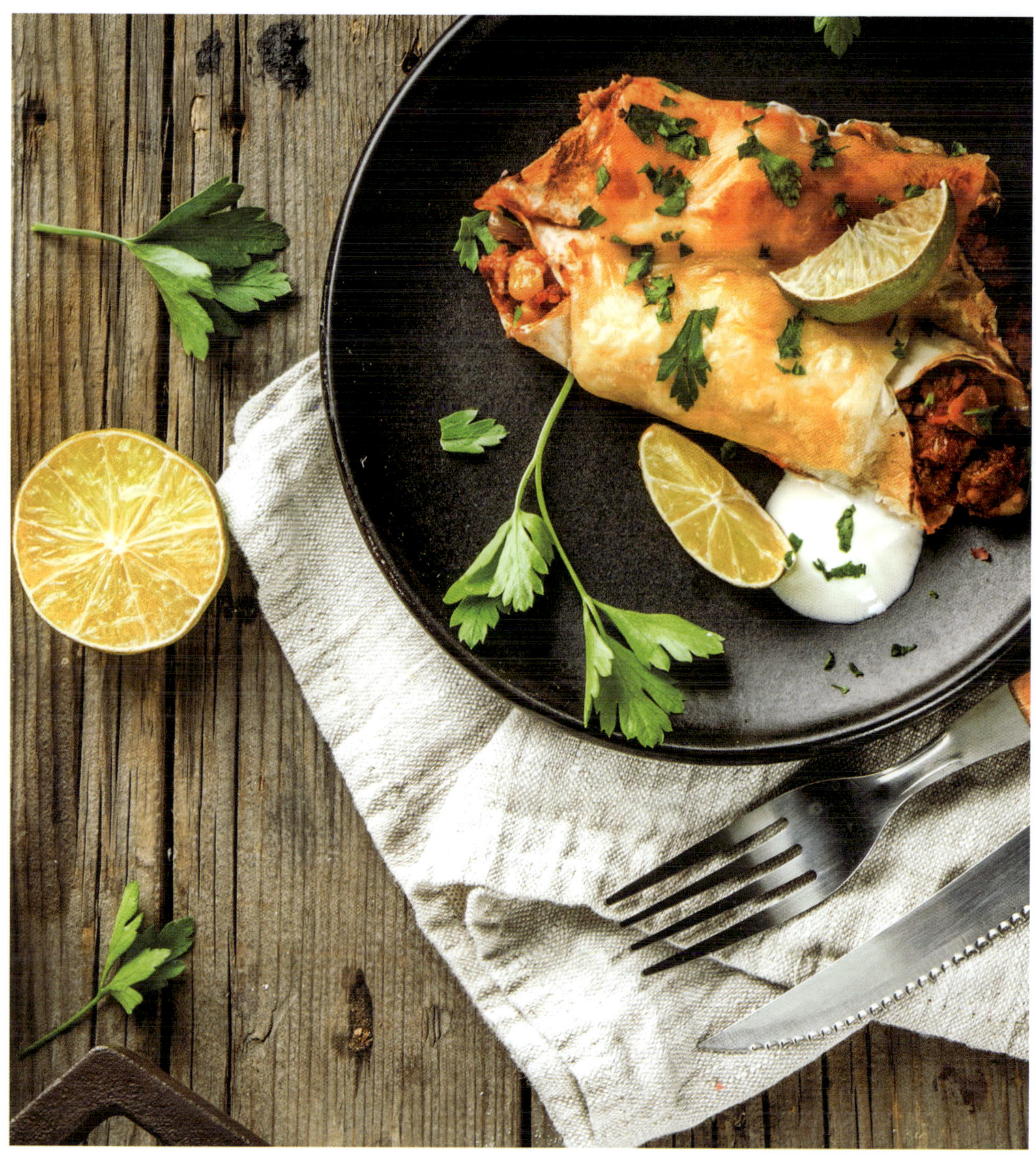

Enchiladas

SERVES 3

COOK TIME: LOW 7-8 HRS + OVEN 25-30 MINS

ENCHILADAS

500g piece shin beef, boned
2 tbsps tomato paste
1 tsp dried oregano
1 tsp ground cumin
½ tsp ground coriander
¼ tsp chilli flakes
1 onion, chopped
4 cloves garlic, thinly sliced
1 x 400g can pinto beans, drained and rinsed
1 x 400g can chopped tomatoes
Salt and pepper to taste
½ cup (10g) coriander leaves, chopped
6 medium flour tortillas
1 cup (125g) grated cheese
Sour cream and lime wedges, to serve

Cut beef into two or three pieces. In a small bowl mix together tomato paste, herbs and spices. Spread over the surface of the meat.

Place the meat into the slow cooker. Add onion, garlic, beans and tomatoes. Season with salt and pepper. Cover and cook on low for 7-8 hours, until the meat falls apart.

Remove the meat from the cooker. Place on a plate and cut into bite-size pieces. Use a slotted spoon to scoop out beans and onions from cooker and add to the meat along with chopped coriander.

Preheat oven to 200°C.

Warm the tortillas according to packet directions. Spoon meat and bean mixture onto a tortilla and roll up. Place in a greased lasagne-style dish. Repeat with remaining tortillas, fitting them together snugly. Pour over the remaining sauce from slow cooker and scatter over grated cheese. Bake for 25-30 minutes until cheese is melted and golden and filling hot. Serve with sour cream and lime wedges.

Beef Brisket Ragu

SERVES 8

COOK TIME: HIGH 4 HRS/LOW 8 HRS

GLUTEN FREE • DAIRY FREE

3 tbsps olive oil
1kg beef brisket, cut into 3cm chunks
1 large onion, finely chopped
2 medium carrots, finely diced
1 stalk celery, finely diced
2 bay leaves
2 tbsps dried oregano
1 tbsp chilli flakes
3 cloves garlic, crushed
¾ cup (185ml) beef stock
¼ cup (60ml) red wine
¼ cup (60g) tomato passata
2 tbsps tomato paste
Salt and pepper to taste
2 tbsps chopped parsley, to serve

Heat 1 tablespoon of the oil in a large frying pan over high heat. Cook the beef in batches for 3 minutes until browned, using another tablespoon of oil as needed. Transfer browned beef to the slow cooker.

Heat the remaining oil in the same frying pan over medium-high heat. Add the onion, carrots, celery, bay leaves, oregano and chilli and cook for 3-5 minutes or until the onion is soft and translucent. Add the garlic and fry for a further minute until fragrant. Transfer to the slow cooker.

Stir together the stock, wine, passata and tomato paste in a small bowl. Pour over the beef in the cooker and stir through.

Cover and cook on low for 8 hours or on high for 4 hours until beef is tender. Season to taste. Discard bay leaves before serving.

Scatter with fresh parsley and serve with pasta or rice.

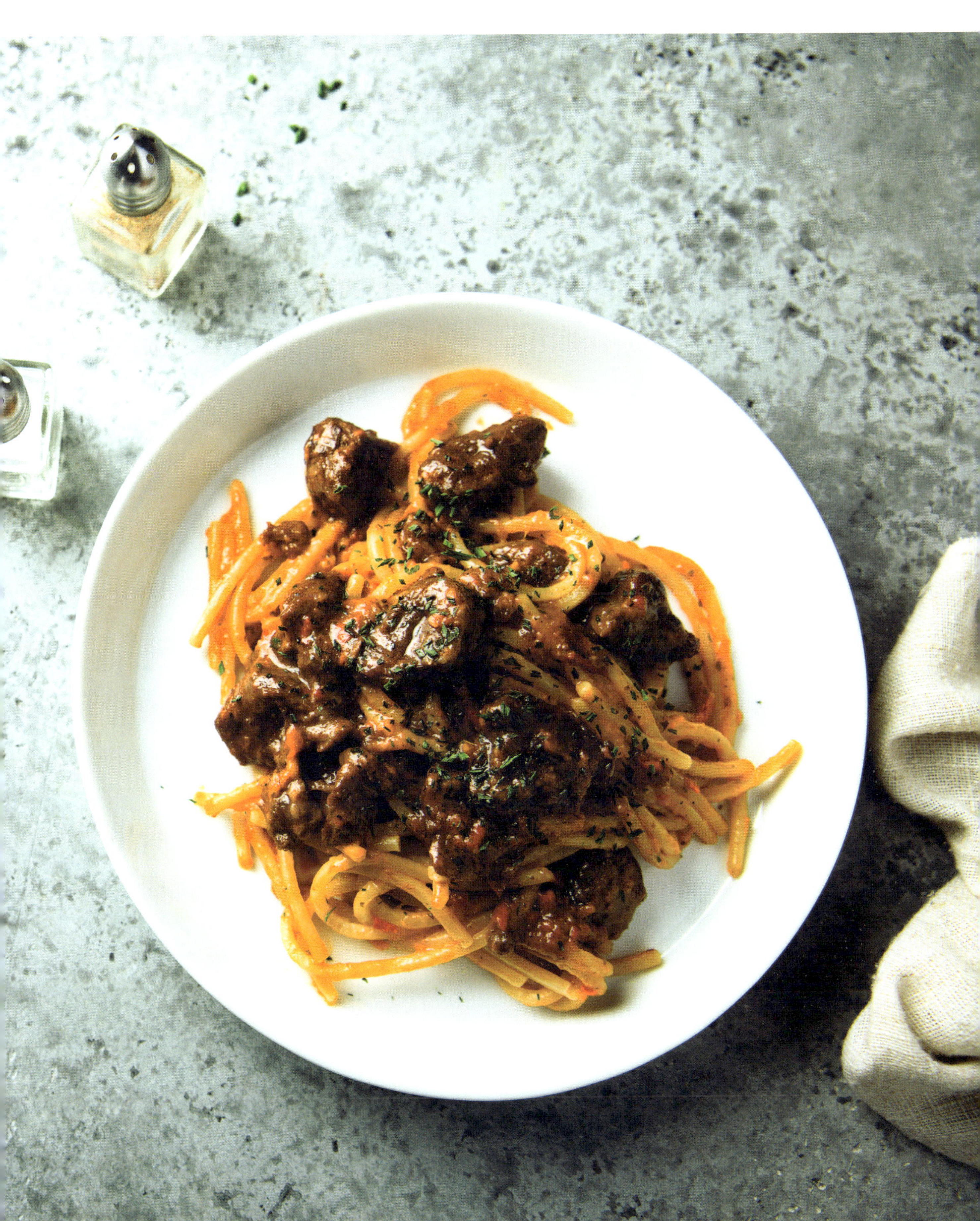

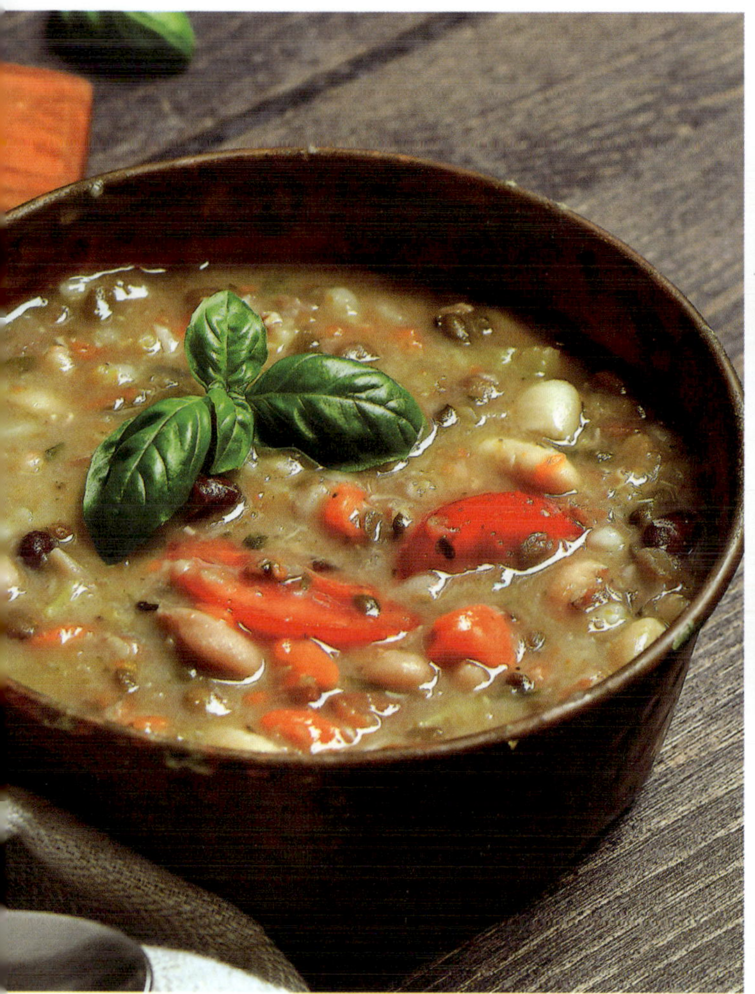

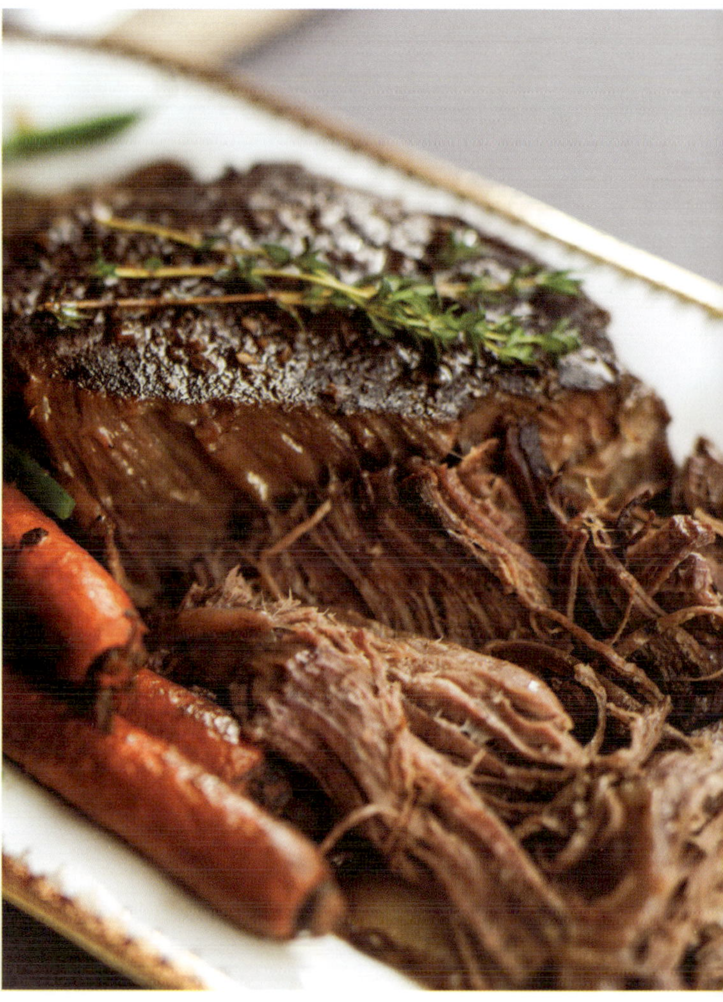

Bean and Ham Soup

SERVES 4

COOK TIME: HIGH 4 HRS/LOW 8 HRS

GLUTEN FREE • DAIRY FREE

Beef Pot Roast

SERVES 4

COOK TIME: HIGH 4 HRS/LOW 8 HRS

GLUTEN FREE

BEAN AND HAM SOUP

2 tbsps olive oil
1 onion, finely chopped
2 cloves garlic, chopped
1 large carrot, chopped
1 large stalk celery, chopped
1 x 400g can cannellini beans, drained and rinsed
1 x 400g can kidney beans, drained and rinsed
500g smoked ham hocks
1 sprig rosemary
½ tsp dried oregano
½ tsp red chilli flakes (optional)
4 cups (1L) chicken stock
2 tomatoes, quartered
Salt and pepper to taste

Heat oil in a frying pan over medium heat. Add onion, garlic, carrot and celery. Cook for 10 minutes, stirring regularly, until vegetables are tender.

Transfer vegetables to slow cooker with remaining ingredients. Cook on low for 8 hours. Ladle into bowls, shredding the ham as needed, to serve.

BEEF POT ROAST

1kg beef chuck roast
Salt and pepper to taste
1 tsp garlic powder
4-5 sprigs thyme
2 tsps butter
2 tsps olive oil
1 tbsp cornflour
1 tbsp water
8 shallots, peeled
14 baby carrots, peeled
2 tbsps Worcestershire sauce

Generously season roast with salt, pepper and garlic powder and scatter with thyme. Rub seasoning into roast on all sides.

Heat a large frying pan over medium-high heat. When pan is hot add butter and oil. Place roast in pan and brown for 4-5 minutes on each side.

Whisk cornflour and water until smooth.

Place shallots and carrots in the slow cooker. Season with salt and pepper and drizzle with cornflour mixture. Toss to coat.

Add meat to the slow cooker. Drizzle with Worcestershire sauce. Cover and cook for 4 hours on high or 8 hours on low.

Allow to rest for 10 minutes before slicing.

Lamb and Pumpkin Curry

SERVES 4

COOK TIME: HIGH 4 HRS/LOW 6 HRS + 30 MINS ON HIGH

GLUTEN FREE • DAIRY FREE

- 2 tbsps vegetable oil
- 600g boneless lamb shoulder, cut into 3cm pieces
- 1 onion, finely chopped
- 1 long green chilli, deseeded, finely chopped
- 2 cloves garlic, crushed
- Small piece ginger, grated
- 1 cinnamon stick
- 1 tsp ground turmeric
- 2 tsps ground cumin
- 1 tsp paprika
- 1 tsp ground coriander
- 1 x 400g can diced tomatoes
- 1 x 400ml can coconut milk
- Salt and pepper to taste
- 500g pumpkin, cut into 3cm pieces
- Chopped fresh coriander, to serve

Heat half the oil in a large frying pan over medium-high heat. Cook the lamb in batches, turning occasionally, for 5 minutes, or until brown all over. Transfer to the slow cooker.

Heat remaining oil in the pan over medium heat. Add onion and cook for 3-5 minutes, stirring, until soft and translucent. Add chilli, garlic, ginger, cinnamon, turmeric, cumin, paprika and ground coriander and cook, stirring, for 1 minute or until fragrant. Add tomatoes and coconut milk and stir to combine. Pour over the lamb. Season with salt and pepper.

Cook for 6 hours on low or 4 hours on high or until lamb is tender. Add pumpkin and cook for a further 30 minutes on high or until tender.

Sprinkle with fresh coriander leaves to serve.

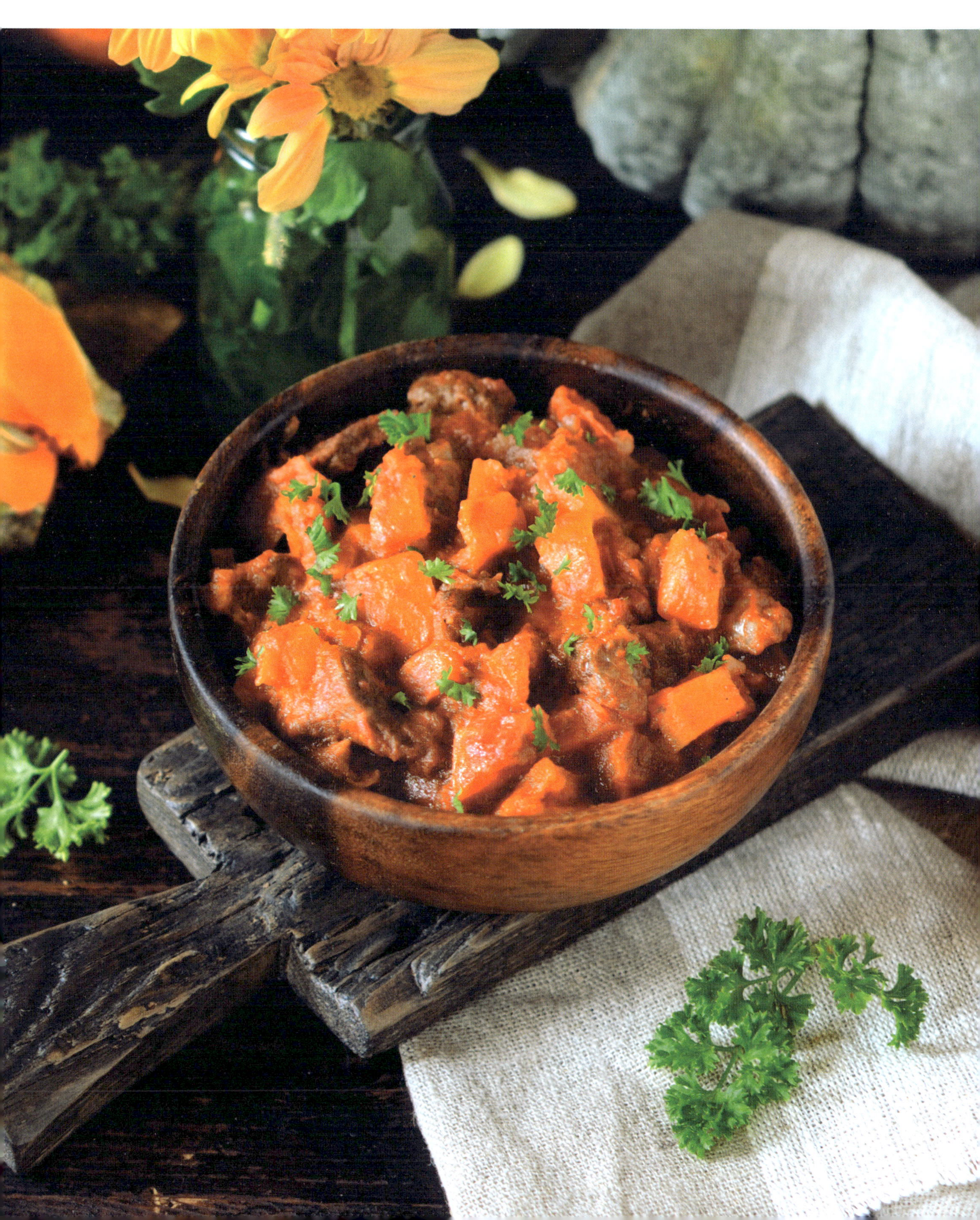

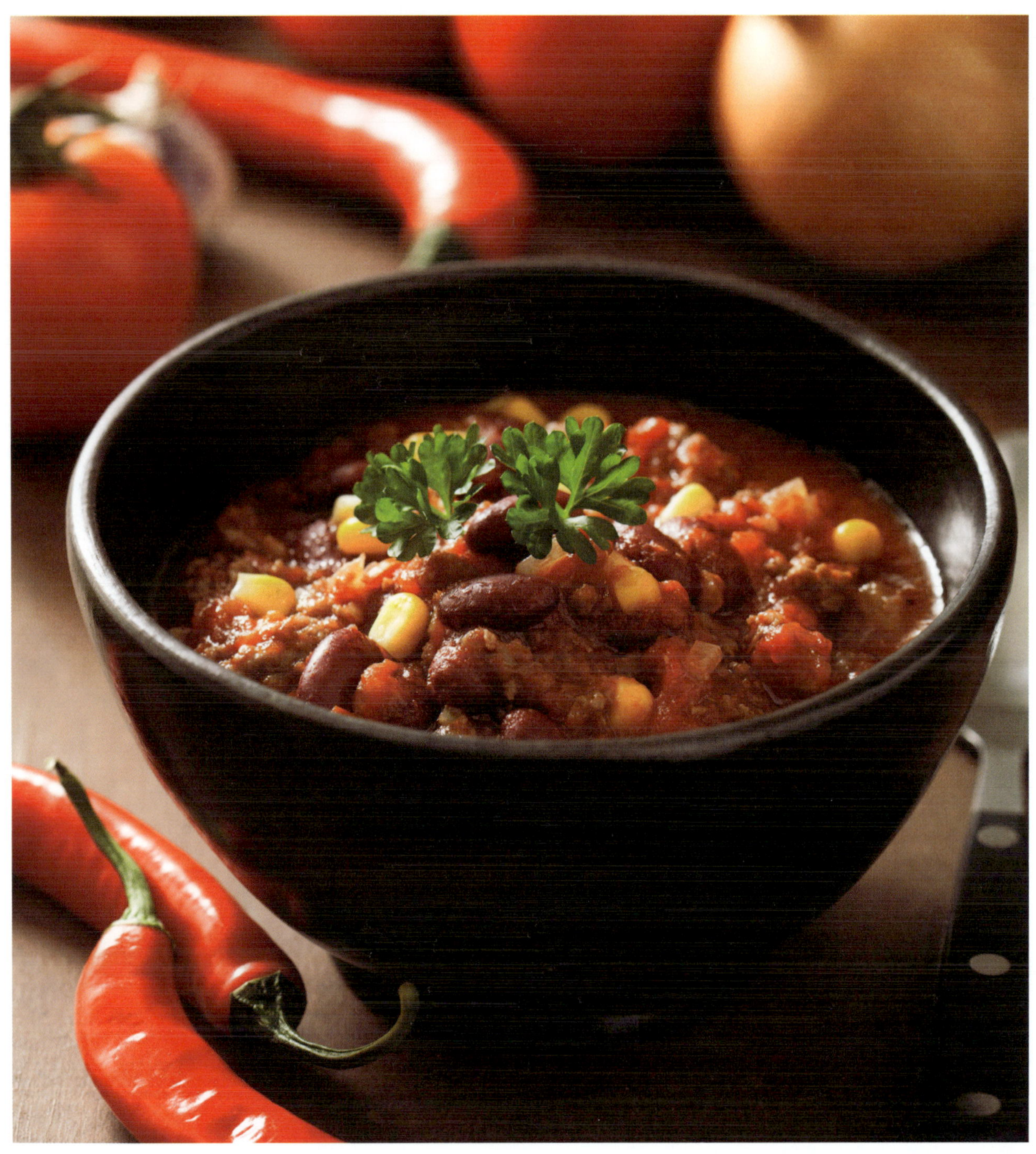

Chilli con Carne

SERVES 4-6

COOK TIME: LOW 8 HRS + 30 MINS ON HIGH

GLUTEN FREE • DAIRY FREE

CHILLI CON CARNE

2 tbsps olive oil
1 onion, finely chopped
1 clove garlic, crushed
450g beef mince
½-1 tsp chilli powder
1 tsp ground cumin
½ tsp paprika
⅔ cup (150ml) beef stock
1 x 400g can chopped tomatoes
3 tbsps tomato paste
25g dark chocolate, broken into pieces (optional)
1 x 400g can red kidney beans, drained and rinsed
½ cup (85g) corn kernels
1 cup (45g) fresh coriander, chopped
Salt and pepper to taste

Heat the oil in a large frying pan. Add onion and cook, stirring, for 3-5 minutes until soft and translucent. Add garlic and cook for 1 minute until fragrant.

Add the beef, chilli powder, cumin and paprika and fry for 5-7 minutes or until well browned, stirring to break up any lumps. Transfer to the slow cooker.

Deglaze the pan with the beef stock, using a spatula to scrape up any brown bits. Pour into slow cooker.

Add chopped tomatoes and tomato paste to slow cooker. Stir to combine.

Cover and cook on low for 8 hours.

Stir in the chocolate, if using, kidney beans, corn and coriander. Season with salt and pepper.

Cook, covered, on high for 30 minutes or until hot.

Pomegranate Lamb Shanks

SERVES 6

COOK TIME: LOW 8 HRS

GLUTEN FREE • DAIRY FREE

6 large lamb shanks, trimmed
Salt and pepper to taste
2 tbsps olive oil
3 cups (750ml) light red wine
2 onions, cut into quarters
6 cloves garlic, thinly sliced
2 large oranges, halved and sliced, skin on
2 finely chopped tbsps rosemary
1 tsp ground fennel
¼ cup (10g) shredded mint leaves
1 tsp whole black peppercorns
1 cup (250ml) pomegranate juice
1 cup (250ml) orange juice
1 large pomegranate, seeded

Season each shank with salt and pepper. Heat oil in a large frying pan over medium-high heat. Add the shanks, two at a time, and brown for 2 minutes on all sides. Remove from heat and place in slow cooker.

Deglaze the pan with the wine, using a spatula to scrape up any brown bits. Pour into the slow cooker.

Add onions, garlic, orange slices, rosemary, ground fennel, 2 tablespoons mint, peppercorns and 1 teaspoon salt to the slow cooker.

Cover and cook on low for 8 hours until lamb is tender.

Half an hour before the shanks are ready to come out of the slow cooker, bring pomegranate and orange juices to a boil in a small saucepan. Reduce the heat and simmer for 20 minutes. Once the shanks are ready, pour the juices over the lamb and stir into the remaining liquid in the slow cooker.

Serve sprinkled with pomegranate seeds and fresh mint.

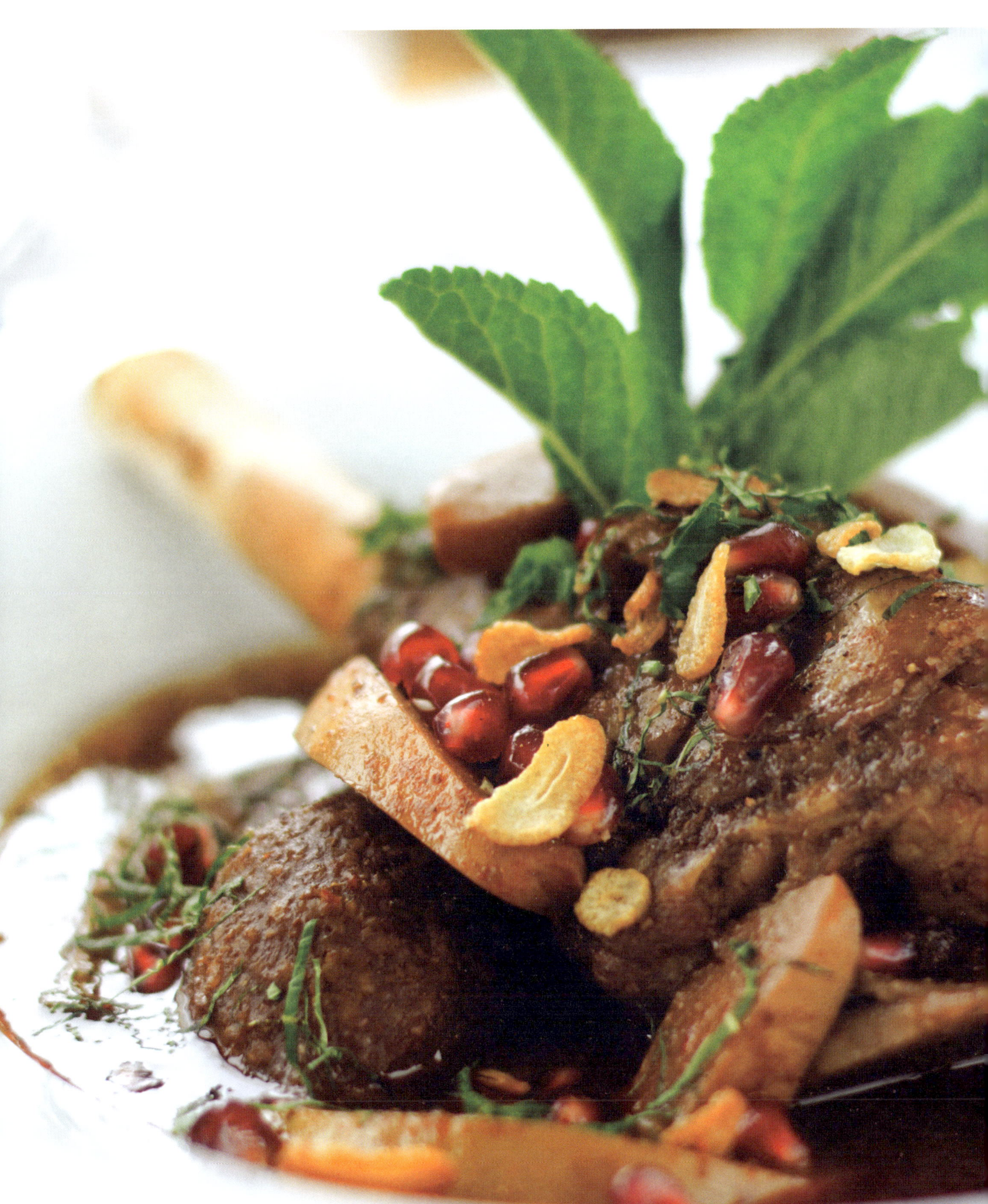

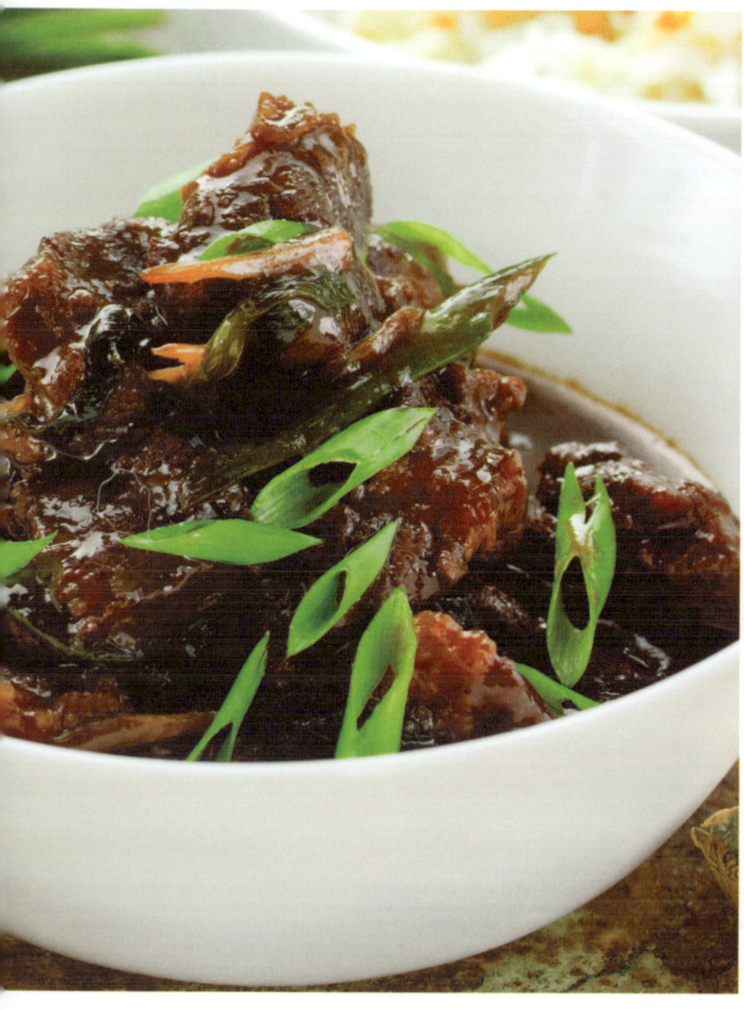

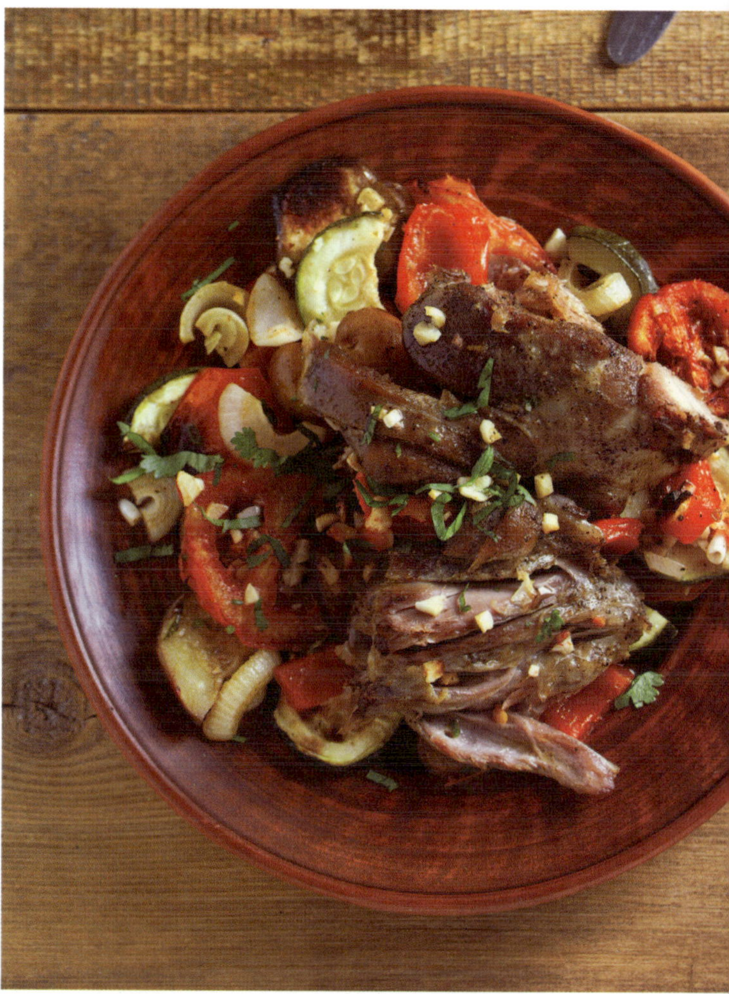

Mongolian Beef

SERVES 8

COOK TIME: HIGH 3 HRS/LOW 5 HRS

GLUTEN FREE • DAIRY FREE

Lamb Shoulder Pot Roast

SERVES 6

COOK TIME: LOW 8 HRS

GLUTEN FREE • DAIRY FREE

MONGOLIAN BEEF

1kg skirt steak, cut into thin strips
¼ cup (30g) arrowroot flour
½ tsp salt
½ tsp pepper
2 tbsps sesame oil
2 cloves garlic, minced
½ tsp grated fresh ginger
¾ cup (185ml) soy sauce (or tamari)
¾ cup (185ml) vegetable stock
¾ cup (120g) brown sugar
3 carrots, grated
4 spring onions, sliced on the diagonal

Add the meat, flour, salt and pepper to a large bowl. Toss to coat.

Add the sesame oil, garlic, ginger, soy sauce, stock, brown sugar, carrots and half the spring onions to the slow cooker and stir to combine.

Add the steak slices and stir through to combine.

Cook on high for 3 hours or low for 5 hours or until steak is cooked through and tender.

Serve over rice or noodles, garnished with remaining spring onion slices.

LAMB SHOULDER POT ROAST

1.5-2kg lamb shoulder
5 cloves garlic, thinly sliced
2 tbsps olive oil
1 tsp salt
½ tsp pepper
1 tsp dried parsley
1 tsp dried oregano
½ tsp dried rosemary
1 capsicum, roughly chopped
1 eggplant, thinly sliced
2 zucchinis, sliced
2 onions, thinly sliced
400g Roma tomatoes, sliced
1 cup (250ml) chicken or lamb stock
½ cup (125ml) white wine
¼ cup (5g) parsley leaves, chopped, to serve

Use a small sharp knife to cut slits all over the lamb. Fill the slits with thinly sliced garlic.

In a small bowl combine olive oil with salt, pepper and dried herbs. Rub all over lamb.

Place capsicum, eggplant, zucchini, onion and tomatoes in base of slow cooker. Pour over stock and wine. Place lamb on top. Cover and cook on low for 8 hours until lamb is tender.

Allow lamb to rest for 10 minutes then slice, scatter with chopped parsley and serve with vegetables and cooking juices.

Lamb Tagine with Chickpeas

SERVES 6
COOK TIME: LOW 8 HRS + 30 MINS
GLUTEN FREE

1kg lamb, cut into 2.5cm cubes
2 tsps cinnamon
Salt and pepper to taste
2 tbsps olive oil
1 onion, diced
4 cloves garlic, minced
1 tbsp grated fresh ginger
1 tsp ground cumin
1 tsp ground coriander
2½ cups (625ml) chicken stock
1 tomato, chopped
1 cup (190g) dried apricots, chopped
¼ cup (30g) flaked almonds
1 x 400g can chickpeas, drained and rinsed
1¼ cups (300g) Greek yoghurt
½ cup (20g) fresh coriander, roughly chopped

Toss the lamb with 1 teaspoon cinnamon and a good seasoning of salt and pepper.

Heat the oil in a large frying pan with high sides over medium-high heat. Cook the lamb in batches, frying for 4 minutes per batch until brown on all sides. Transfer to slow cooker.

Add the onion to the pan and fry for 3-5 minutes until soft and translucent. Add garlic, ginger and spices and cook for 1 minute until fragrant. Transfer to slow cooker.

Deglaze the pan with the stock, using a spatula to scrape up any brown bits. Pour into slow cooker.

Add tomato, apricots and half the almonds.

Cover and cook on low for 8 hours.

Add chickpeas and cook, covered, on high for 30 minutes.

Serve hot with a spoonful of yoghurt and a scattering of fresh coriander and almonds for garnish.

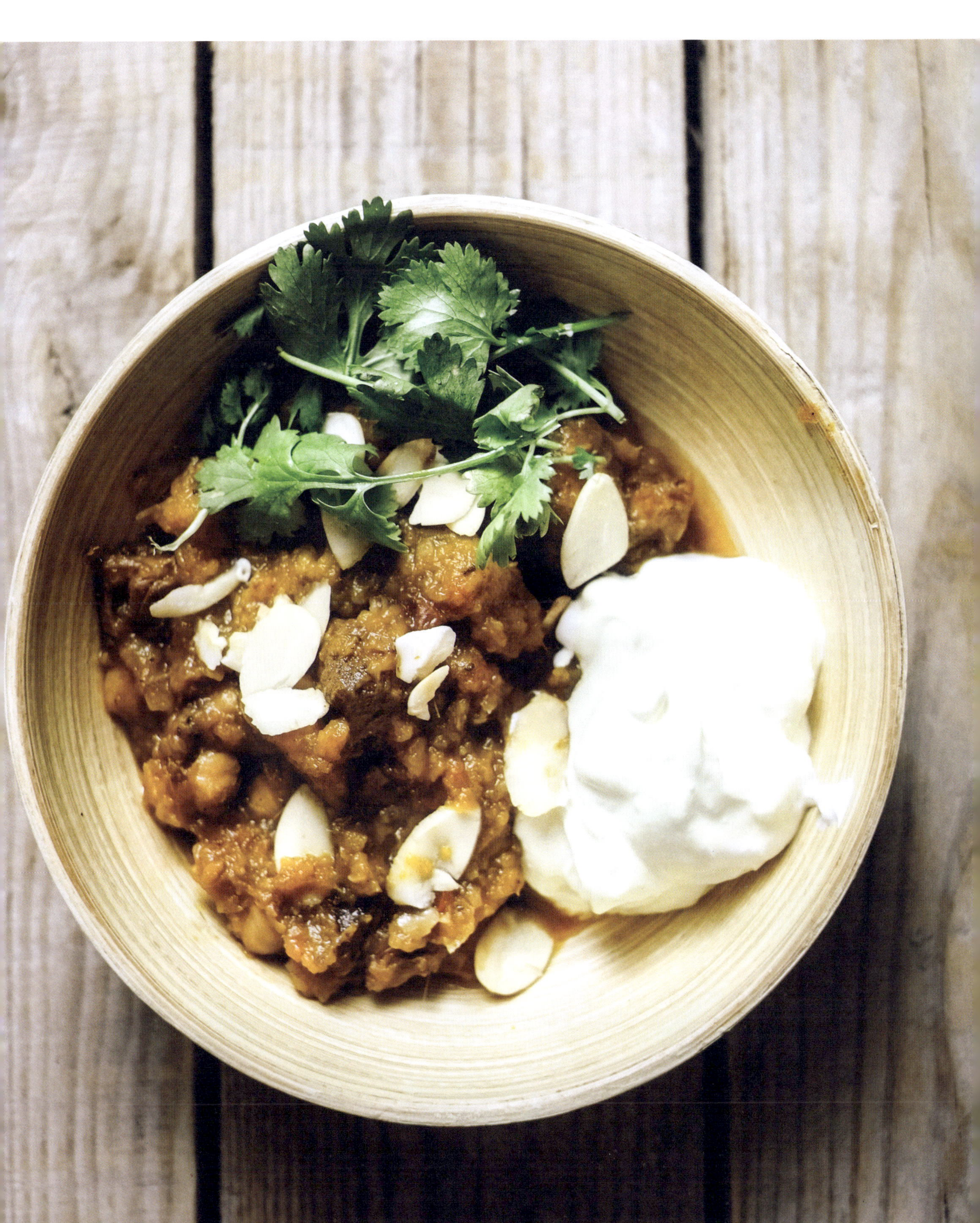

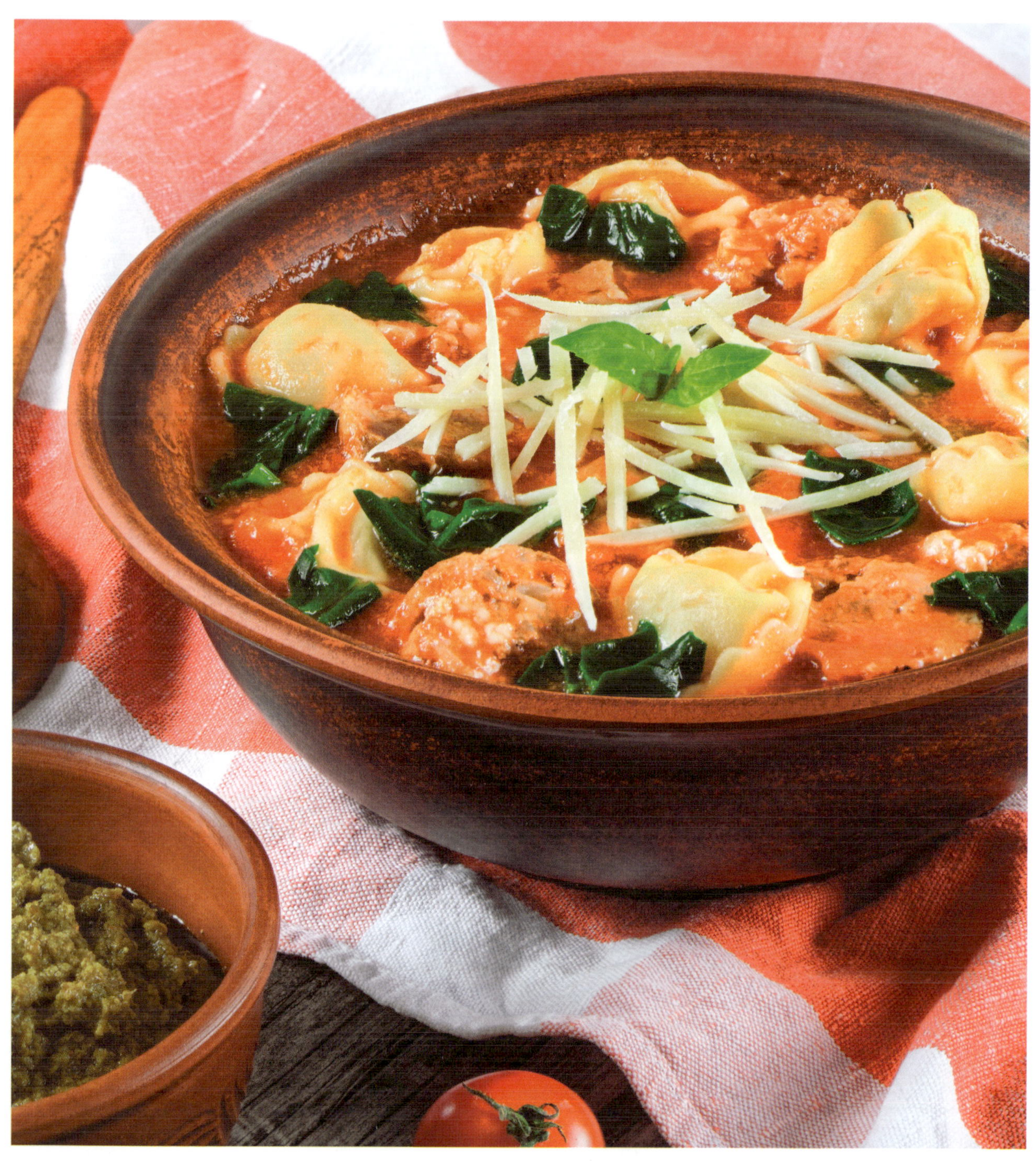

Sausage and Tortellini Soup

SERVES 6

COOK TIME: LOW 6 HRS

SAUSAGE AND TORTELLINI SOUP

2 tbsps olive oil
455g beef sausage, sliced
2 stalks celery, diced
1 onion, diced
2 carrots, diced
2 cloves garlic, minced
1½ tsps salt + more to taste
½ tsp pepper + more to taste
1 tsp paprika
4 cups (1L) vegetable stock
2 x 400g cans diced tomatoes
4 tbsps tomato paste
1 bay leaf
¾ cup (25g) basil, roughly chopped + extra to garnish
¾ cup (75g) Parmesan cheese, grated + extra to garnish
½ cup (125ml) thickened cream
330g frozen tortellini
½ bunch silverbeet, stems removed and leaves chopped

Heat 1 tablespoon oil in large frying pan over a medium-high heat. Add sausage and cook, stirring, for 3-4 minutes until browned. Drain and set aside.

Wipe pan clean with paper towel and heat remaining oil. Add celery, onion and carrots and cook for 4-5 minutes until almost soft. Add garlic, salt, pepper and paprika and cook for a further 1 minute until aromatic. Place the onion mixture, sausage, stock, tomatoes, tomato paste, bay leaf and basil in the slow cooker and stir to combine.

Cover and cook on low for 6 hours. Remove bay leaf and discard. Remove sausage slices and set aside. Puree the soup with a stick blender (or puree in batches using a stand blender). Add cheese and cream and stir to combine. Season to taste.

Increase slow cooker to a high setting. Return sausages to the slow cooker. Add tortellini and cook for 10 minutes, then add silverbeet. Continue cooking for 5 minutes until silverbeet has wilted.

Serve garnished with extra Parmesan and basil.

COCOA-RUBBED BABY BACK RIBS

3 tbsps brown sugar, firmly packed
3 tbsps unsweetened cocoa powder
2 tsps mild chilli powder
1kg beef baby back ribs, cut to fit slow cooker
1 cup (250ml) beef stock
2 tbsps tomato paste
½ cup (125ml) apple cider vinegar
Brussels sprouts and carrots, to serve

Mix the brown sugar, cocoa powder and chilli powder in a bowl. Rub the spice evenly onto the ribs.

Whisk together the stock and tomato paste in a small bowl.

Add the apple cider vinegar to the bottom of the slow cooker followed by the ribs. Pour over the stock and tomato paste mix.

Cook covered on high for 4 hours or low for 8 hours. Serve with Brussels sprouts and carrots.

VEAL AND MUSHROOM CASSEROLE

⅓ cup (40g) plain flour
Salt and pepper to taste
1kg boneless veal shoulder, cut into 5cm pieces
1 tbsp olive oil
1 onion, chopped
2 cups (500ml) red wine
1 cup (250ml) beef stock
500g button mushrooms, sliced
4 bay leaves
2 tbsps chopped fresh parsley, to serve

Place flour in a large bowl and season with salt and pepper. Add veal and toss to coat.

Heat oil in a large frying pan over medium-high heat. Add onion and cook for 3-5 minutes until soft and translucent. Add veal and cook until browned. Transfer to slow cooker.

Deglaze the pan with ½ cup wine. Use a spatula to scrape up any brown bits. Pour into slow cooker with remaining wine and stock. Add mushrooms and bay leaves and stir gently.

Cover and cook on low for 8 hours.

Remove bay leaves and sprinkle with fresh parsley to serve.

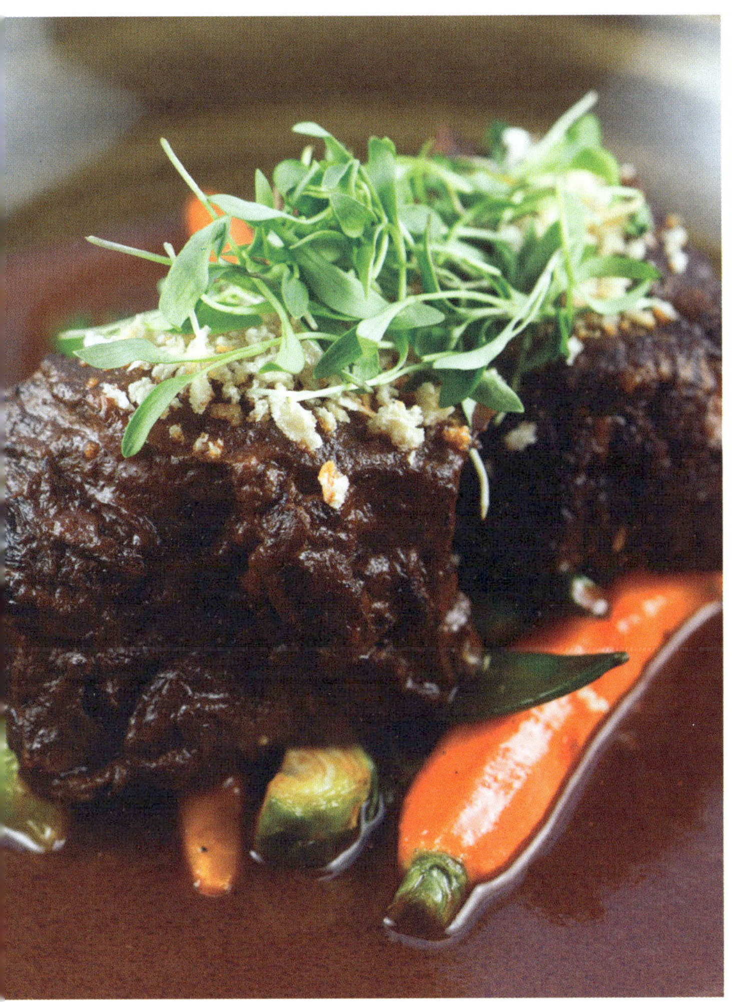

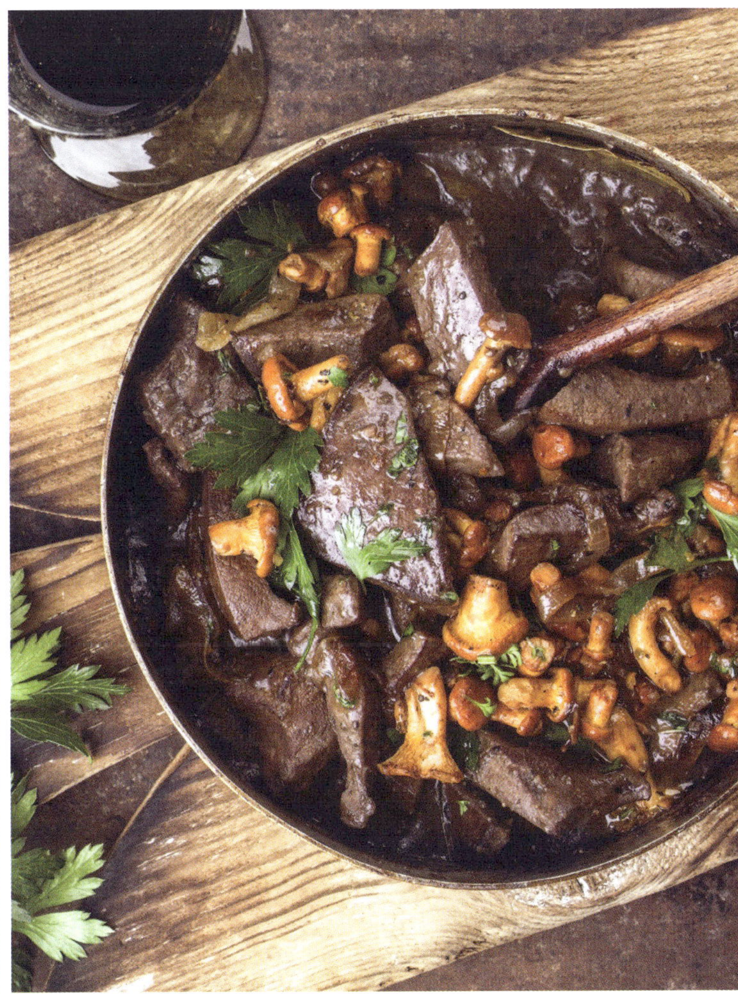

Cocoa-Rubbed Baby Back Ribs

SERVES 4

COOK TIME: HIGH 4 HRS/LOW 8 HRS

GLUTEN FREE • DAIRY FREE

Veal and Mushroom Casserole

SERVES 4

COOK TIME: LOW 8 HRS

DAIRY FREE

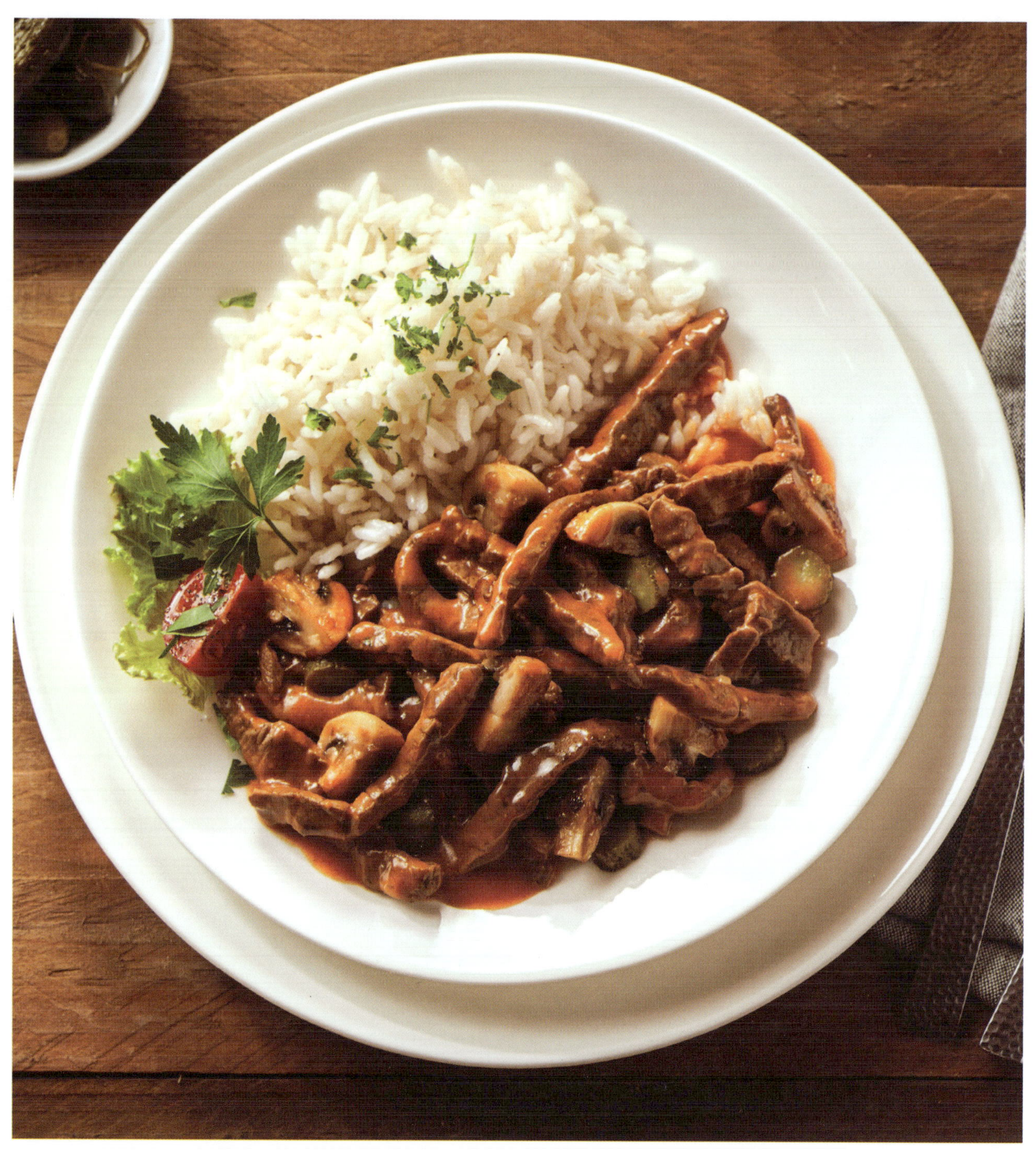

Beef Stroganoff

SERVES 6

COOK TIME: HIGH 4 HRS 30 MINS

BEEF STROGANOFF

800g trimmed beef brisket, cut into 3cm pieces
Salt and pepper to taste
2 tbsps olive oil
2 onions, thinly sliced
500g button mushrooms, halved
4 cloves garlic, thinly sliced
2 tbsps plain flour
1 tbsp sweet paprika
1½ cups (375ml) beef stock
1 tbsp tomato paste
1 tbsp Worcestershire sauce
2 tbsps sour cream
2 large dill pickles, sliced
2 tbsps parsley, to garnish

Season the beef with salt and pepper. Heat 1 tablespoon of oil in a large frying pan over high heat. Add the beef in batches and brown quickly all over. Transfer to the slow cooker.

Heat the remaining oil in the same pan over a medium-high heat. Add the onion and mushrooms and cook, stirring occasionally, for 5 minutes. Next add the garlic and flour and cook, stirring constantly, for 1 minute. Sprinkle with paprika and transfer the mixture to the slow cooker.

Combine the stock, tomato paste and Worcestershire sauce in a jug until smooth. Pour liquid over the beef and stir to combine. Cover and cook on high for 4½ hours or until beef is tender.

Stir in the sour cream and dill pickles. Season with salt and pepper.

Serve with pasta, mashed potatoes or rice and garnish with parsley.

Osso Bucco

SERVES 4
COOK TIME: LOW 8 HRS
DAIRY FREE

4 cross-cut, bone-in beef or veal shanks

1 cup (125g) flour

Salt and pepper to taste

Olive oil, for frying

1 onion, diced

2 carrots, diced

1 stalk celery, diced

2½ tbsps tomato paste

4 cloves garlic, minced

½ cup (125ml) dry white wine

1 cup (250ml) chicken stock

1 tbsp balsamic vinegar

1 tbsp oregano

2 sprigs rosemary

2 bay leaves

Pat meat dry using a paper towel. Place flour on a plate. Season beef with salt and pepper and dredge in the flour, shaking off excess.

Heat oil in a large frying pan over medium-high heat. Add meat in batches and cook for 3- 5 minutes on each side, until browned. Transfer to the slow cooker.

Add onion, carrots and celery to pan and cook, stirring occasionally, for 5 minutes until just soft. Add tomato paste and garlic and cook for a further minute, until aromatic. Add wine and stir, using a spatula to scrape up any brown bits. Transfer to the slow cooker.

Add stock, vinegar, oregano, rosemary sprigs and bay leaves to the slow cooker. Season with salt and pepper.

Cover and cook on low for 8 hours until meat is tender.

Remove and discard rosemary sprigs and bay leaves before serving.

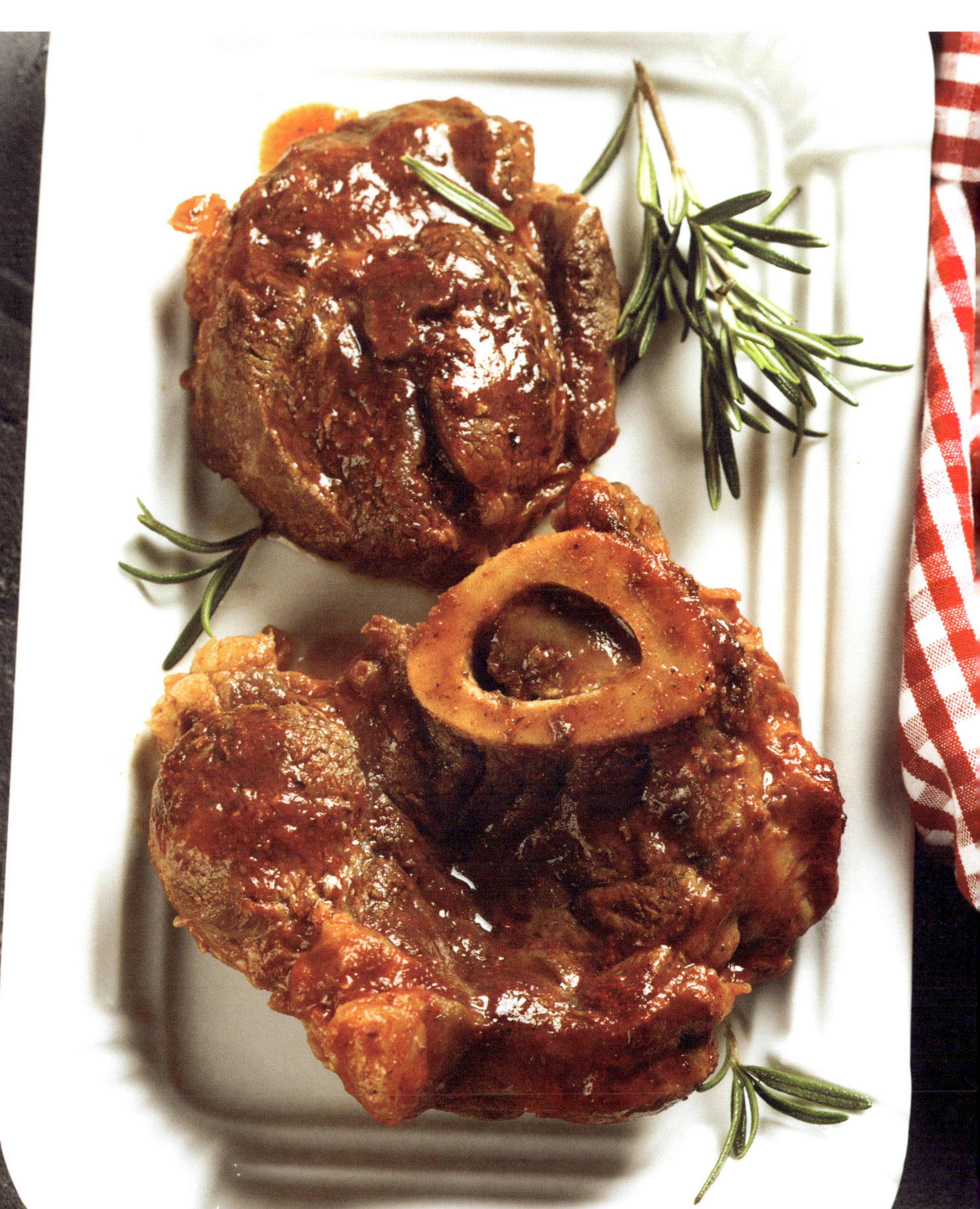

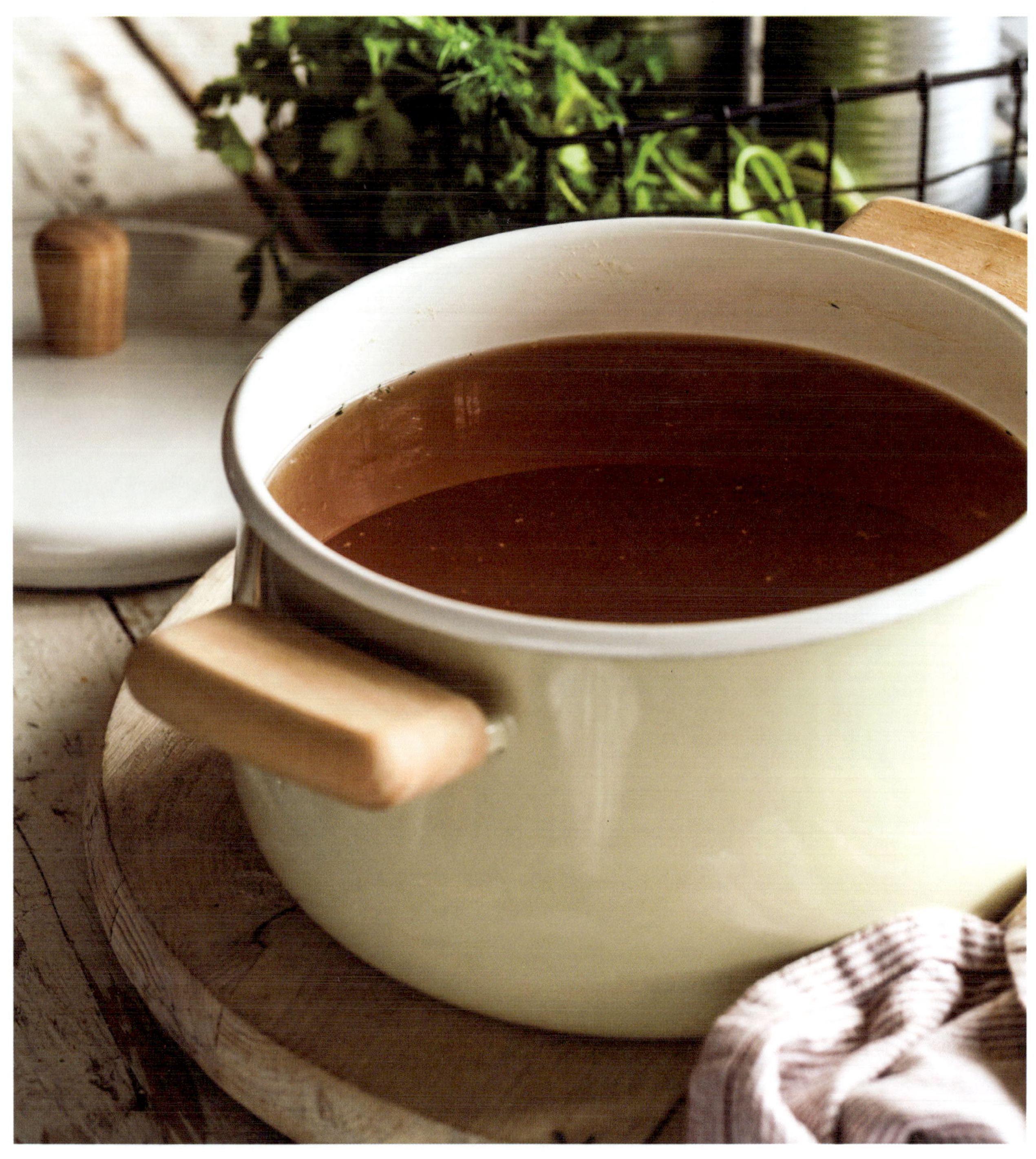

Beef Bone Broth

SERVES 6

COOK TIME: LOW 24 HRS

GLUTEN FREE • DAIRY FREE

BEEF BONE BROTH

2kg beef bones (mix of marrow, knuckle and meat bones)

2 tbsps apple cider vinegar

1 onion, quartered

1 head garlic, cut in half

2 carrots, chopped

2 stalks celery, chopped

2 bay leaves

2 sprigs parsley

2 sprigs thyme

Water as needed

Preheat oven to 200°C. Place bones on a roasting tray. Roast for 30 minutes.

Transfer to slow cooker with vinegar, vegetables and herbs. Fill the slow cooker with water.

Cook on low for 24 hours, adding more water if necessary to keep the bones covered.

Strain stock through a fine mesh sieve into a large bowl and discard solids.

Use immediately or cool slightly then refrigerate to cool completely. Remove and discard fat from top.

Store broth in glass jars in the fridge for up to 1 week or in the freezer for up to a month. Use as a drink on its own or as a base for soups and stews.

Madras Beef Curry

SERVES 6
COOK TIME: LOW 8 HRS
GLUTEN FREE • DAIRY FREE

5 cloves garlic, crushed
Small piece ginger, minced
2 tsps pepper
½ tsp cinnamon
2 tsps garam masala
2 tsps ground turmeric
¼ cup (30g) ground coriander
2 tsps brown mustard seeds
2 tbsps ground cumin
¼ cup (60ml) malt vinegar
1 tbsp oil or ghee
1kg chuck beef, cubed
1 onion, sliced
2 tbsps tomato paste
1 tsp chilli powder
1 whole red chilli
4 curry leaves
1 x 400g can chopped tomatoes
1 cup (250ml) beef stock

In a small bowl combine garlic, ginger, pepper, cinnamon, garam masala, turmeric, coriander, mustard seeds, cumin and vinegar. Mix well.

Heat oil or ghee in a frying pan over high heat. Add the beef and brown quickly. Remove from pan and set aside.

In the same frying pan, add the spice paste and cook over medium heat for 3-5 minutes, stirring regularly, until fragrant.

Transfer the beef and curry paste to the slow cooker. Add onion, tomato paste, chilli powder, whole chilli, curry leaves, chopped tomatoes and beef stock.

Cook on low for 8 hours or until the beef is tender.

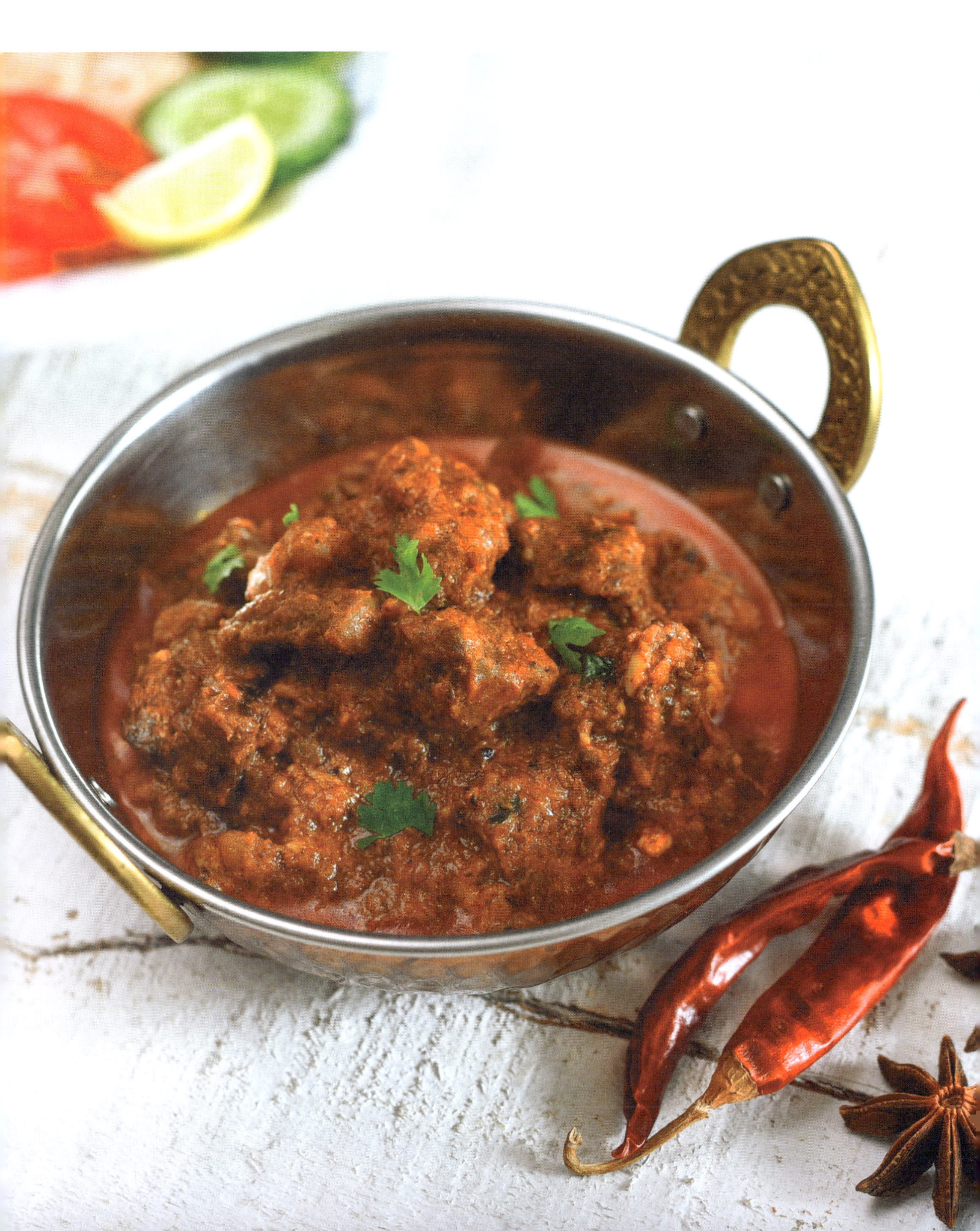

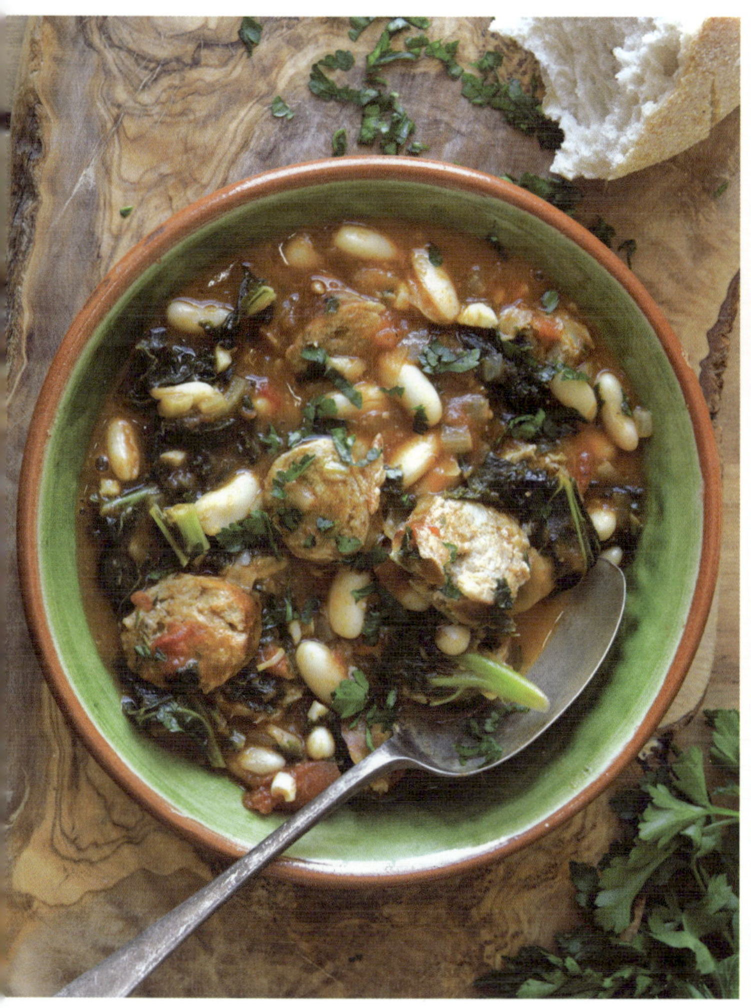

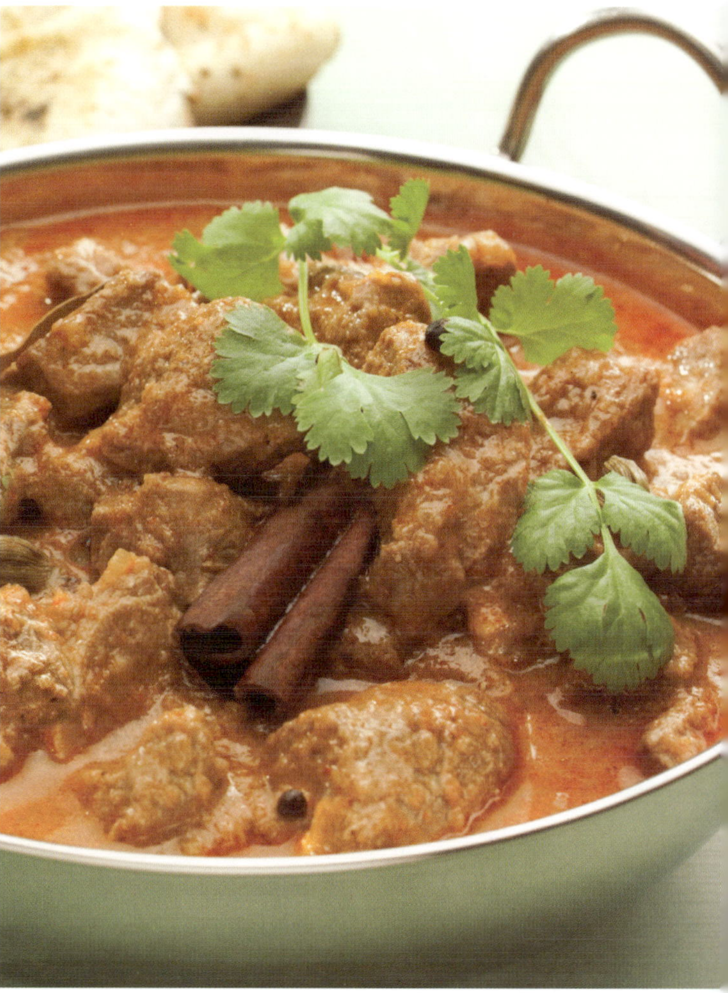

Sausage, Bean and Kale Stew

SERVES 8

COOK TIME: HIGH 2½ HRS/LOW 5 HRS

+ HIGH 45 MINS/LOW 1½ HRS

GLUTEN FREE • DAIRY FREE

Lamb Rogan Josh

SERVES 4

COOK TIME: LOW 7 HRS

GLUTEN FREE • DAIRY FREE

SAUSAGE, BEAN AND KALE STEW

500g pork sausage, sliced
1 tbsp olive oil
2 x 400g cans cannellini beans
2 cups (500ml) chicken stock
1 x 400g can chopped tomatoes
1 onion, diced
1 carrot, peeled and chopped
2 stalks celery, diced
4 cloves garlic, minced
1 tsp dried oregano leaves
½ tsp ground fennel
4 cups (270g) kale, stems removed and chopped
Salt and pepper to taste

Place sausages and oil in a frying pan over medium heat. Cook for 10 minutes, turning regularly until browned. Set aside to cool then slice into 1cm slices.

Place sausage, beans, stock, tomatoes, onion, carrot, celery, garlic, oregano and fennel into slow cooker. Stir gently. Cook for 2½ hours on high or 5 hours on low.

Add kale and stir through. Cook for a further 45 minutes on high or 1½ hours on low.

Season with salt and pepper and serve.

LAMB ROGAN JOSH

2-3 tbsps oil
800g lamb fillets, diced
1 medium onion, chopped
¾ cup (210g) rogan josh paste
2 small green capsicums, diced
2 x 400g cans crushed tomatoes
4 green cardamom pods, crushed
2 cinnamon sticks
2 bay leaves
Sprigs of coriander, to garnish

Heat 1 tablespoon oil in a large frying pan over high heat. Add lamb in batches, adding more oil as needed, and cook for 4-5 minutes until slightly browned. Remove from heat and set aside.

Add another tablespoon oil to same pan over medium-high heat. Add onion and cook for 3-5 minutes until soft and translucent. Reduce heat to medium. Add curry paste and cook for 2-3 minutes, stirring regularly, until fragrant.

Transfer to slow cooker with lamb, capsicum, tomatoes and spices.

Cover and cook on low for 7 hours. Serve with rice or naan and garnish with coriander.

BEEF AND DUMPLINGS

1 cup (125g) flour

½ tsp sweet paprika

Salt and pepper to taste

750g gravy steak, diced into 2cm pieces

2 tbsps olive oil

1 clove garlic

¼ cup (70g) tomato paste

1 cup (250ml) beef stock

1 tsp bicarbonate of soda

½ cup (125ml) milk

Fresh basil, to garnish

Mix a quarter of the flour with paprika and season with salt and pepper. Toss the steak pieces in the seasoned flour.

Heat 1 tablespoon of olive oil in a frying pan. Cook the garlic until fragrant then add to the slow cooker. Add the rest of the olive oil to the frying pan, add the meat and cook over a high heat until the meat is browned. Place the meat in the slow cooker.

In a large bowl mix the tomato paste with the beef stock and pour over the beef. Add to the slow cooker, cover and cook on low for 6 hours.

To make the dumplings, place the remaining flour, bicarb and ½ teaspoon salt in a mixing bowl. Pour in the milk and combine thoroughly to form a soft dough. Form into dumplings using your fingers. Add these to the slow cooker after 5 hours of cooking, for the final hour.

Serve with fresh basil as a garnish.

OXTAIL STEW

2 tbsps plain flour

Salt and pepper to taste

1kg oxtail pieces

2 tbsps olive oil

1 large onion, coarsely chopped

4 carrots, coarsely chopped

½ cup (125ml) red wine

1½ cups (375ml) beef stock

1 tbsp tomato paste

1 bay leaf

Spring onions, sliced, to garnish

Place the flour on a plate. Season the oxtail pieces then roll them in flour, shaking off the excess.

Heat the oil in a large frying pan over a medium-high heat. Cook the oxtail pieces for 2 minutes until browned all over – cook in batches if necessary. Transfer the meat to the slow cooker.

Add the onion, carrot, wine, stock, tomato paste and bay leaf (if using) to the slow cooker. Cover with the lid and cook on low for 4 hours or high for 8 hours, or until oxtail meat is tender. Garnish with spring onion to serve.

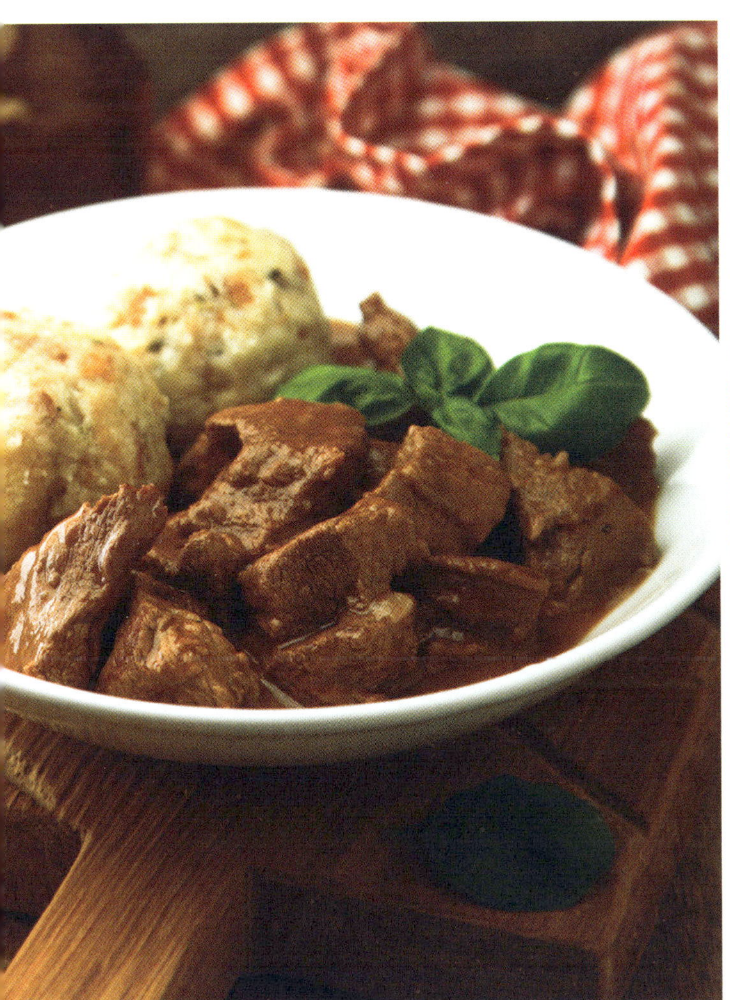

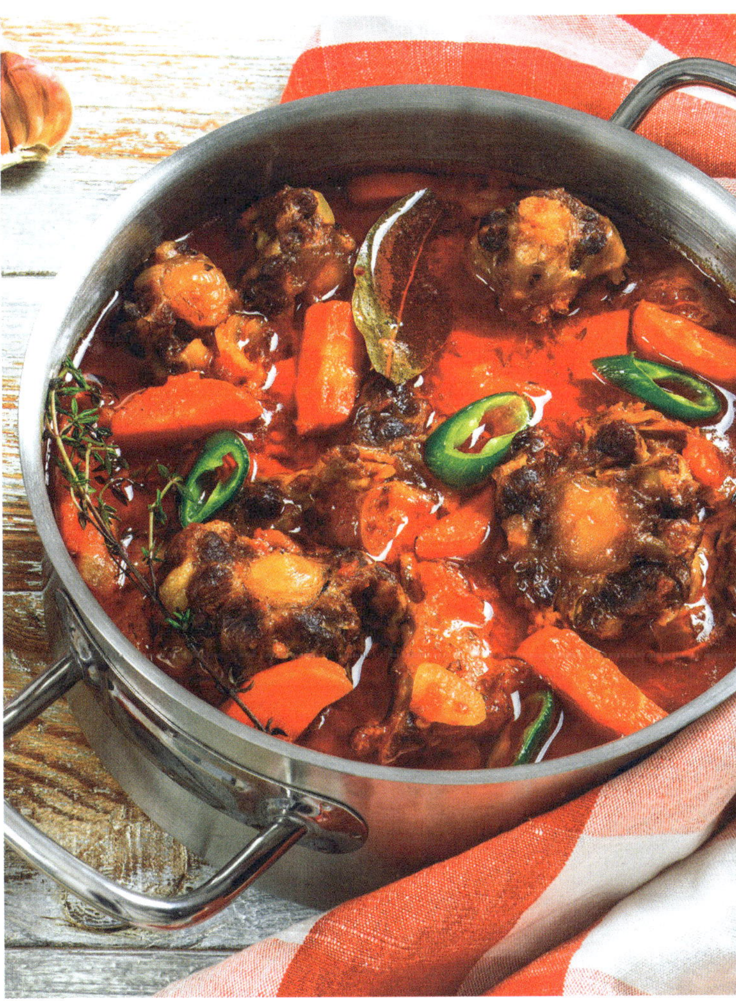

Beef and Dumplings

SERVES 4

COOK TIME: LOW 6 HRS

Oxtail Stew

SERVES 4

COOK TIME: HIGH 4 HRS/LOW 8 HRS

DAIRY FREE

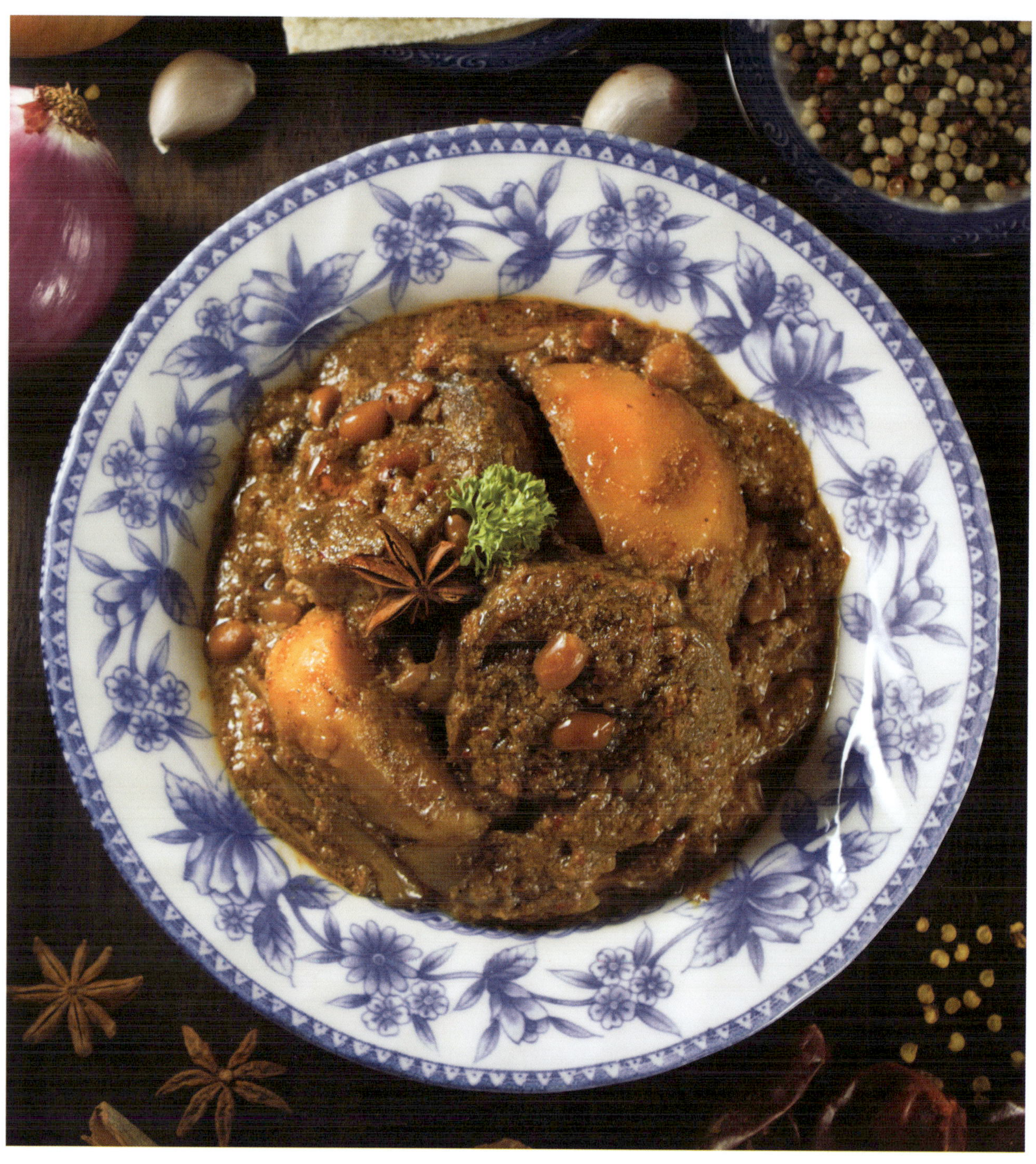

Massaman Curry

SERVES 6

COOK TIME: LOW 6 HRS

GLUTEN FREE • DAIRY FREE

MASSAMAN CURRY

2 tbsps canola oil

1kg chuck beef, cubed

1½ tsps arrowroot flour

Salt and pepper to taste

1 large onion, sliced

3 large waxy potatoes, peeled and cut into chunks

1⅔ cups (400ml) beef stock

1 x 400ml can coconut milk, shaken

2 tbsps lime juice

Chopped coriander leaves, star anise and cardamom, to garnish

MASSAMAN PASTE

1 red onion, chopped

2 small red chillies, deseeded and roughly chopped

2 tsps ground coriander

2 tsps ground cumin

1 star anise

½ tsp cardamom seeds

3 cloves garlic, crushed

2 stalks lemongrass, white part finely chopped

2 tsps chopped ginger

1 tsp shrimp paste

3 tsps fish sauce

1 tsp palm sugar

10 sprigs coriander

Salt and pepper to taste

Place all the paste ingredients in a food processor or use a stick blender to process into a paste.

Heat half the oil in a large pan over medium-high heat. Toss the beef in the arrowroot flour with some salt and pepper.

Cook the beef in batches for 3 minutes until browned, using the rest of the oil as needed. Transfer browned beef to the slow cooker. Add the paste and stir to coat the beef.

Add in the onion, potatoes, beef stock and coconut milk and stir through. Cover and cook on low for 6 hours.

Just before serving, stir through the lime juice.

Serve with a sprinkling of chopped coriander leaves, some star anise and cardamom for garnish.

Lasagne

SERVES 4

COOK TIME: LOW 5 HRS

1 tbsp olive oil
1 onion, finely chopped
1 clove garlic, chopped
2 carrots, diced
1 stalk celery, diced
550g beef mince
1 tbsp fresh or dried thyme (or oregano)
1 x 680g jar passata
Salt and pepper to taste
2 tbsps butter
2 tbsps plain flour
2 cups (500ml) milk
½ cup (60g) grated Parmesan cheese
375g lasagne sheets
¾ cup (90g) grated mozzarella cheese

Heat oil in a large saucepan over medium-high heat. Add onion and garlic and saute for 5 minutes, until soft and translucent. Add carrots and celery and cook, stirring, for 2-3 minutes until starting to soften. Add beef mince and herbs and cook, stirring, for 3-4 minutes until browned.

Pour in the passata and season with salt and pepper to taste. Stir to combine, then cover and allow to simmer for 15 minutes.

Heat butter in a saucepan over a low heat. Add flour and mix until a smooth thick paste forms. Gradually add the milk and gently bring to the boil, stirring constantly. Add the Parmesan and stir through until melted.

Assemble in slow cooker, starting with the meat sauce, then cheese sauce, then lasagne sheets. Repeat to form two more layers finishing with cheese sauce. Scatter the mozzarella cheese over the top.

Cover and cook on low for 5 hours.

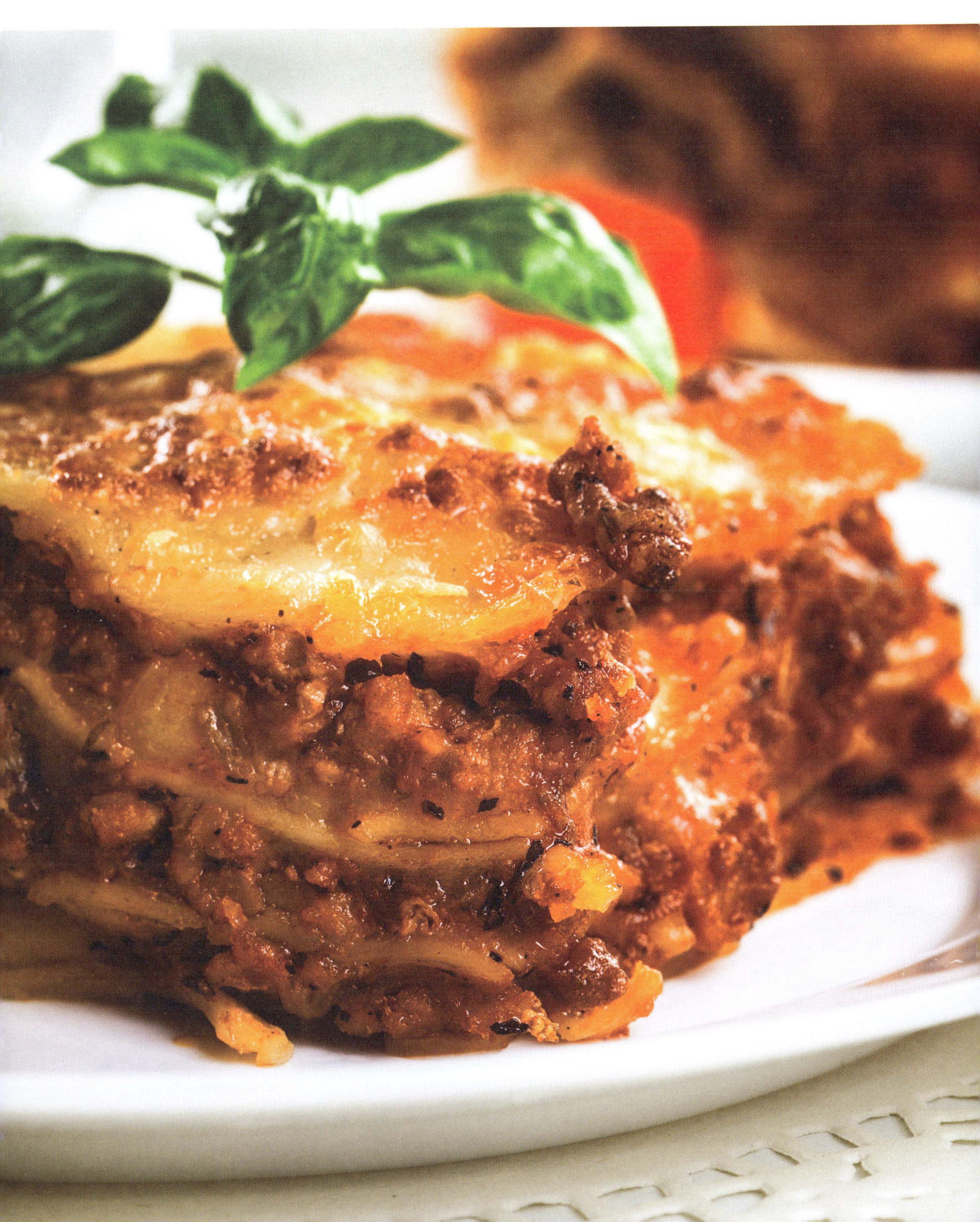

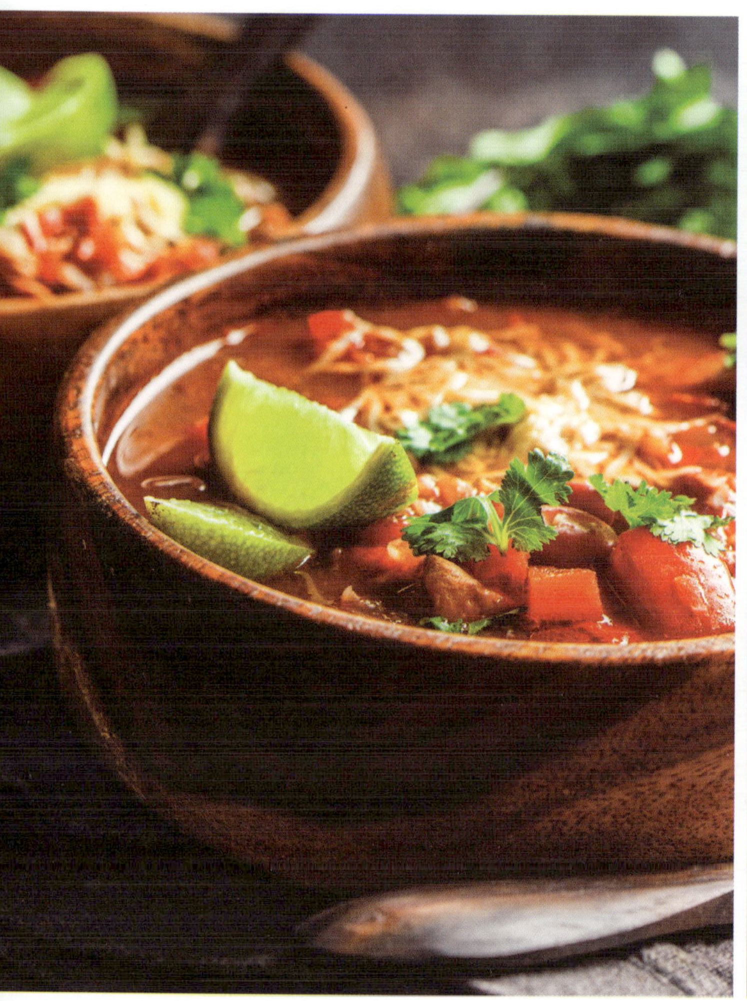

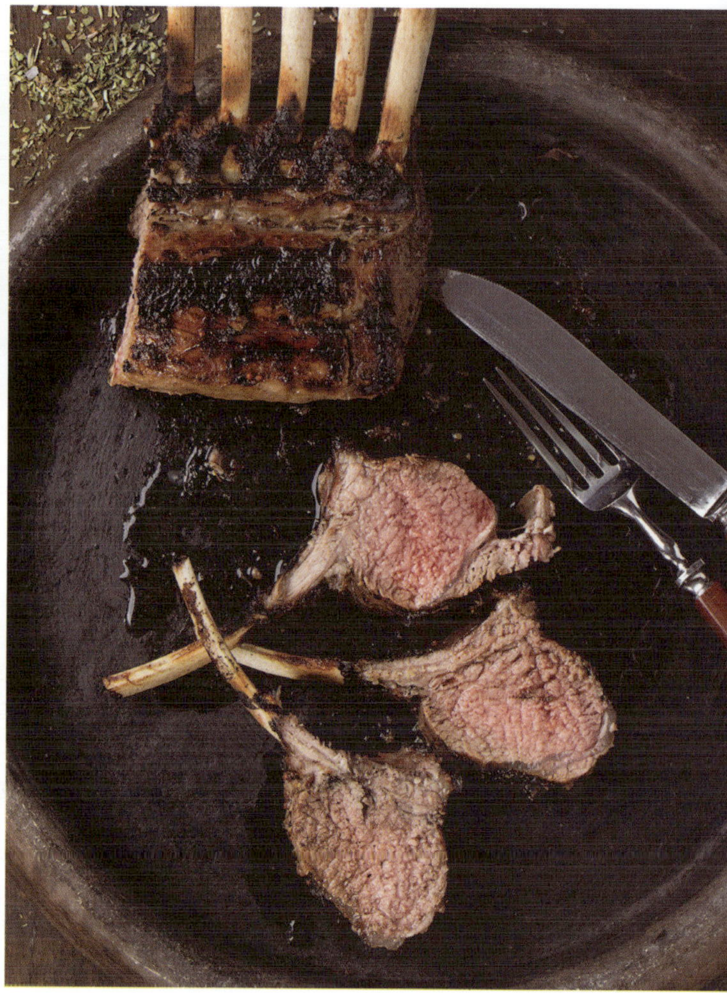

Beef and Bean Stew

SERVES 6
COOK TIME: LOW 5-6 HRS
GLUTEN FREE

Lamb Rack

SERVES 4
COOK TIME: HIGH 4 HRS/LOW 8 HRS
GLUTEN FREE • DAIRY FREE

BEEF AND BEAN STEW

1 tbsp olive oil
1 red onion, finely diced
500g beef mince
2 cloves garlic, minced
2 red chillies, finely sliced
3 tsps ground cumin
2 tsps ground coriander
2 tsps chilli powder
1 large red capsicum, diced
1 x 400g canned diced tomatoes
4 medium tomatoes, roughly chopped
4 cups (1L) beef stock
Salt and pepper to taste
2 x 400g cans kidney beans, drained and rinsed
Grated Cheddar cheese and fresh coriander, to serve

Heat oil in a large pan over medium heat. Add onion and cook for 3 minutes until soft. Transfer to slow cooker.

Add mince to pan and cook, stirring, until browned. Transfer to slow cooker with garlic, spices, capsicum, tomatoes and stock. Season with salt and pepper. Cook for 5-6 hours on low. Add beans, stir and cook for 10 minutes more. Serve with cheese and coriander.

LAMB RACK

2 lamb racks (about 1.2kg)
Salt and pepper to taste
2 tbsps olive oil
1⅓ cups (350ml) red wine
2 cloves garlic, minced
2 tbsps fresh rosemary, chopped
1 tsp dried thyme
100g plum jam

Season lamb all over with salt and pepper.

Heat oil in a frying pan over high heat. When hot, sear the lamb on all sides, turning to ensure lamb is browned evenly. Remove lamb from pan and set aside on a plate.

Use wine to deglaze the pan, scraping up any brown bits with a spatula. Pour into slow cooker.

In a small bowl combine garlic, rosemary, thyme and jam.

Spread evenly over lamb and place in slow cooker.

Cover and cook on low for 8 hours or high for 4 hours, turning the racks 1 or 2 times and spooning over the marinade.

Allow the lamb to rest for 10 minutes before slicing.

MUTTON AND ONION STEW

700g lamb shoulder, cubed
1 cup (125g) plain flour
1 tsp salt
½ tsp pepper
2 tbsps olive oil
1 large onion, roughly chopped
1 tsp dried rosemary
2 cups (500ml) water
2 quinces, peeled and cut into wedges
Fresh dill, roughly chopped, to garnish

Place the lamb in a mixing bowl with the flour, salt and pepper, and toss until coated.

Heat the oil in a large frying pan over a medium-high heat, and brown the lamb in batches for about 3-4 minutes. Transfer the lamb to the slow cooker.

Reduce the heat to medium and cook the onion for 3-4 minutes or until softened. Add the rosemary and water, stirring well. Add the liquid and quinces to the slow cooker and cook on high for 4 hours or low for 8 hours.

Serve with a garnish of fresh dill.

SAUSAGES WITH ONIONS AND MUSHROOMS

1 tbsp olive oil
12 pork sausages
3 red onions, sliced
1 tbsp brown sugar
2 tbsps plain flour
1 tbsp passata
2 cups (500ml) beef stock
2 bay leaves
350g mushrooms, sliced
Salt and pepper to taste
Handful fresh parsley leaves, chopped

Heat oil in a large frying pan over medium-high heat. Add sausages to pan and brown quickly for 2 minutes on each side. Transfer to slow cooker.

Discard all but about 1 tablespoon of fat from pan. Add onions and sugar to pan and cook for 5 minutes, stirring regularly, until soft and translucent. Add flour and passata. Cook, stirring, for 1 minute, then add stock; stir well to remove any lumps. Bring to boil then pour into slow cooker along with bay leaves and mushrooms.

Cover and cook for 8 hours on low or 4 hours on high.

Season with salt and pepper and sprinkle with parsley.

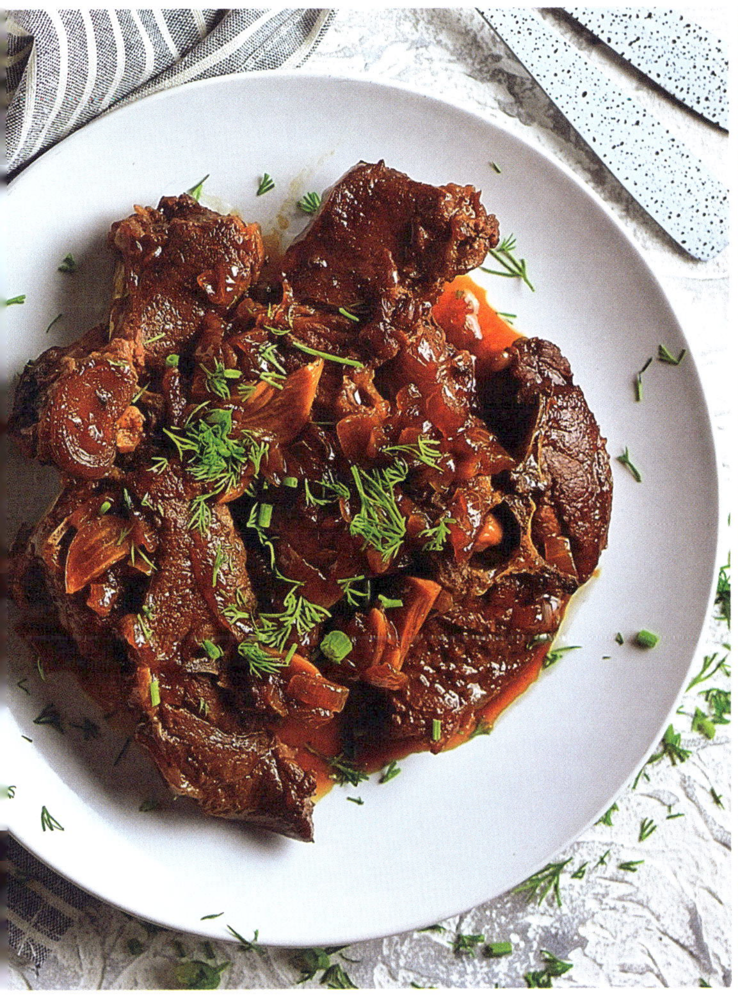

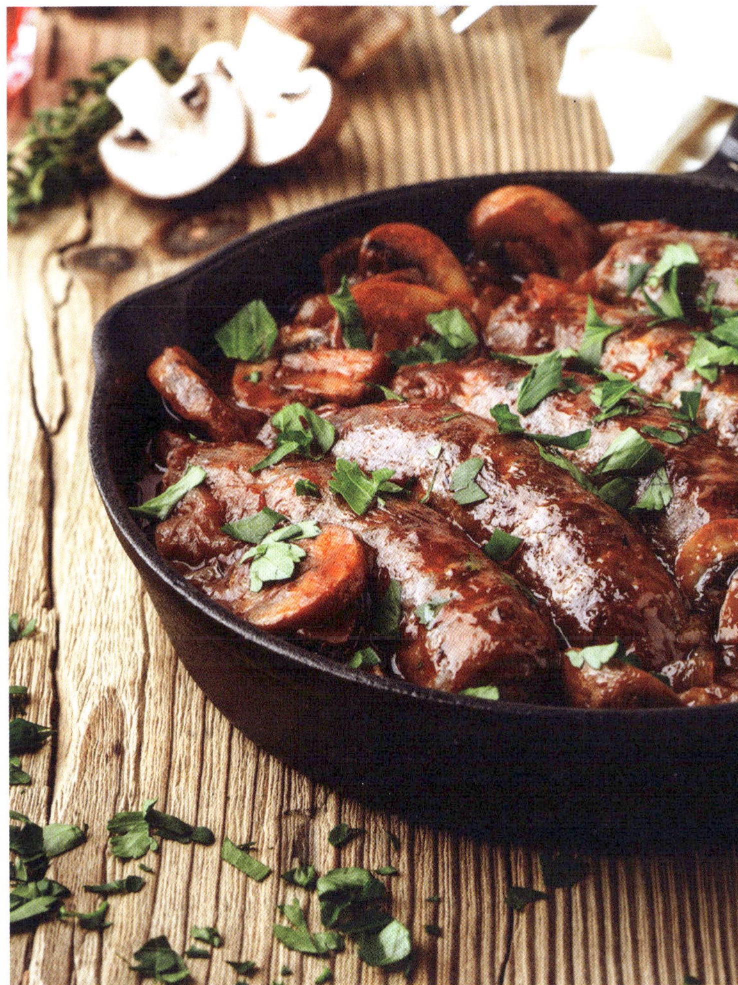

Mutton and Onion Stew

SERVES 4

COOK TIME: HIGH 4 HRS/LOW 8 HRS

DAIRY FREE

Sausages with Onions and Mushrooms

SERVES 4

COOK TIME: HIGH 4 HRS/LOW 8 HRS

DAIRY FREE

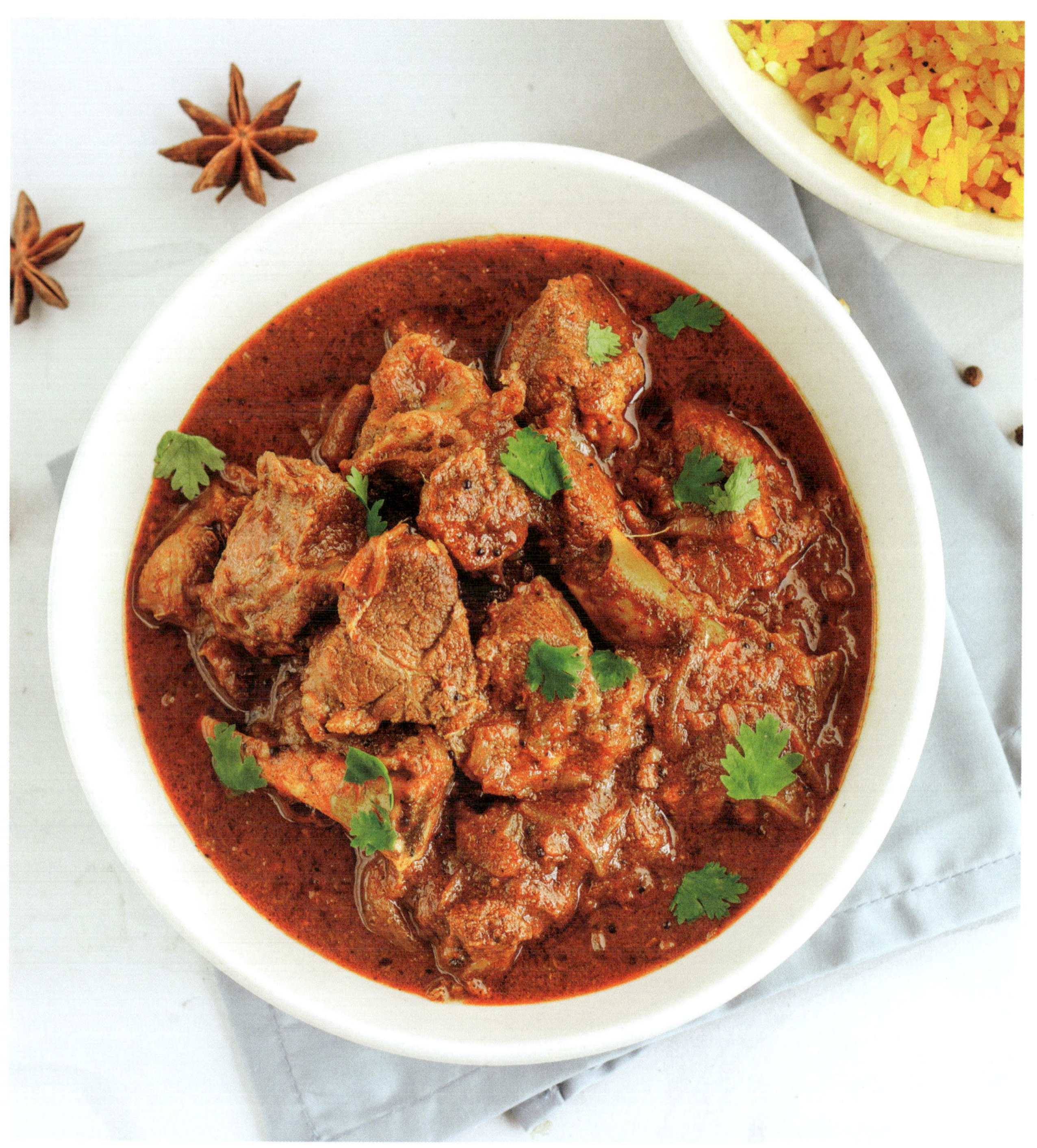

Lamb Vindaloo

SERVES 6

COOK TIME: LOW 6-7 HRS

GLUTEN FREE • DAIRY FREE

LAMB VINDALOO

1kg lamb shoulder on the bone, cut into medium-sized pieces

3 tbsps ghee or vegetable oil

2 onions, finely chopped

1 cup (250ml) water

1 sprig curry leaves

Salt and pepper to taste

¼ cup (10g) chopped fresh coriander leaves

VINDALOO PASTE

15 dried red Kashmiri chillies (use less for a milder curry)

10 cloves garlic

Medium piece ginger, roughly chopped

1 tbsp coriander seeds

1½ tsps cumin seeds

7 cloves

3 green cardamom pods

10 black peppercorns

1 cinnamon stick

½ tsp ground turmeric

2 tsps tamarind pulp

3 tbsps apple cider vinegar

3 tbsps water

Place vindaloo paste ingredients into a food processor and blend until smooth. Add to a large bowl with lamb. Coat evenly then cover and refrigerate overnight.

Heat oil in a frying pan over medium-high heat. Add onions to pan and cook for 5 minutes, stirring regularly, until soft.

Transfer onions to slow cooker with lamb and marinade. Add water and curry leaves. Season with salt and pepper.

Cover and cook on low for 6-7 hours until tender. Discard curry leaves.

Sprinkle with chopped coriander leaves to serve.

Meatball Soup

SERVES 6

COOK TIME: HIGH 4 HRS/LOW 8 HRS

MEATBALLS

3-4 slices white bread, crusts removed

2 cups (500ml) water

500g beef mince

2 eggs

½ cup (50g) grated Parmesan cheese

1 tsp dried parsley

1 tsp dried oregano

1 tsp salt

1 clove garlic, minced

2 tbsps olive oil, for frying

SOUP

2 carrots, chopped

1 small onion, chopped

2 stalks celery, chopped

2 medium potatoes, chopped

3 ripe tomatoes, deseeded and chopped

2 tbsps finely chopped fresh dill or basil

½ tsp dried basil

½ tsp dried oregano

4 cups (1L) vegetable stock

¾ cup (160g) spaghetti, broken into small pieces

In a small bowl soak bread in water for 1 minute, then squeeze out moisture and crumble.

In a medium bowl combine bread crumble mixture with remaining meatball ingredients and combine well.

Roll to form into small balls.

Heat oil in a medium frying pan and brown meatballs on all sides.

Using a slotted spoon transfer the meatballs to the slow cooker, then add the carrots, onion, celery, potatoes, tomatoes, herbs and stock.

Cover and cook on high for 4 hours or on low for 8 hours.

Add spaghetti and cook on high for 15 minutes.

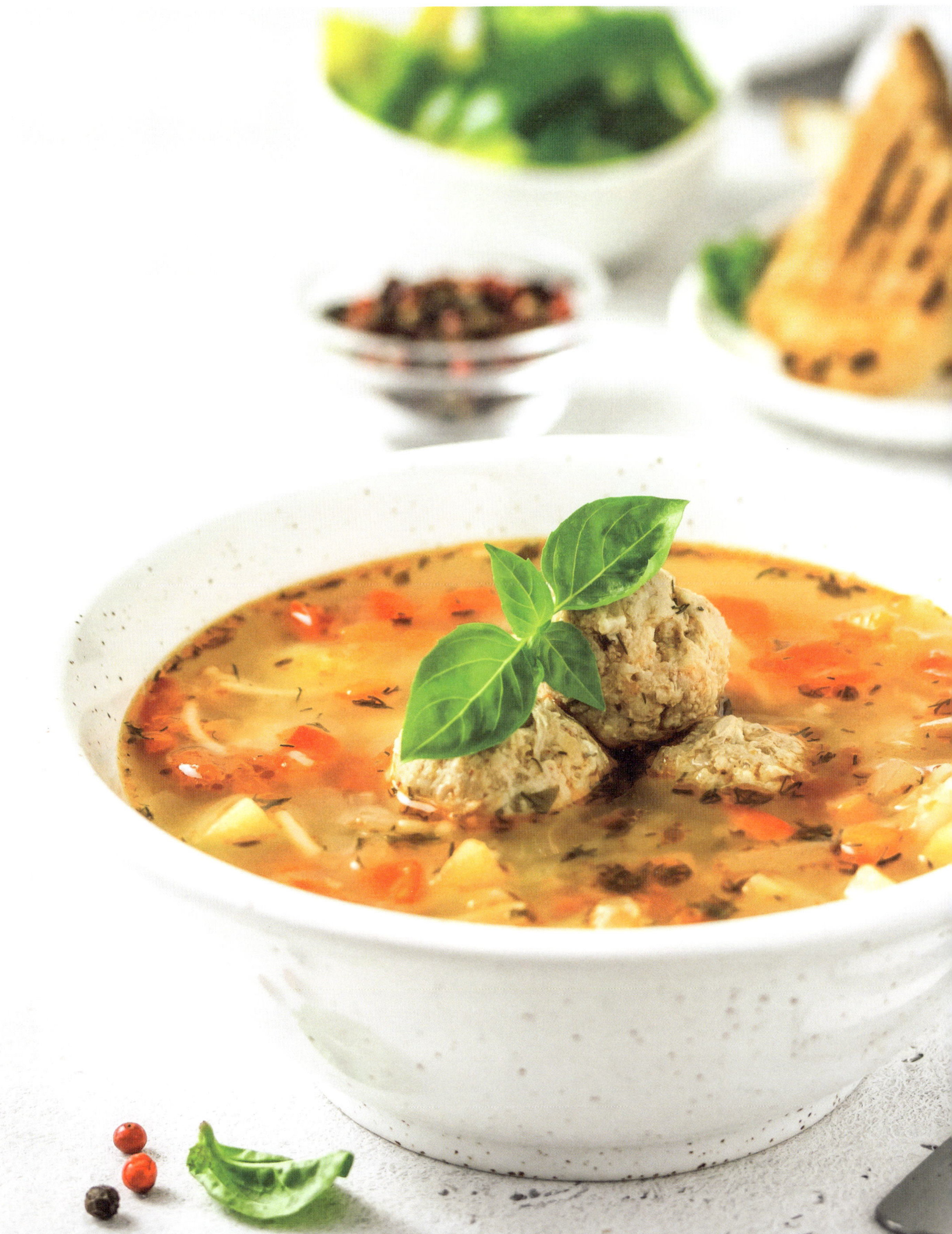

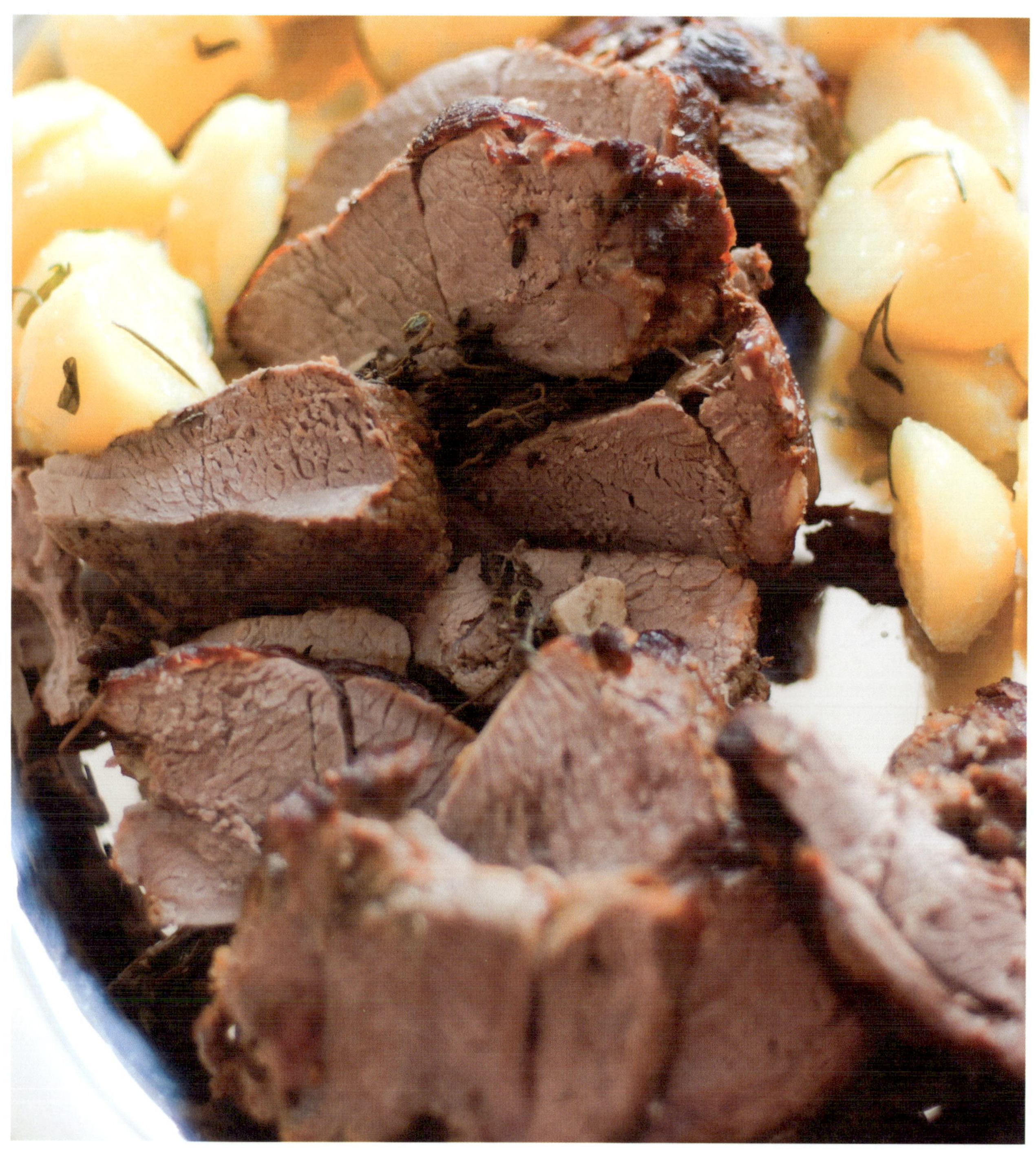

Herb and Quince Stuffed Lamb Shoulder

SERVES 4

COOK TIME: LOW 10 HRS

GLUTEN FREE

HERB AND QUINCE STUFFED LAMB SHOULDER

6 tbsps olive oil

1 onion, finely chopped

2 tbsps fresh rosemary, roughly chopped, plus extra to garnish

20g unsalted butter

100g pickled quinces (or quince paste)

Rind of 1 lemon, grated

2 tbsps fresh thyme, roughly chopped, plus extra to garnish

Salt and pepper to taste

1kg lamb shoulder, small enough to fit slow cooker

Baby potatoes, to serve

Heat 2 tablespoons of olive oil in a large frying pan over a medium-high heat. Add the onion and rosemary and cook until caramelised – about 5 minutes. Set aside in a mixing bowl.

Add another 2 tablespoons of olive oil to the pan with the butter. Over a high heat, saute the quinces until golden in colour, then add to the onion and rosemary mixture.

Add the lemon rind and thyme and season well with salt and pepper. Mix well.

Spread out the lamb shoulder on a clean surface. Place the stuffing in the centre and tie it up with string as if it were a parcel, keeping the stuffing in place.

Heat the rest of the olive oil in the frying pan and sear the lamb on all sides until browned. Place in the slow cooker and cook on low for 10 hours, or until the lamb is cooked through and tender.

Serve with cooked baby potatoes and extra rosemary and thyme as a garnish.

BEEF STEW WITH BEER AND ROSEMARY

2 tbsps olive oil
1.5kg chuck steak, cubed
2 stalks celery, roughly chopped
2 cups (500ml) dark beer
2 tbsps tomato paste
Salt and pepper to taste
300g potatoes (such as Desiree), roughly chopped
2 sprigs rosemary, chopped

Heat half of the oil in a large saucepan over a medium-high heat. Brown the beef in batches, adding more oil if necessary. Remove the beef from the saucepan and place in the slow cooker.

Heat the rest of the oil in the saucepan and add the celery. Cook while stirring for 3 minutes or until the celery is softened. Add to the slow cooker with the beer, tomato paste and salt and pepper, and stir well.

Cook on high for 4 hours or low for 8 hours or until the beef is tender. Add potatoes and rosemary with 30 minutes to go.

LAMB KHOOR CURRY

2 tbsps olive oil
4 lamb shanks
1 tsp garam masala
1 tsp chilli powder
2 tsps paprika
1 tsp ground cumin
2 cups (500ml) beef stock
1 cup (250ml) water
Fresh coriander, to garnish

Heat the olive oil in a large frying pan over a medium-high heat. Add the lamb shanks and sear on all sides for about 5 minutes or until browned.

Add the lamb to the slow cooker with garam masala, chilli powder, paprika, cumin, stock and water.

Cook on low for 6 hours or until lamb is tender. Serve with a garnish of coriander leaves.

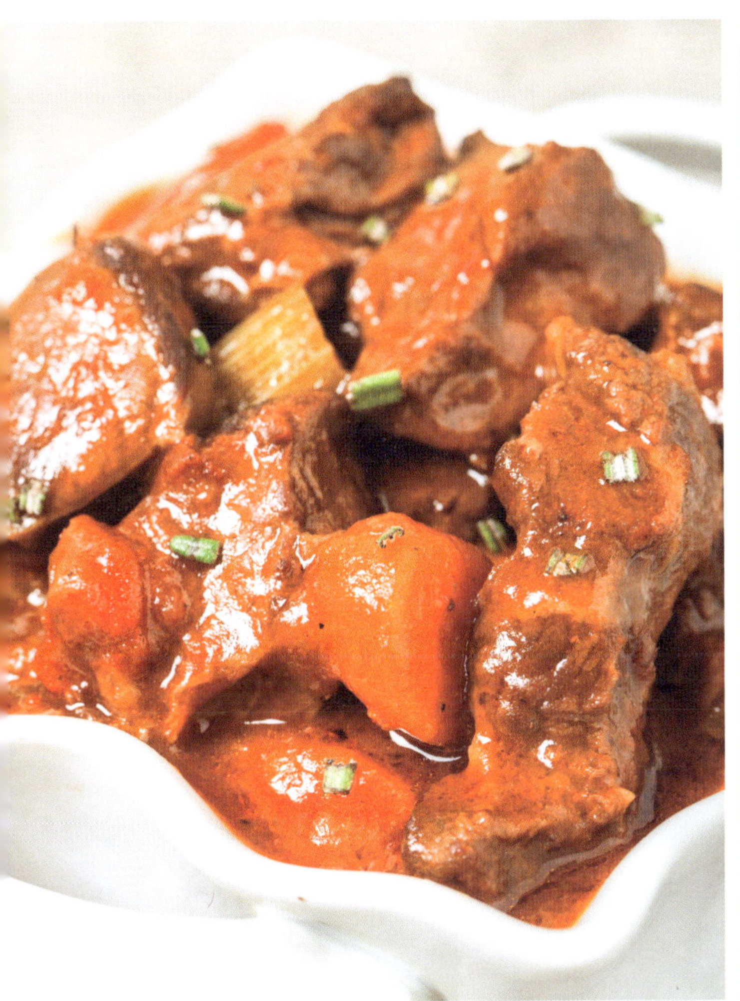

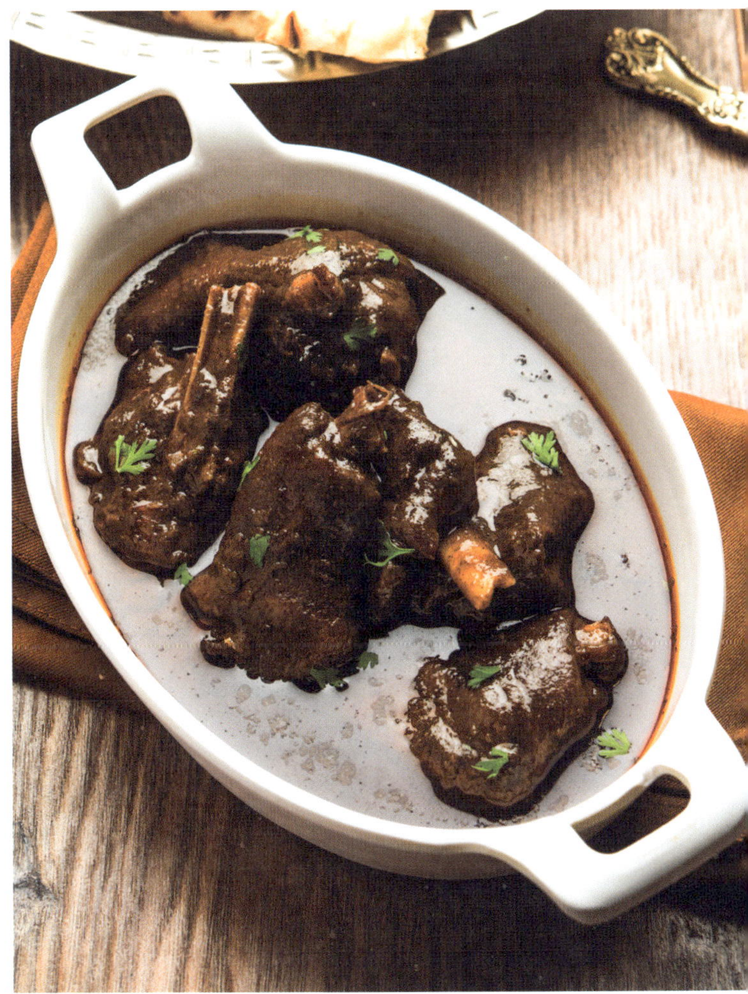

Beef Stew with Beer and Rosemary

SERVES 4

COOK TIME: HIGH 4 HRS/LOW 8 HRS

DAIRY FREE

Lamb Khoor Curry

SERVES 4

COOK TIME: LOW 6 HRS

GLUTEN FREE • DAIRY FREE

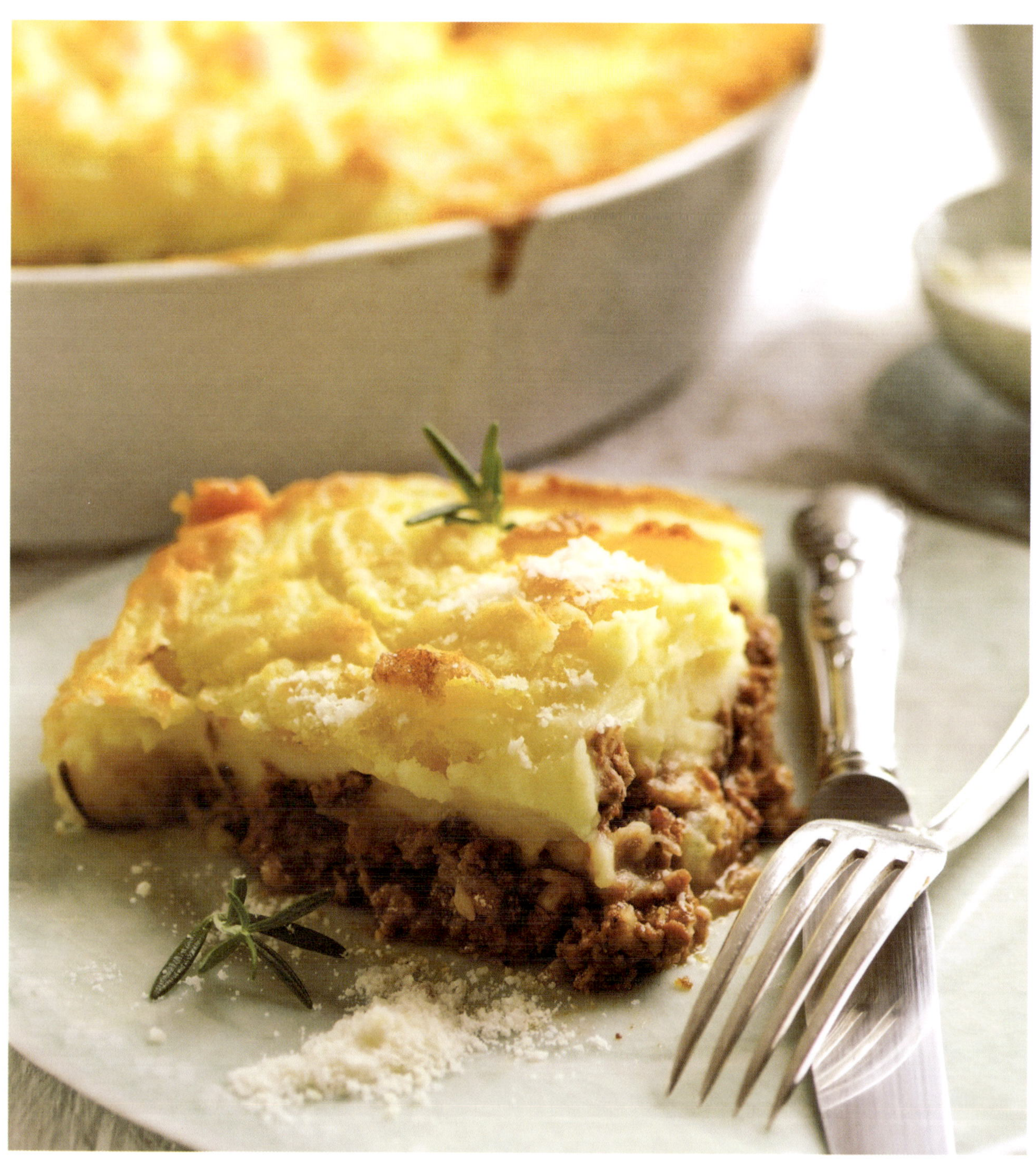

Shepherd's Pie

SERVES 4-6

COOK TIME: LOW 5 HRS

GLUTEN FREE

SHEPHERD'S PIE

900g potatoes, peeled and cut into chunks

2 tbsps creme fraiche

25g butter

Salt and pepper to taste

1 tbsp olive oil

1 onion, finely chopped

2 carrots, finely diced

2 stalks celery, finely diced

2-3 rosemary sprigs

750g lamb mince

1 tbsp dried mixed herbs

1 tbsp passata

1 tsp Worcestershire sauce

1½ cups (375ml) beef stock

¼ cup (25g) grated Parmesan cheese

Place potatoes in a pan of salted water. Bring to the boil then reduce heat and simmer for 12-13 minutes or until cooked through. Drain well, then mash with the creme fraiche, butter, salt and pepper. Set aside.

Heat the oil in a large frying pan over medium-high heat. Add the onion and fry for 3-5 minutes, stirring, until soft and translucent. Add carrots and celery and rosemary and fry for a further 2 minutes.

Add the lamb and herbs and fry for 8 minutes until the lamb is browned, using a wooden spoon to break up the lamb. Add passata and Worcestershire sauce. Stir to combine. Transfer to slow cooker.

Deglaze the pan with beef stock, using a spatula to scrape up any brown bits. Pour into slow cooker and stir to combine.

Spoon mashed potato on top of the mince mixture and spread out evenly with a fork. Sprinkle with Parmesan cheese. Cook on low for 5 hours. The mixture should be bubbling at the sides when it is ready.

Roast Lamb with Garlic and Rosemary

SERVES 6

COOK TIME: HIGH 4-5 HRS/LOW 9-10 HRS

GLUTEN FREE • DAIRY FREE

1 tsp salt

½ tsp pepper

8 cloves garlic, peeled and crushed

6 sprigs fresh rosemary, leaves chopped

1.5kg boneless leg of lamb, trimmed and tied

2 tbsps olive oil

½ cup (125ml) vegetable stock (or water)

Preheat the slow cooker on a high setting for 20 minutes.

In a small bowl, combine the salt, pepper, garlic and rosemary together to form a paste. Rub all over the lamb.

Heat the olive oil in a large frying pan over a medium-high heat. Add the lamb and cook for 3-4 minutes, turning, to ensure even browning. Place browned roast into the slow cooker.

Deglaze the pan with the stock, using a spatula to scrape up any brown bits. Transfer to the slow cooker.

Cover and cook for 4-5 hours on high or 9-10 hours on low.

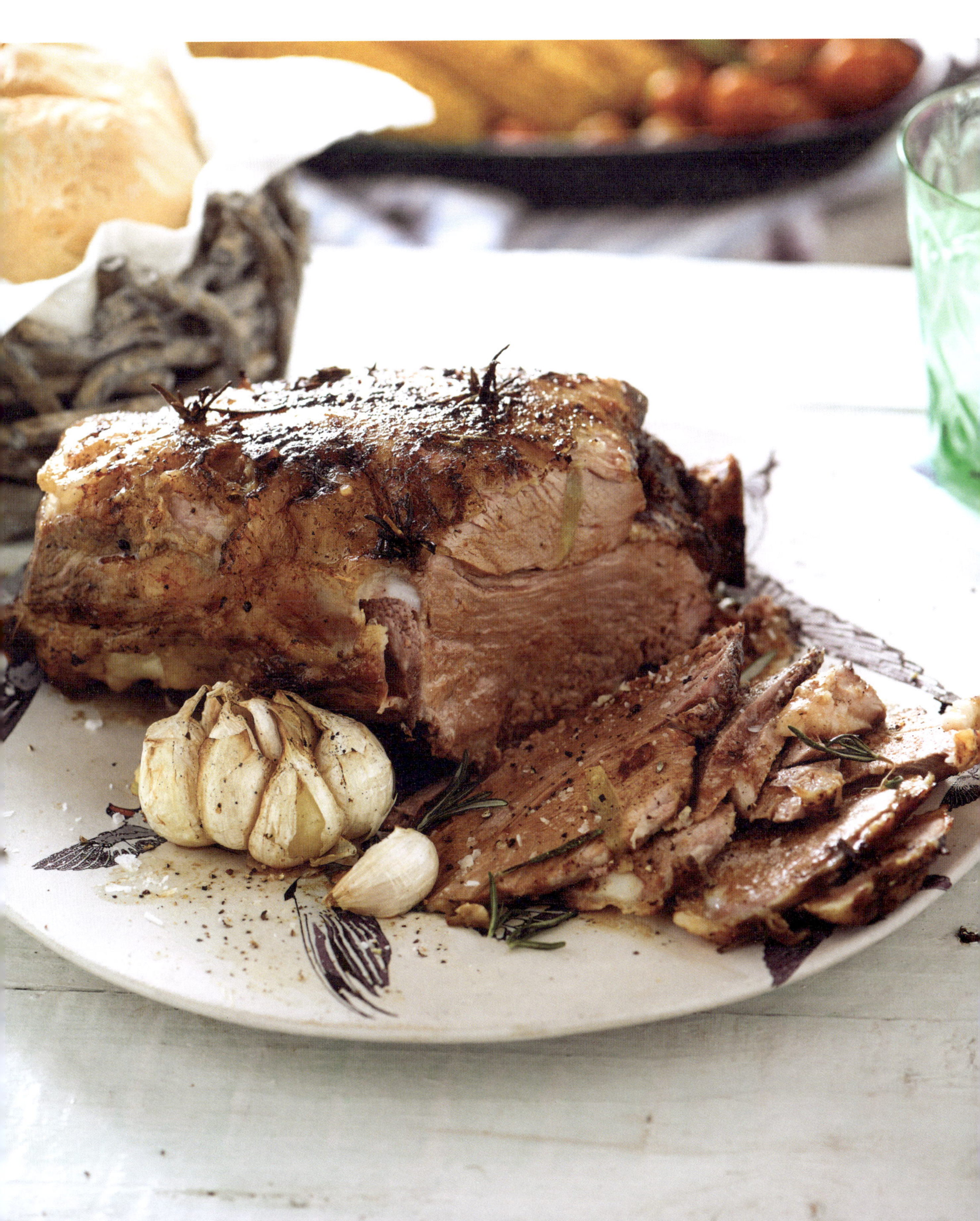

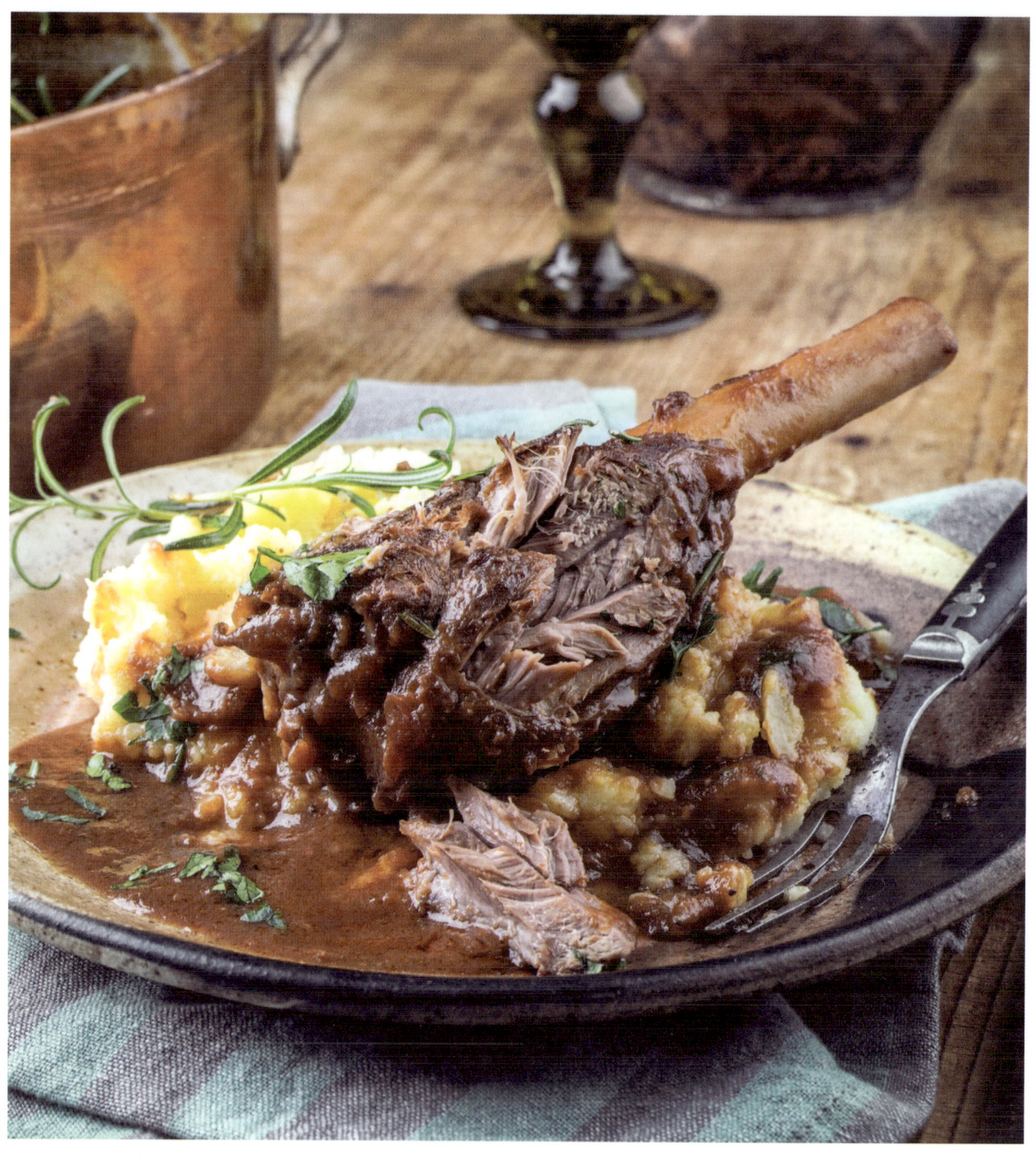

Lamb Shanks in Red Wine Sauce

SERVES 4

COOK TIME: LOW 8 HRS

GLUTEN FREE • DAIRY FREE

LAMB SHANKS IN RED WINE SAUCE

2 tbsps olive oil
4 lamb shanks
1 cup (250ml) beef stock
⅔ cup (150ml) red wine
2 tbsps tomato paste
1 bay leaf
Salt and pepper to taste
1 tbsp cornflour
Mashed potato, to serve

Heat the olive oil in a large frying pan over a medium-high heat. Brown the lamb shanks on all sides, then place in the slow cooker with the stock, wine, tomato paste and bay leaf. Stir well and sprinkle with salt and pepper to taste. Cook on low for 8 hours.

When cooking is complete, remove the lamb shanks from the cooker and place in a dish. Cover with silver foil to keep warm.

Pour the liquid from the slow cooker into a saucepan, add the cornflour, and stir well over a low heat until the sauce has thickened slightly. Remove the lamb shanks from the foil, pour on the sauce and serve with a side of mashed potato.

Bulgur with Beef Ragu

SERVES 4
COOK TIME: LOW 5 HRS
DAIRY FREE

1kg beef mince
Salt and pepper to taste
3 tbsps olive oil
2 carrots, finely copped
2 stalks celery, peeled and finely chopped
1 tbsp tomato paste
1 cup (250ml) beef stock
3½ cups (875ml) water
1½ cups (270g) medium-grain bulgur
Fresh basil, roughly chopped, to garnish

In a large bowl season the beef mince to taste.

Place 1 tablespoon of oil in a large frying pan over a medium-high heat. Cook the beef in batches until browned, splashing in some more oil between batches as needed. Use a draining spoon to transfer the meat to the slow cooker, leaving the oils and juices in the pan.

Add the carrots and celery to the frying pan and reduce to a low heat. Cook for 15 minutes or until softened. Add the tomato paste and cook for 1 minute more, then pour the mixture into the slow cooker with the stock and ½ cup of water. Cook for 5 hours on low until the meat is tender.

About 30 minutes before serving, place the bulgur in a large saucepan with 3 cups of water. Bring to the boil, cover, and reduce the heat to simmer for 10-12 minutes or until tender. Drain if necessary.

Serve with a garnish of chopped basil.

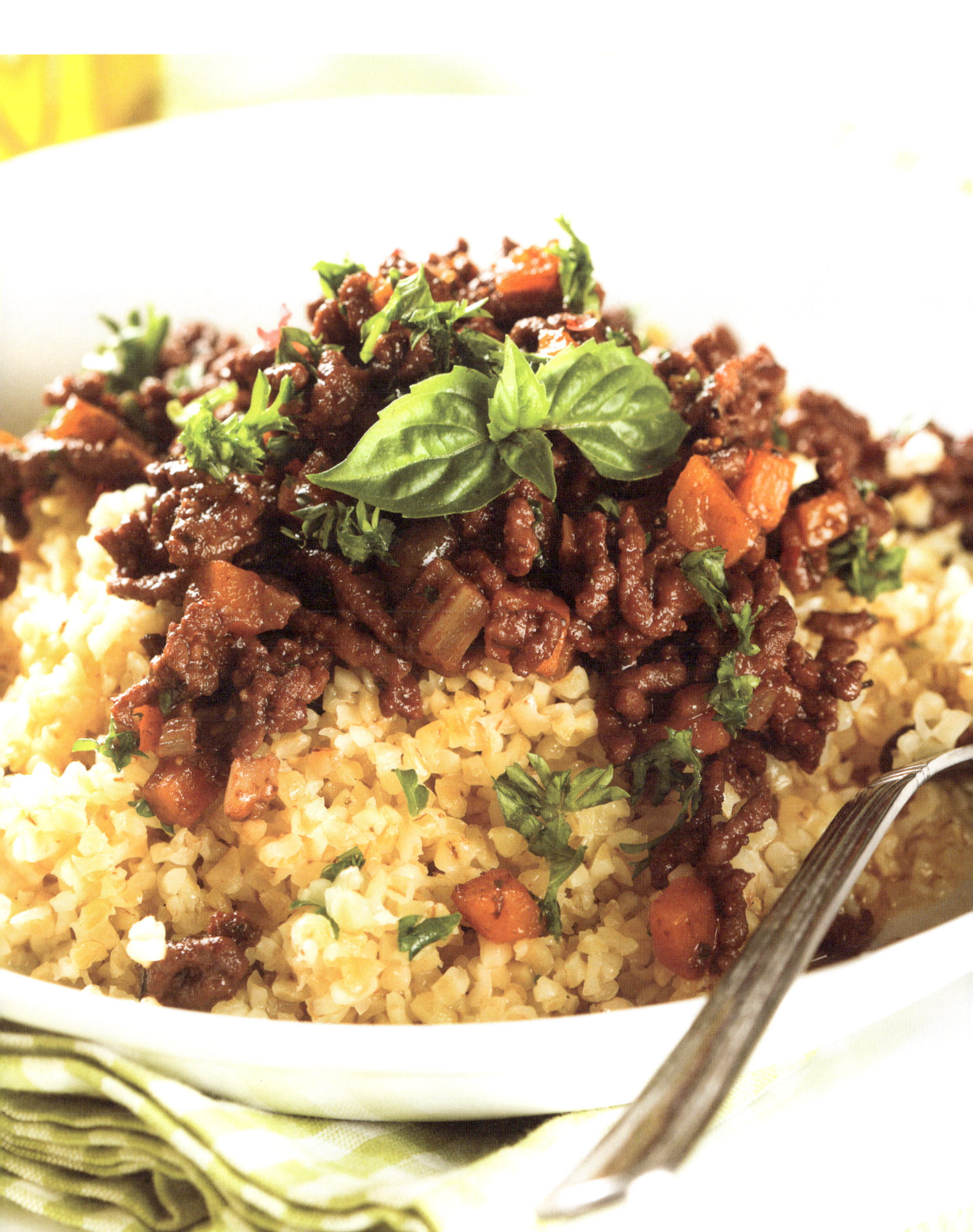

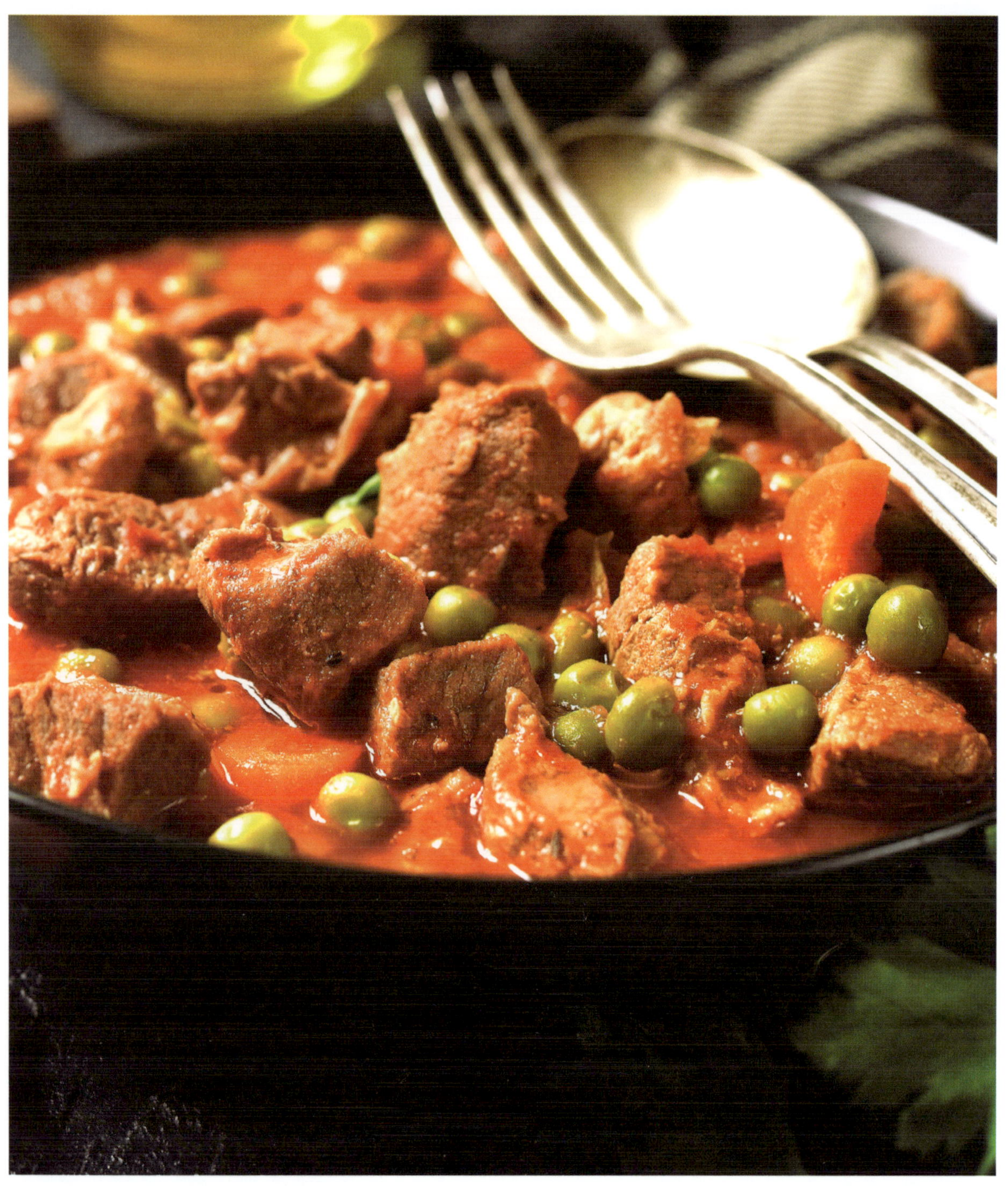

Veal and Pea Casserole

SERVES 4

COOK TIME: HIGH 4 HRS/LOW 8 HRS

DAIRY FREE

VEAL AND PEA CASSEROLE

2 tbsps olive oil
1kg veal, cut into cubes
Pepper to taste
1 onion, roughly chopped
1 small green capsicum, roughly chopped
¼ cup (30g) plain flour
2 cups (500ml) chicken stock
1 x 400g can chopped tomatoes
2 cups (340g) peas, fresh or frozen
Flat-leaf parsley, to garnish

Heat the oil in a large frying pan over a medium-high heat. Season the veal with pepper and cook in batches for 4-5 minutes or until browned on all sides.

Place the veal, onion and capsicum in the slow cooker. Sprinkle with flour and toss well to coat.

Stir in the stock and chopped tomatoes. Cover and cook on high for 4 hours or low for 8 hours, adding the peas with 1 hour or 2 hours to left to cook respectively (depending on your temperature setting).

Serve with a garnish of flat-leaf parsley.

Chapter Two

Pork and Chicken

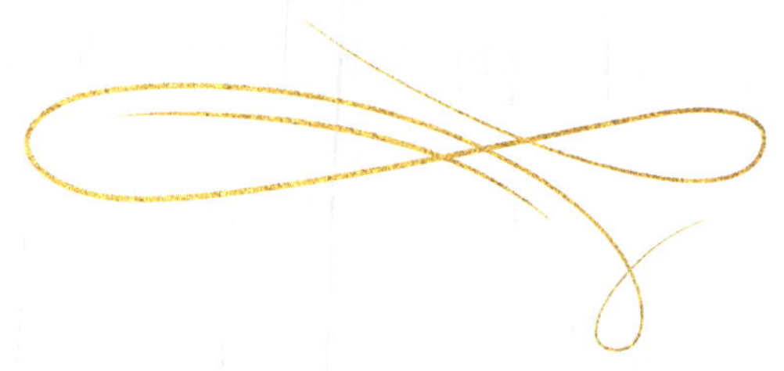

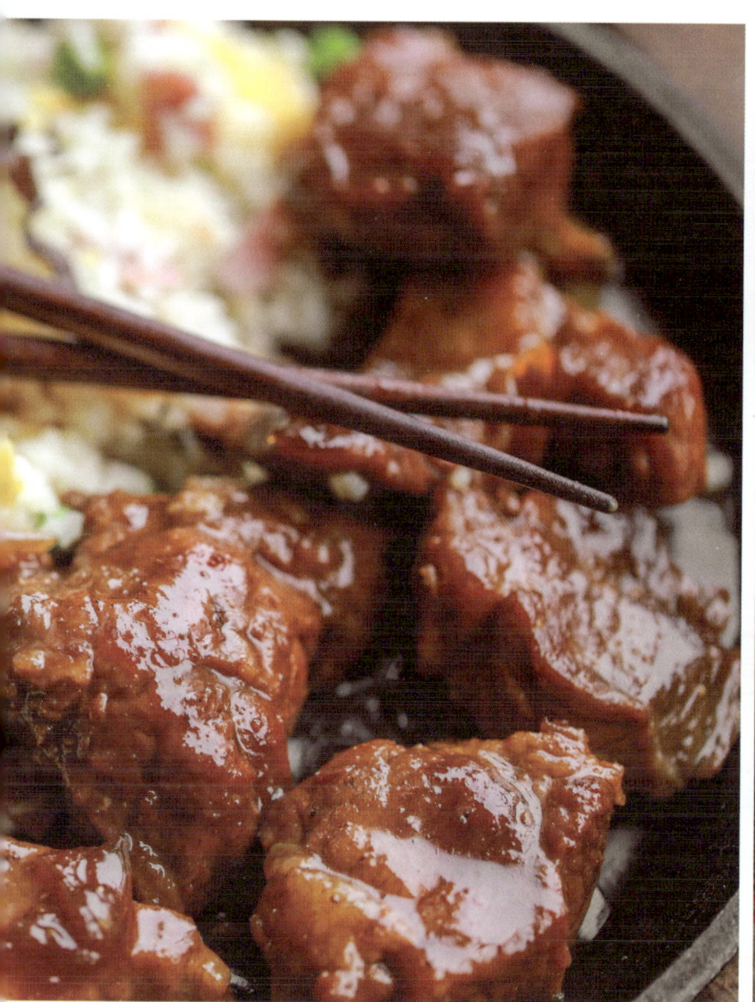

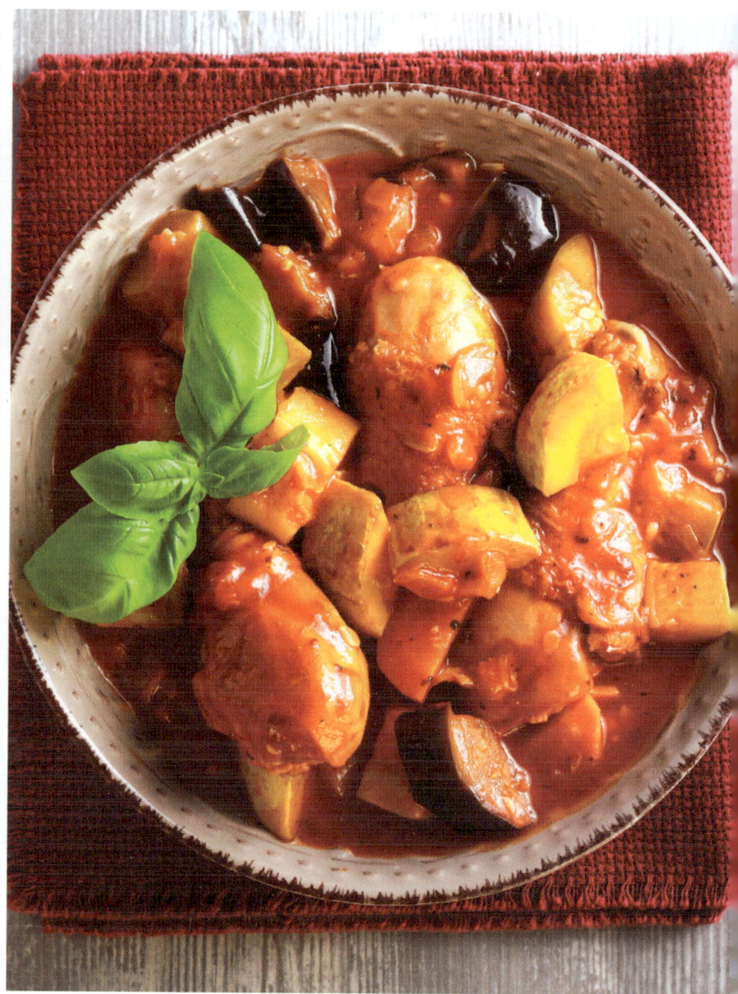

Caramelised Pork

SERVES 4

COOK TIME: HIGH 4 HRS/LOW 8 HRS

GLUTEN FREE • DAIRY FREE

Chicken and Tomato Casserole

SERVES 4

COOK TIME: LOW 6 HRS

GLUTEN FREE • DAIRY FREE

CARAMELISED PORK

1kg rindless pork belly cut into 1cm-thick slices
4 cups (1L) chicken stock, hot
Medium piece ginger, finely chopped
3 cloves garlic, peeled and chopped in half

GLAZE

2 tbsps vegetable oil
Pinch of salt and pepper
Large piece ginger, peeled and minced
1 red chilli, finely chopped
2 tbsps honey
2 tbsps brown sugar
3 tbsps dark soy sauce (or tamari)
1 stalk lemongrass, soft part only, finely chopped

Add pork belly, chicken stock, ginger and garlic to the slow cooker. Cover and cook on low for 8 hours or on high for 4 hours. Remove pork and chop into bite-size chunks.

Heat oil in a pan over high heat and add pork, salt and pepper. Fry until golden.

Mix the remaining glaze ingredients in a small bowl. Pour glaze over pork and cook until pork looks dark and sticky. Serve with fried rice.

CHICKEN AND TOMATO CASSEROLE

2 tbsps olive oil
4 chicken drumsticks and 4 chicken thighs on the bone
1¼ cups (300ml) red wine
1 onion, sliced
1 red capsicum, diced
4 cloves garlic, sliced
½ tsp dried chilli flakes
2 cups (500g) cherry tomatoes, halved
1 cup (250ml) chicken stock
1 tbsp passata
2 sprigs fresh thyme
2 sprigs fresh rosemary
Salt and pepper to taste

Heat oil in a large frying pan. Cook chicken in batches over high heat until browned all over. Transfer to slow cooker.

Use wine to deglaze pan. Use a spatula to scrape up brown bits. Pour into slow cooker.

Add remaining ingredients to slow cooker and season with salt and pepper. Stir to combine.

Cook, covered, on low for 6 hours.

Pulled Pork

SERVES 6
COOK TIME: HIGH 8 HRS/LOW 10 HRS
GLUTEN FREE • DAIRY FREE

- 2 small onions, diced
- 2 cloves garlic, crushed
- ½ tsp ground cumin
- ¼ tsp ground cinnamon
- 1 tbsp chilli powder
- 2 tsps dried thyme
- ½ tsp salt
- ¼ cup (40g) brown sugar
- 1 tbsp Dijon mustard
- 2kg pork shoulder roast
- 1 cup (250ml) barbecue sauce
- ½ cup (125ml) apple cider vinegar
- ½ cup (125ml) chicken stock

Place onions and garlic in the bottom of the slow cooker.

Place cumin, cinnamon, chilli powder, thyme, salt, brown sugar and mustard in a small bowl and stir to combine.

Pat the pork dry with paper towel. Rub with the spice rub all over the pork and place into the slow cooker on top of the onions.

Pour over the barbecue sauce, apple cider vinegar and chicken stock. Cover and cook for 10 hours on low or 8 hours on high, until the meat shreds easily with a fork.

Remove meat from the slow cooker and transfer to a chopping board. Shred the meat using two forks. Return the shredded pork to the slow cooker and stir the meat into the juices.

Serve inside toasted burger buns.

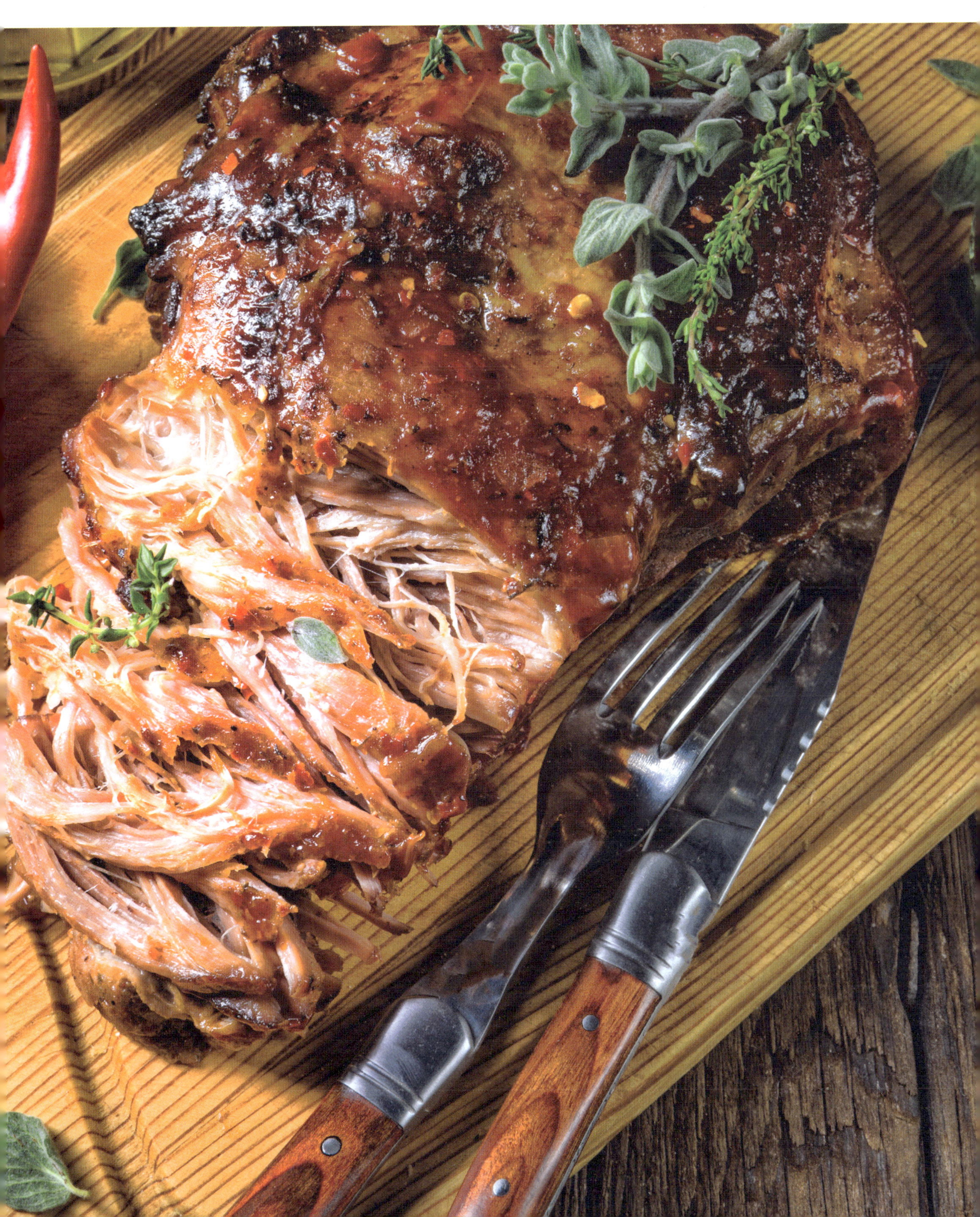

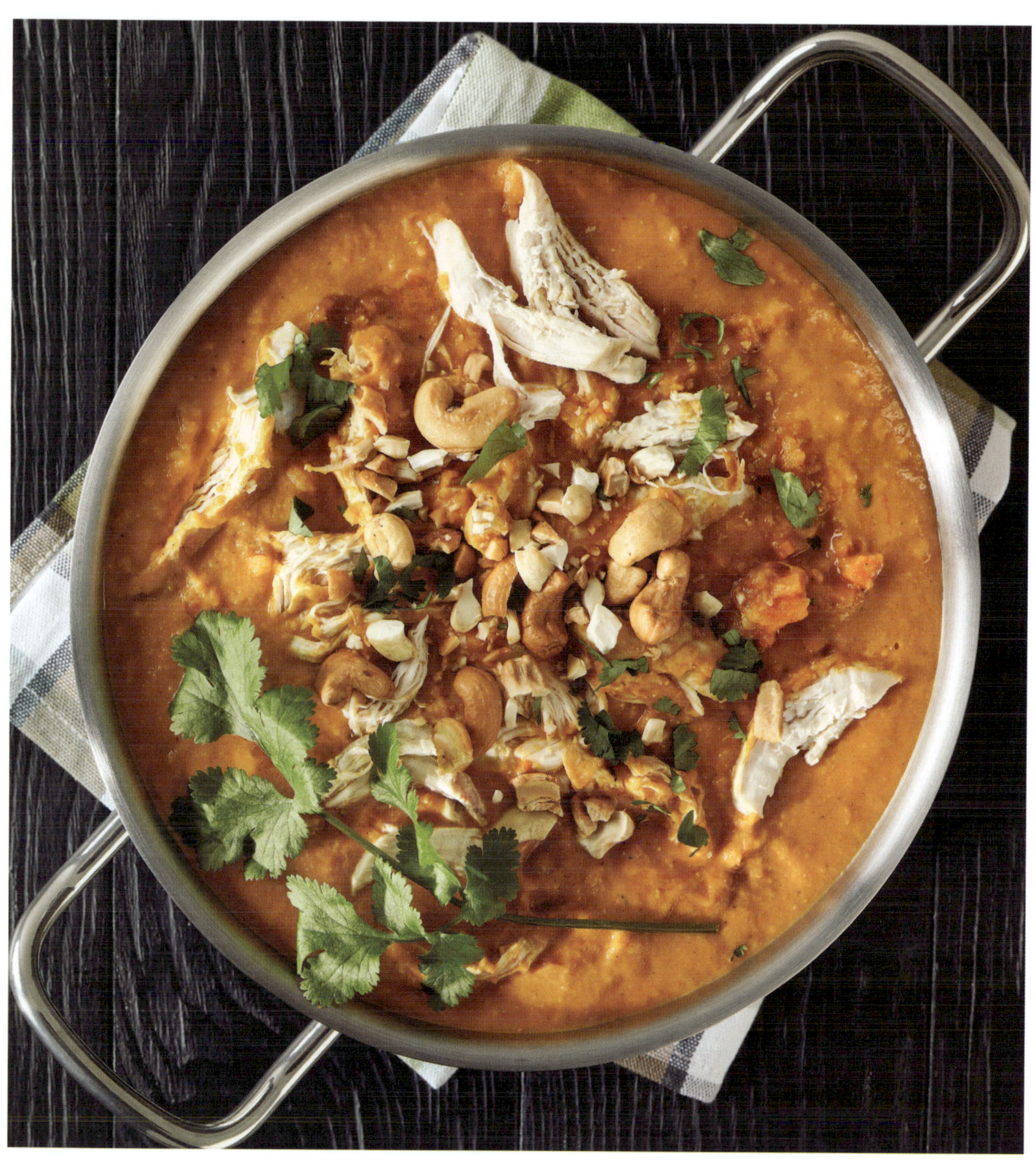

Chicken Mulligatawny

SERVES 8

COOK TIME: LOW 4-5 HRS

CHICKEN MULLIGATAWNY

3 tbsps butter
2 onions, chopped
4 carrots, chopped
1 stalk celery, minced
Small piece ginger, grated
4 cloves garlic, minced
1 tbsp tomato paste
1 tbsp curry powder
2 tsps garam masala
Salt and pepper to taste
¼ tsp cayenne pepper
⅓ cup (40g) plain flour
5 cups (1.25L) chicken stock
750g boneless, skinless chicken thighs
1 x 400ml can coconut milk
½ cup (90g) brown lentils
¼ cup (30g) cashew nuts, roughly chopped
Fresh coriander leaves, chopped

Melt butter in large saucepan over medium heat. Add onions, carrots and celery and cook, stirring, for 10-14 minutes until onions are soft and just beginning to brown.

Add ginger, garlic, tomato paste, curry powder, garam masala, 1 teaspoon salt, and cayenne pepper. Cook for about 30 seconds until fragrant. Stir in flour and cook for 1 minute. Stir in stock, scraping up any browned bits. Transfer to slow cooker. Stir in chicken, coconut milk, and lentils.

Cover and cook on low for 4-5 hours until chicken and lentils are tender. Remove chicken with a slotted spoon and shred with two forks.

Season soup with salt and pepper to taste. Scatter with shredded chicken, cashews and coriander to serve.

BUTTER CHICKEN

½ cup (125ml) chicken stock
¾ cup (170g) tomato paste
2 tsps curry powder
1 tsp garam masala
1 tsp ground turmeric
Salt and pepper to taste
1kg boneless, skinless chicken thighs, cut into 3cm chunks
1 onion, diced
3 cloves garlic, minced
Small piece ginger, grated
½ cup (125ml) cream
2 tbsps fresh lime juice
1½ tsps light brown sugar
Chopped coriander, to serve

In a small bowl, whisk together chicken stock, tomato paste, curry powder, garam masala, turmeric and ½ teaspoon each of salt and pepper.

Place chicken, onion, garlic and ginger into the slow cooker. Stir in chicken stock mixture.

Cover and cook on low for 4 hours. Stir in cream, lime juice and brown sugar. Season with salt and pepper to taste.

Scatter with coriander leaves to serve.

CHICKEN STOCK

1 chicken carcass (left over from a roast)
1 tbsp apple cider vinegar
2 onions, quartered
3 carrots, roughly chopped
4 stalks celery, roughly chopped
½ bunch parsley, torn
10 peppercorns
1-2 bay leaves
Water, to cover

Place the chicken carcass into slow cooker. Add all of the other ingredients and enough water to fully cover.

Cover and cook on low for at least 12 hours or up to 24 hours.

Sieve the stock through a fine mesh sieve. Discard the vegetables and retain the stock.

Store in jars in the fridge or freezer.

Can be served as a soup, heated through with cooked carrots and other root vegetables.

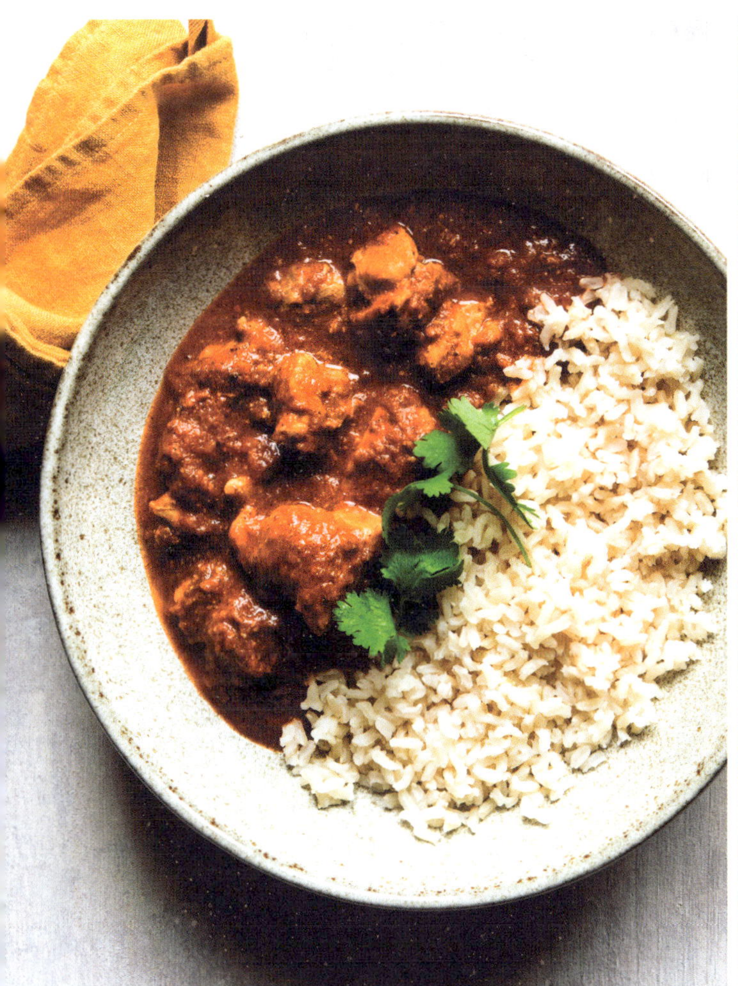

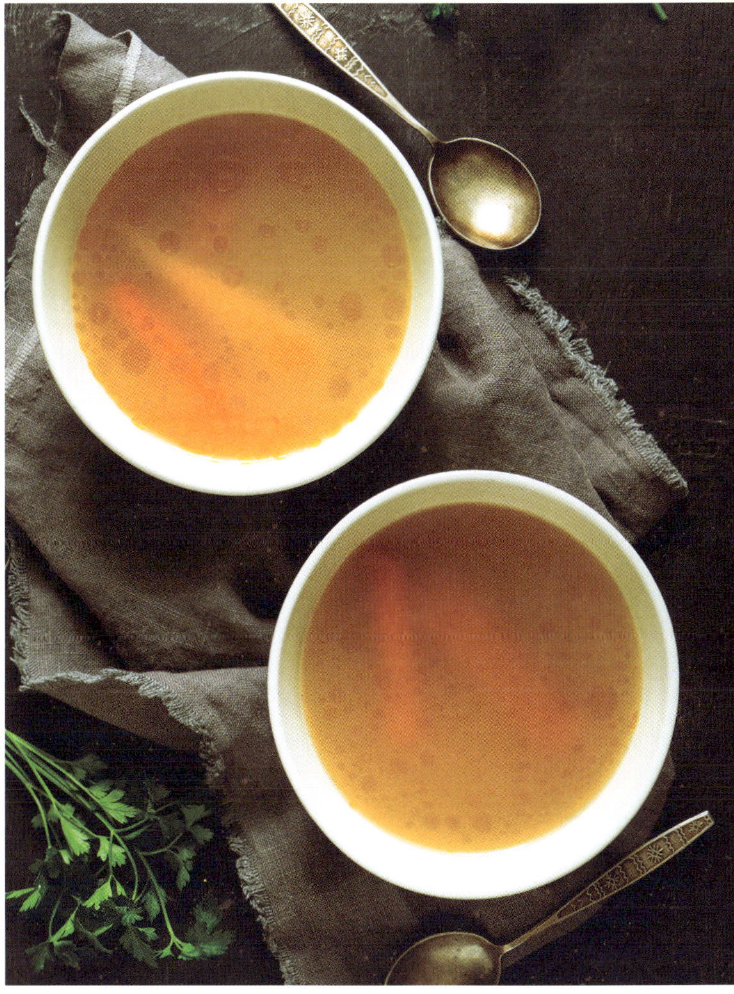

Butter Chicken

SERVES 6

COOK TIME: LOW 4 HRS

GLUTEN FREE

Chicken Stock

SERVES 6

COOK TIME: LOW 12-24 HRS

GLUTEN FREE • DAIRY FREE

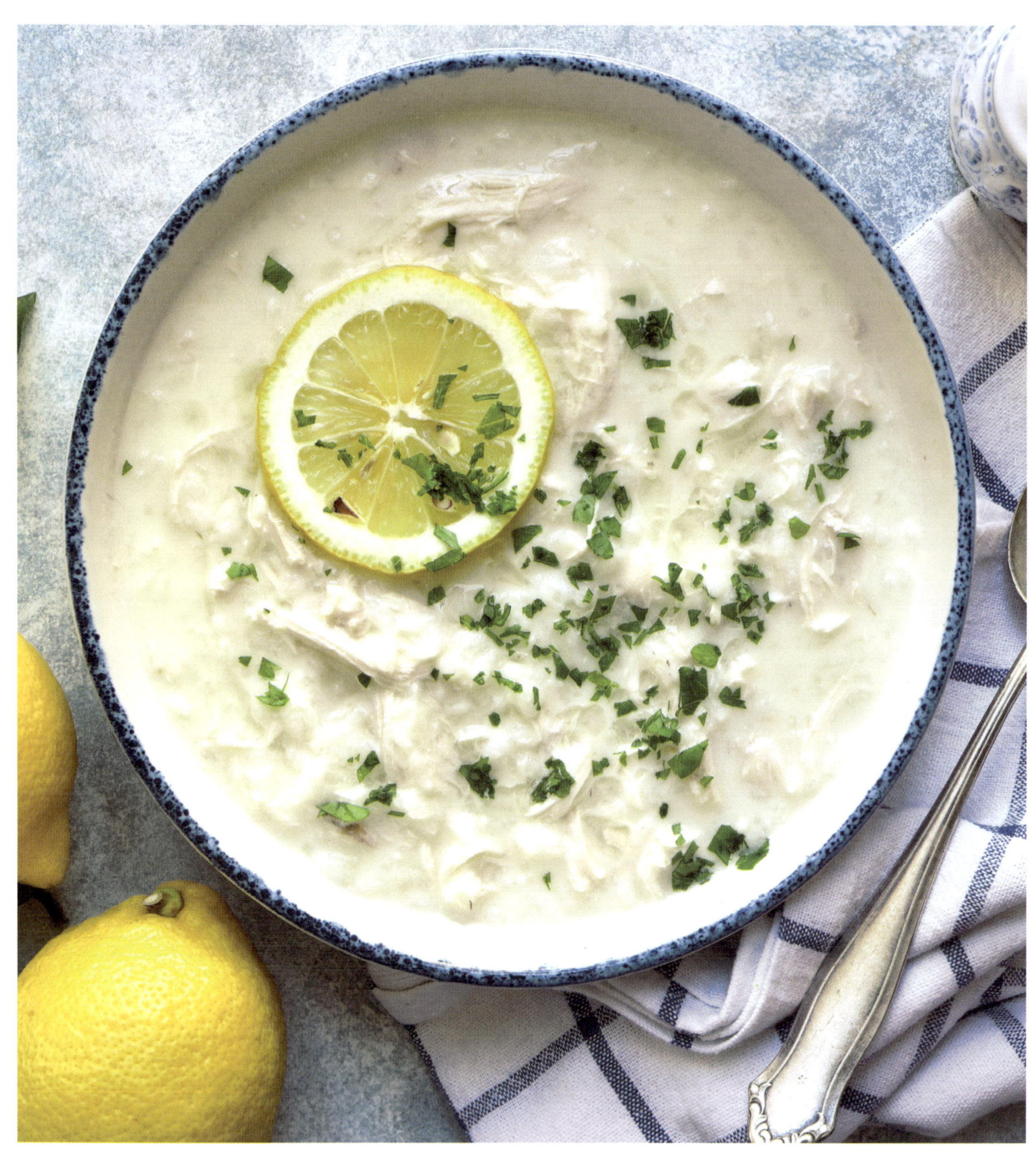

Greek Chicken Soup

SERVES 4

COOK TIME: HIGH 3 HRS/LOW 6 HRS

GLUTEN FREE • DAIRY FREE

GREEK CHICKEN SOUP

600g chicken breasts
5 cups (1.25L) chicken stock
3½ cups (900ml) water
2 bay leaves
2 cloves garlic, crushed
⅔ cup (100g) medium-grain white rice
2 eggs
¼ cup (60ml) lemon juice
Lemon slices, to serve
¼ cup (10g) chopped fresh flat-leaf parsley, to serve

Place chicken breasts, stock, water, bay leaves, garlic and rice in the slow cooker. Cover and cook on low for 6 hours or high for 3 hours or until chicken is tender.

Transfer chicken to a bowl and shred with two forks.

Discard bay leaves.

Whisk together eggs and lemon juice in a small bowl. Add ½ cup of the hot stock mixture to eggs, whisking as you do so.

Return chicken to the soup. Stir in egg mixture. Cook, stirring, on high for 5 minutes or until soup thickens slightly. Season with salt and pepper.

Serve soup topped with lemon slices and parsley.

CREAMY CHICKEN WITH SPINACH AND PEAS

1kg chicken breasts or boneless thigh fillets, cut into 5cm pieces

Salt and pepper to taste

1 tbsp olive oil

1 cup (250ml) dry white wine

5 cloves garlic, crushed

1 cup (250ml) chicken stock

3 sprigs fresh thyme

1 tbsp cornflour

1 tbsp water

¼ cup (25g) grated Parmesan cheese

¼ cup (60ml) thickened cream

1 cup (170g) green peas

50g baby spinach

Season chicken with salt and pepper. Heat oil in a large frying pan over medium-high heat. Add chicken and cook until both sides are golden brown. Arrange in a single layer on bottom of slow cooker.

Deglaze the pan with wine, using a spatula to scrape up any brown bits. Pour into slow cooker.

Add garlic, chicken stock and thyme to slow cooker. Cover and cook on high for 4 hours.

Twenty minutes before serving, mix together cornflour and water with a whisk to make a slurry. Pour the slurry, Parmesan cheese and cream into the slow cooker and stir to combine. Add peas and spinach and mix well. Cover and cook on high for 20 minutes.

Season to taste and serve.

SUGAR-GLAZED PORK

1 tsp ground sage

½ tsp salt

¼ tsp pepper

1 clove garlic, crushed

1kg pork loin roast

1 cup (250ml) water

½ cup (80g) brown sugar

1 tbsp cornflour

¼ cup (60ml) balsamic vinegar

2 tbsps soy sauce (or tamari)

Combine sage, salt, pepper and garlic.

Rub over pork. Place in slow cooker with ½ cup water.

Cook on low for 6-8 hours.

One hour before end of cooking time, combine brown sugar, cornflour, balsamic vinegar, ½ cup water and soy sauce in a small saucepan over medium low heat. Cook, stirring, for about 5 minutes, until mixture thickens.

Brush pork with glaze two or three times during the last hour of cooking.

Serve pork shredded with remaining glaze on the side.

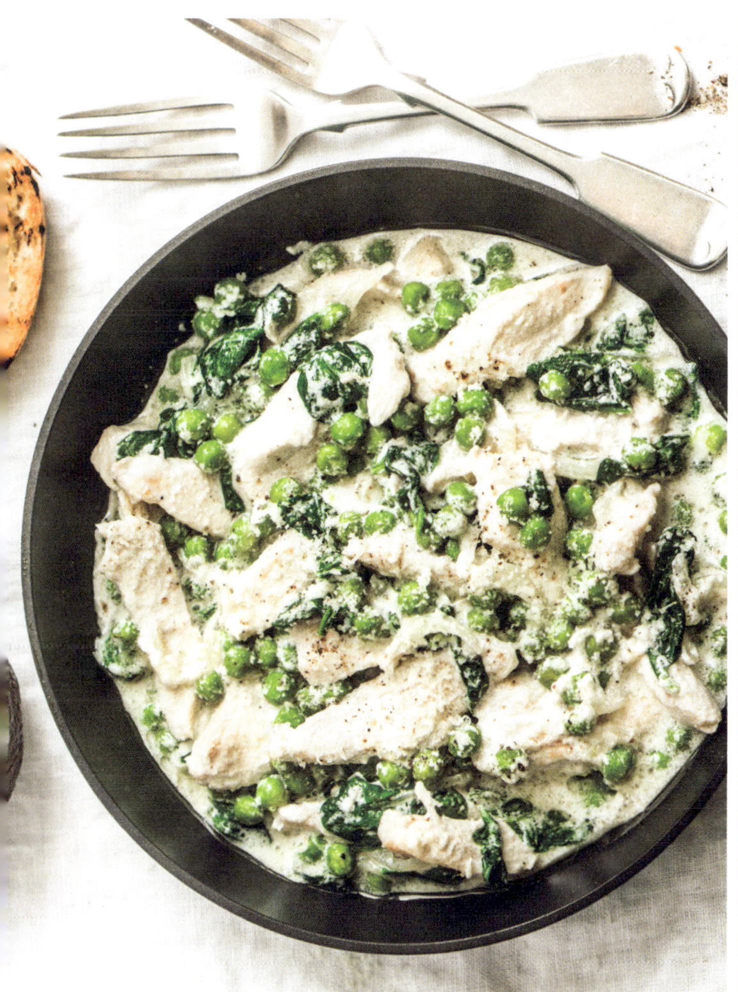

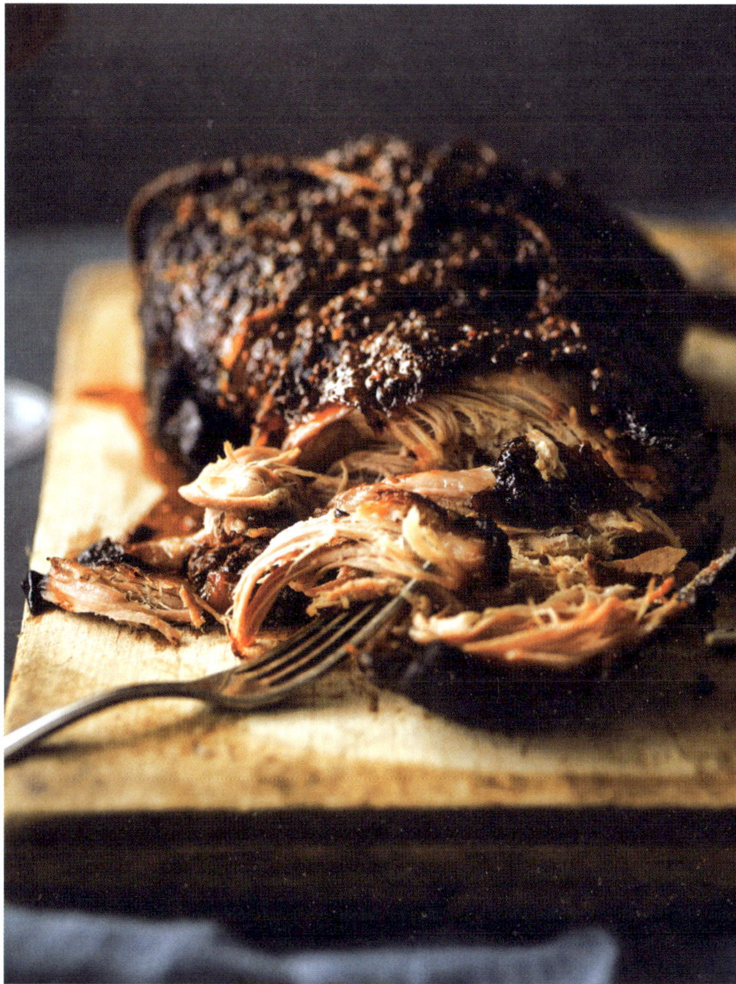

Creamy Chicken with Spinach and Peas

SERVES 4

COOK TIME: HIGH 4 HRS

GLUTEN FREE

Sugar-Glazed Pork

SERVES 6

COOK TIME: LOW 6-8 HRS

GLUTEN FREE • DAIRY FREE

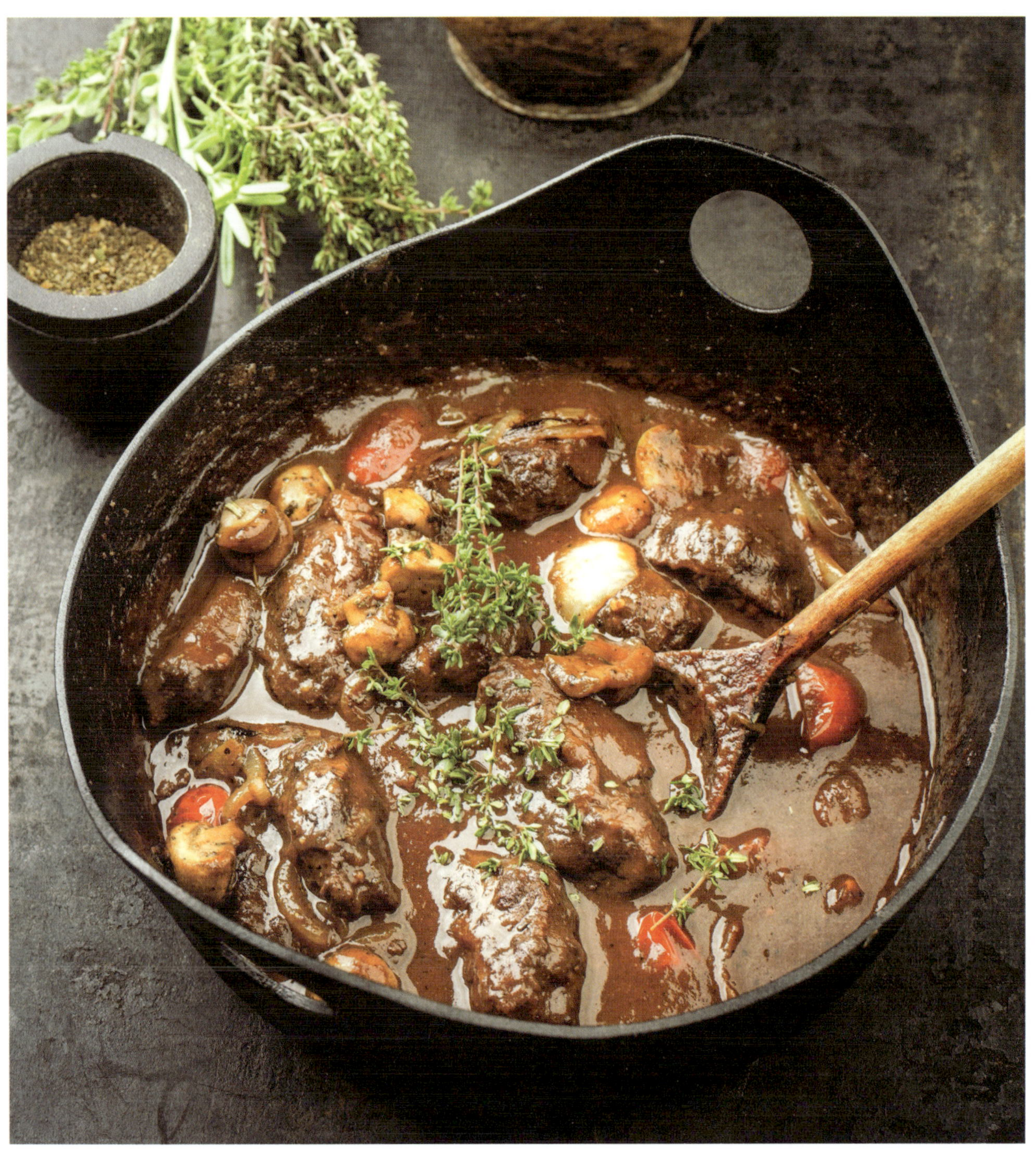

Braised Pork Cheeks

SERVES 4

COOK TIME: HIGH 4 HRS/LOW 8 HRS

BRAISED PORK CHEEKS

8 pork cheeks

Salt and pepper to taste

½ cup (60g) plain flour for dredging, or as needed

2 tbsps butter

1 tbsp olive oil

1 onion, sliced

1 carrot, diced

1 stalk celery, diced

2 tbsps apple cider vinegar

2 cups (500ml) cider

2 cups (500ml) chicken stock

1 tsp finely chopped fresh sage leaves

1 tsp finely chopped fresh rosemary leaves

3 thyme sprigs

150g cherry tomatoes, halved

300g button mushrooms

Season both sides of pork cheeks with salt and pepper.

Place flour in a shallow dish. Dip meat in flour and toss to coat thoroughly.

Heat butter and oil in a large frying pan over medium-high heat. Sear meat on both sides until richly browned. Transfer to the slow cooker.

Remove all but 2 tablespoons fat from the pan. Add onion, carrot and celery to pan. Cook, stirring, for 3-5 minutes until tender. Add vinegar and ½ cup of cider. Stir to deglaze the pan, scraping up any brown bits with a spatula.

Transfer to the slow cooker along with remaining cider, chicken stock, herbs, tomatoes and mushrooms. Season with salt and pepper.

Cover and cook on high for 4 hours or on low for 8 hours.

THAI GREEN CURRY

1kg chicken thighs and drumsticks
2 tbsps Thai green curry paste
2 tbsps fish sauce
2 kaffir limes leaves
2 cloves garlic, minced
Small piece ginger, grated
1 cup (250ml) chicken stock
1 x 400ml can coconut cream
1 tbsp palm sugar or coconut sugar
1 tbsp lime juice
4-6 Thai red and green chillies (optional)
Thai basil leaves, to serve

Place all ingredients in slow cooker. Stir to combine.

Cover and cook on low for 4 hours or on high for 2½ hours.

Stir through basil leaves to serve.

PORK RIBS WITH PRUNES

2⅓ cups (350g) pitted prunes
½ cup (125ml) red wine
2kg pork back ribs
2 tsps salt
½ tsp pepper
1 tbsp flour
2 tbsps butter
1 tbsp olive oil
3 cloves garlic, minced
2 bay leaves
1 cup (250ml) chicken stock
Basil leaves, to serve

In a small bowl, combine prunes and red wine and set aside.

Cuts ribs apart. Toss the ribs with the salt, pepper and flour.

Place the butter and olive oil in a large frying pan over medium high heat. Working in batches, sear the ribs for 2-3 minutes on each side until brown.

Add to slow cooker. Remove prunes from wine and add to slow cooker.

Deglaze pan with the wine, scraping up any brown bits with a spatula. Transfer to slow cooker.

Add garlic, bay leaves and chicken stock to slow cooker. Cover and cook on high for 4 hours or on low for 8 hours. Scatter with basil leaves to serve.

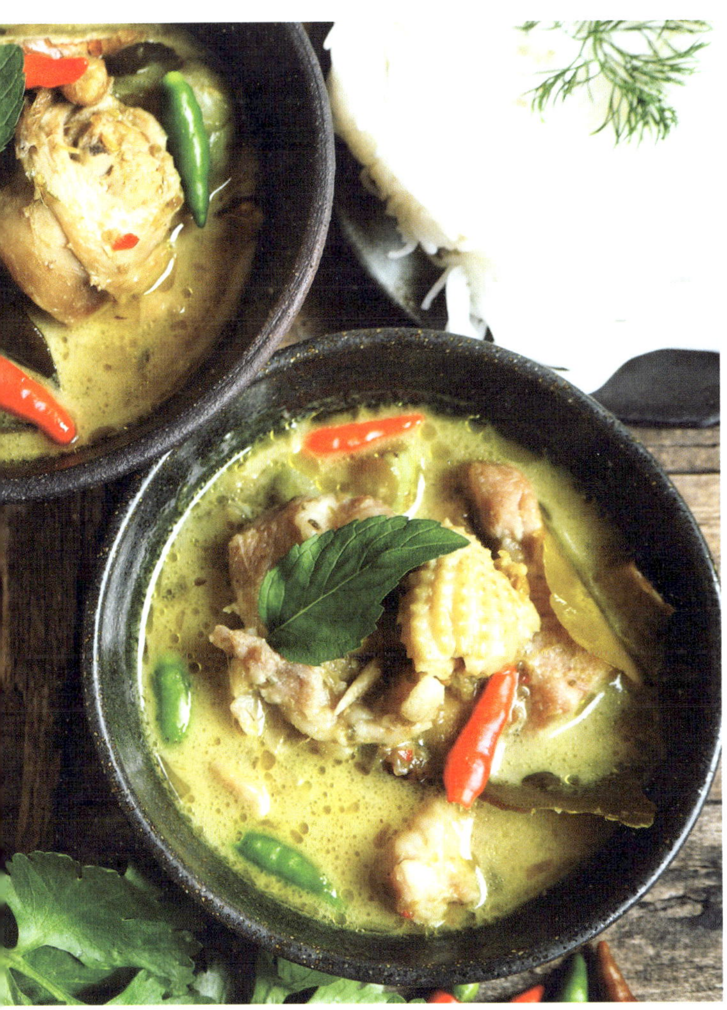

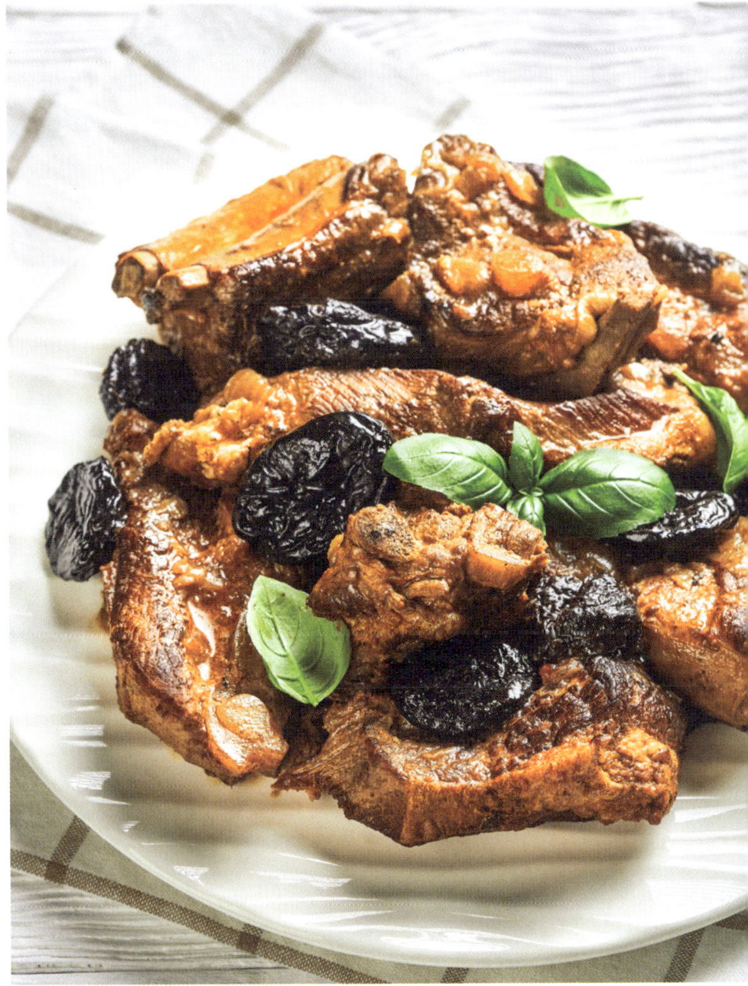

Thai Green Curry

SERVES 4

COOK TIME: HIGH 2 HRS 30 MINS/LOW 4 HRS

GLUTEN FREE • DAIRY FREE

Pork Ribs with Prunes

SERVES 4-6

COOK TIME: HIGH 4 HRS/LOW 8 HRS

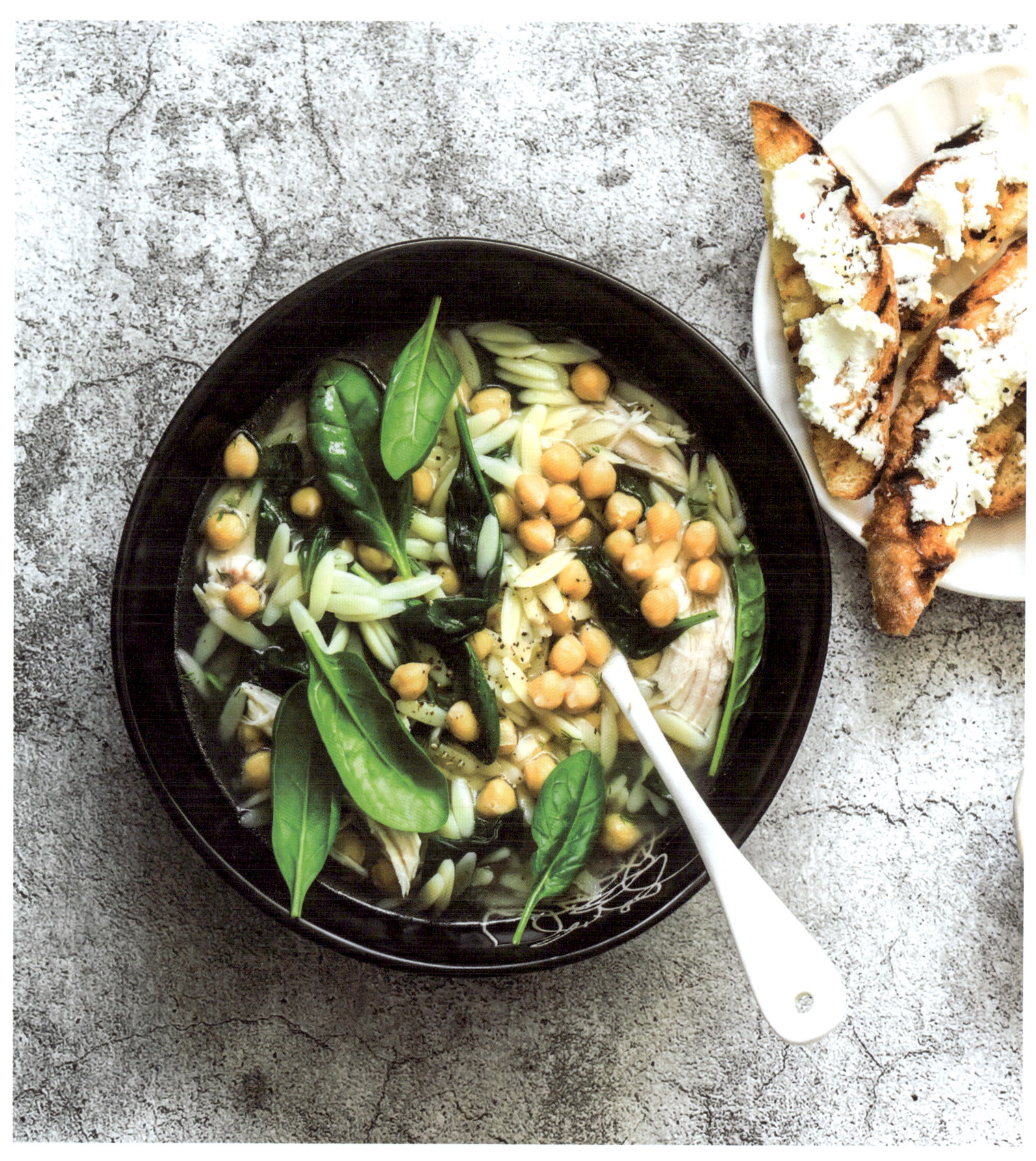

Lemon Chicken Orzo Soup

SERVES 4

COOK TIME: HIGH 2½–3 HRS + 30 MINS

DAIRY FREE

LEMON CHICKEN ORZO SOUP

1 tbsp olive oil
1 medium onion, diced
3 cloves garlic, minced
2 boneless, skinless chicken breasts
8 cups (2L) chicken stock
2 stalks celery, finely sliced
3 carrots, finely chopped
2 sprigs fresh thyme
1 bay leaf
¾ cup (160g) orzo, uncooked
1 x 400g can chickpeas, drained and rinsed
1 tbsp fresh lemon juice
Salt and pepper to taste
100g baby spinach

Heat oil in a medium frying pan over medium-high heat. Add onion and cook for 3-5 minutes, stirring regularly, until soft and translucent. Stir in garlic and cook for 1 minute until fragrant. Transfer to the slow cooker.

Add chicken, chicken stock, celery, carrots, fresh thyme and bay leaf. Cover and cook on high for 2½-3 hours.

Remove the chicken and shred with two forks.

Stir orzo and chickpeas into slow cooker broth. Cover and cook for another 30 minutes on high. Remove the bay leaf and thyme. Stir in the shredded chicken. Squeeze in the lemon juice and season with salt and pepper to taste.

Spoon into bowls then add baby spinach and stir through.

Pork Ramen

SERVES 8

COOK TIME: LOW 8 HRS + 30 MINS

DAIRY FREE

1.5kg boneless pork shoulder, cut into 3 equal pieces

Salt to taste

4 tbsps peanut oil

8 cups (2L) chicken stock

1 onion, coarsely chopped

6 cloves garlic, chopped

Medium piece fresh ginger, peeled and chopped

1 leek, halved lengthwise and coarsely chopped (white and green parts)

Soy sauce (or tamari) to taste

Sesame oil to taste

750g fresh ramen noodles

8 large eggs (optional)

250g shiitake mushrooms

4 spring onions, finely chopped

1 tbsp toasted sesame seeds

Seaweed flakes and pinch of chilli powder, to serve

Season the pork with salt.

Heat 2 tablespoons of oil in a large frying pan over medium-high heat. Working in batches, sear pork pieces for 3-4 minutes on each side. Transfer to slow cooker.

Discard fat from frying pan. Deglaze the pan with 1 cup of stock then pour into slow cooker, then add onion, garlic, ginger, leek and remaining 7 cups of stock and stir to combine. Cover and cook on low for 8 hours.

Transfer pork to a cutting board and slice into thin slices. Strain broth through a sieve into a bowl and discard the solids. Skim off and discard any fat from the surface. Return pork and broth to the slow cooker and season to taste with soy sauce and sesame oil. Cover and cook on low for 30 minutes.

Cook ramen noodles according to the package directions.

Place eggs in boiling water and simmer for 5-6 minutes. Rinse under cold water, peel and halve.

Fry shiitake mushrooms in remaining oil for 5-8 minutes.

Divide noodles evenly among bowls, spoon in broth and top with pork slices, shiitake mushrooms, spring onions, sesame seeds, boiled eggs, seaweed and chilli powder.

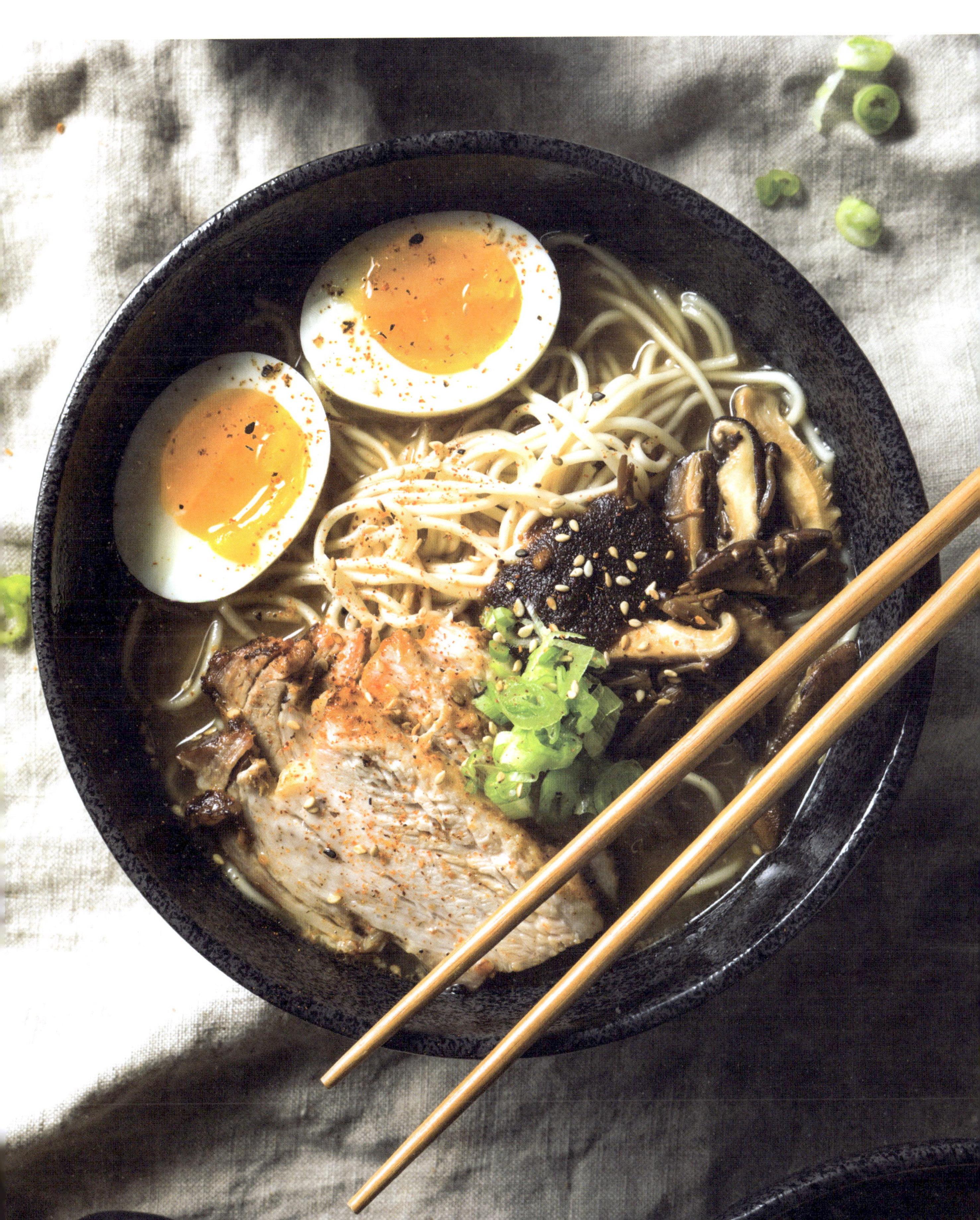

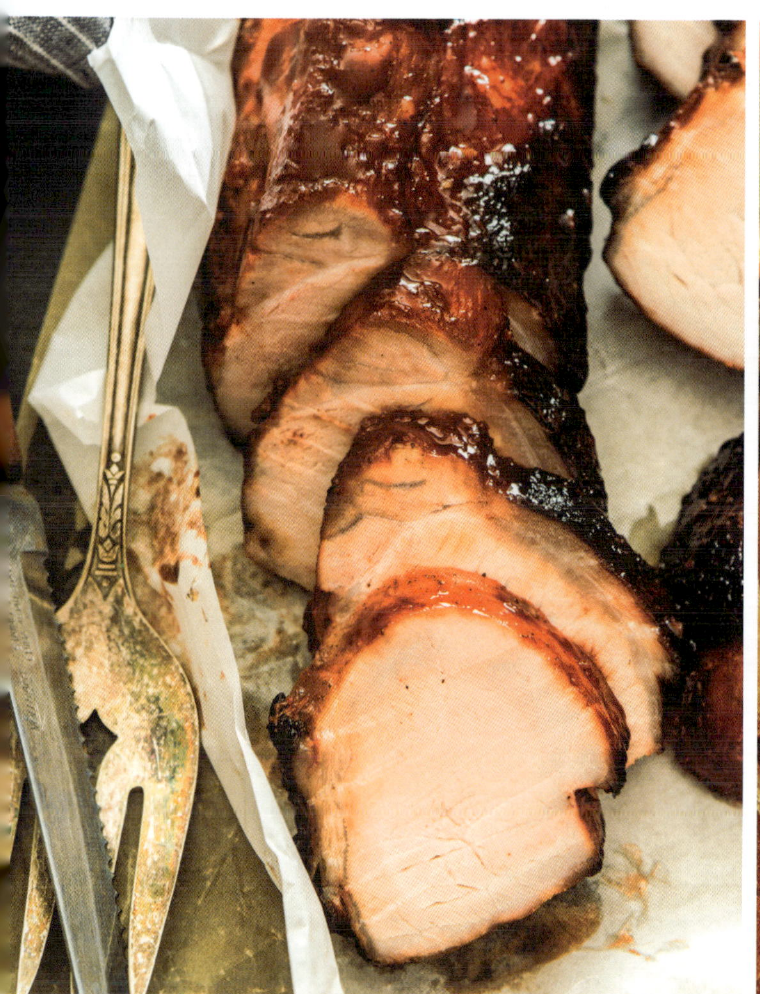

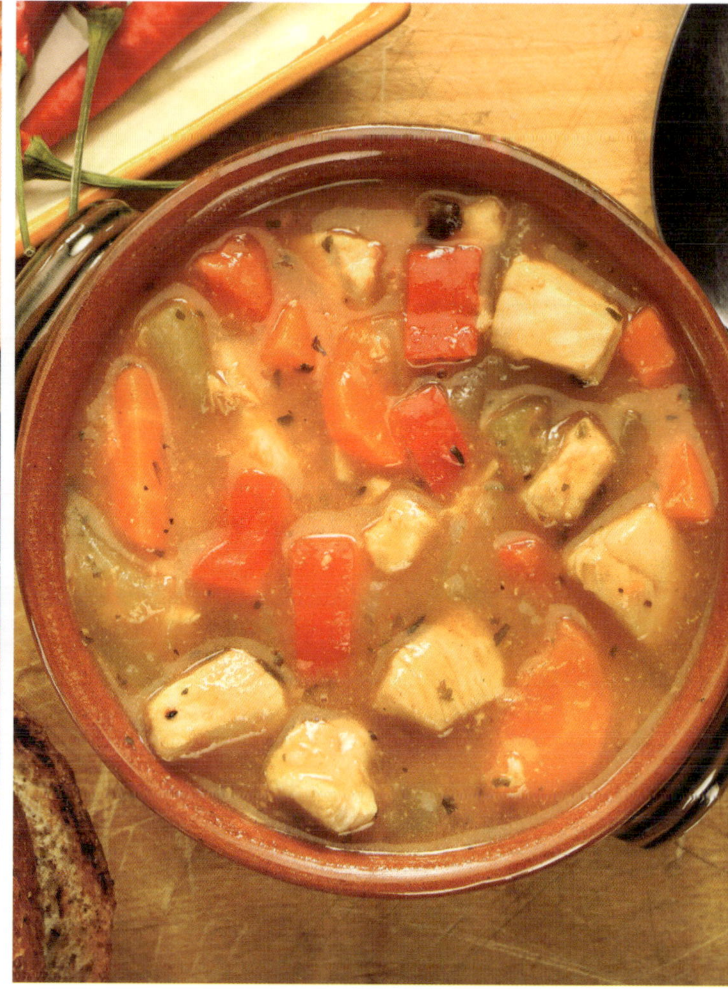

Chinese Roast Pork (Char Siu)

SERVES 8

COOK TIME: LOW 8 HRS

GLUTEN FREE • DAIRY FREE

Chicken and Veg Casserole

SERVES 6

COOK TIME: HIGH 3-4 HRS/LOW 6-7 HRS

DAIRY FREE

CHINESE ROAST PORK (CHAR SIU)

¼ cup (60ml) soy sauce (or tamari)
¼ cup (60ml) hoisin sauce
3 tbsps tomato sauce
3 tbsps honey (or maple syrup)
2 cloves garlic, minced
2 tsps grated ginger
2 tsps dark sesame oil
½ tsp five-spice powder
1kg pork loin roast

Combine soy sauce, hoisin sauce, tomato sauce, honey, garlic, ginger, sesame oil and five-spice powder in a small bowl. Stir with a whisk to combine. Then coat the pork thoroughly with the mixture.

Place in a large ziplock bag and seal. Transfer to the fridge to marinate for 2 hours, turning occasionally.

Place pork and marinade in slow cooker. Cover and cook on low for 8 hours.

Remove pork from slow cooker using a slotted spoon. Place the meat on a cutting board or work surface and slice. Serve with sticky rice and green vegetables.

CHICKEN AND VEG CASSEROLE

750g skinless chicken thighs, cut into 3cm pieces
1 tbsp plain flour
Salt and pepper to taste
1 tbsp olive oil
2 stalks celery, finely chopped
2 leeks, thinly sliced
3 carrots, roughly chopped
2 cloves garlic, minced
2 red capsicums, roughly chopped
1 tsp dried oregano
2 tbsps tomato paste
1 tsp Dijon mustard
1¾ cups (450ml) chicken stock
750g baby potatoes, quartered
Juice of ½ lemon

Toss chicken with flour, salt and pepper in a large bowl.

Heat oil in a large pan over medium heat. Cook chicken for 3-4 minutes, stirring occasionally, until browned.

Add chicken to slow cooker along with remaining ingredients except lemon juice. Stir to combine; cover and cook on high for 3-4 hours or 6-7 hours on low.

Season to taste and stir through lemon juice.

Moroccan Lemon Chicken

SERVES 4

COOK TIME: HIGH 4 HRS/LOW 8 HRS

GLUTEN FREE • DAIRY FREE

6 saffron threads (or 3 tsps ground saffron)

2½ cups (600ml) chicken stock, hot

2 tbsps olive oil

8 chicken pieces (leg, thigh and breast)

1 large onion, chopped

3 cloves garlic, finely chopped

1 tsp ground ginger

1 tsp ground coriander

1 cinnamon stick

16 green olives

1 red chilli, finely diced (optional)

½ cup (10g) coriander leaves (retain some for garnish)

1 large lemon, thinly sliced

Soak the saffron in the jug of hot stock. Set aside.

Heat oil in a large frying pan over medium-high heat. Add chicken and cook for 3 minutes each side, until golden brown. Transfer to the slow cooker.

Add the onion to the frying pan and reduce heat to medium-low. Cook for 5 minutes until soft. Transfer to the slow cooker.

Place the garlic, ginger, ground coriander, cinnamon stick and saffron threads and stock into the slow cooker.

Cover and cook on low for 8 hours or on high for 4 hours.

Thirty minutes before serving, add olives, chilli (if using) and coriander leaves to the slow cooker. Arrange the lemon slices over the top.

Serve garnished with retained coriander.

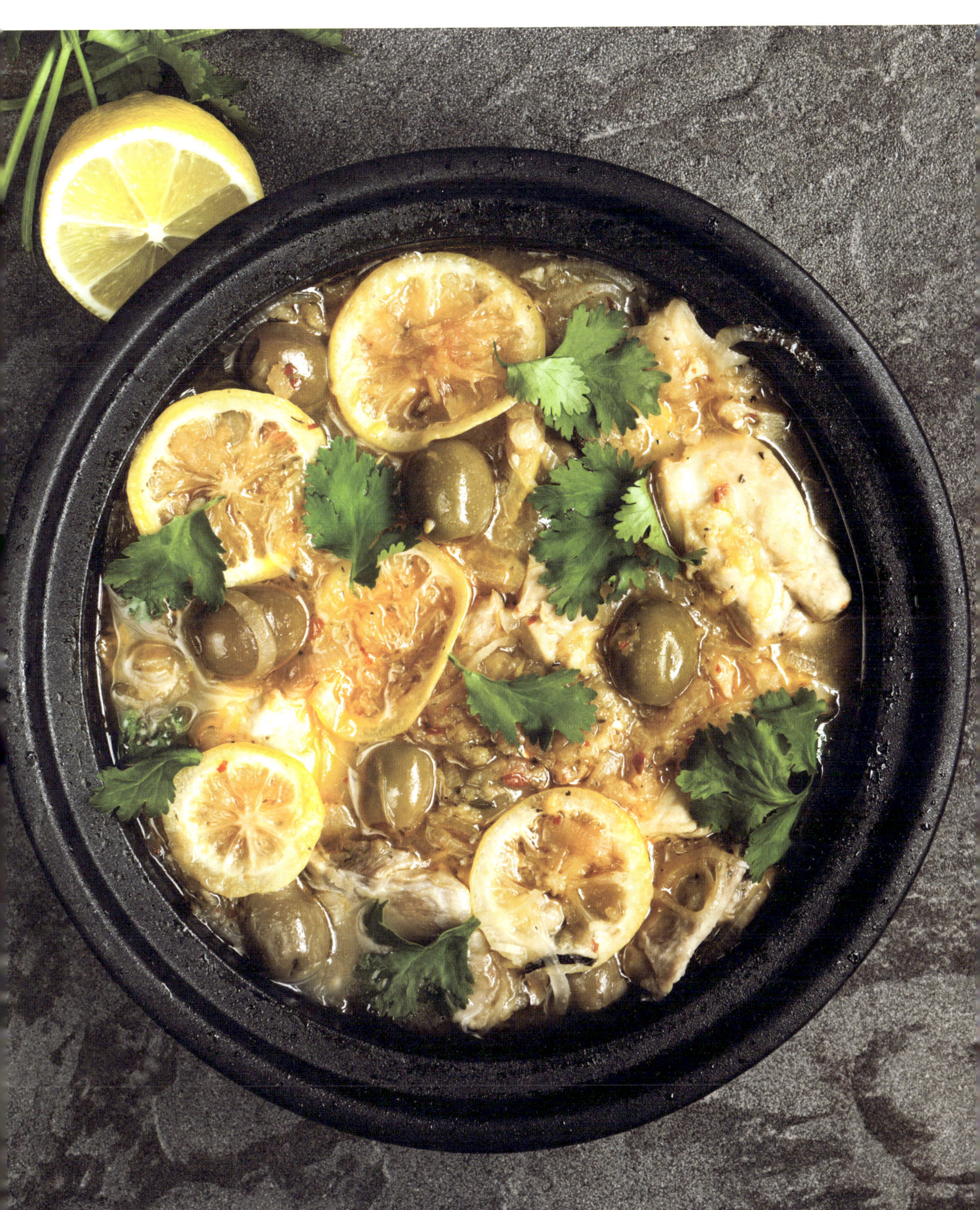

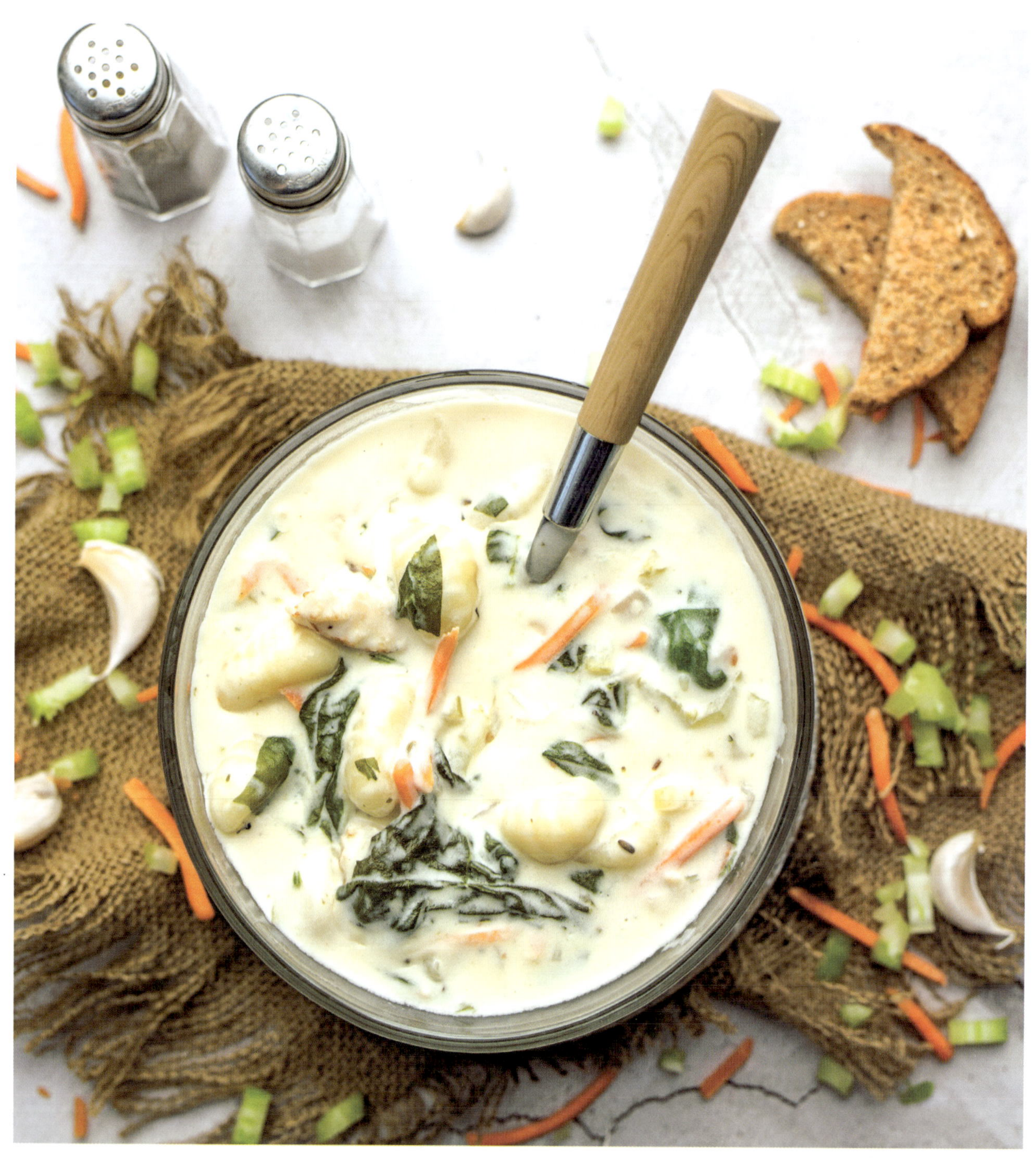

Chicken Gnocchi Soup

SERVES 8-10

COOK TIME: HIGH 4 HRS/LOW 8 HRS + 45 MINS

CHICKEN GNOCCHI SOUP

500g boneless, skinless chicken breasts

1 onion, chopped

2 carrots, julienned

2 stalks celery, finely chopped

2 tsps dried basil

2 tsps Italian seasoning

1 tsp salt

4 cups (1L) chicken stock

3 tbsps cornflour dissolved in 2 tbsps water

2 x 375ml cans evaporated milk

2 x 500g pkts gnocchi (about 4 cups)

1 tsp olive oil

6 rashers bacon, chopped

2-3 cloves garlic, minced

150g baby spinach

Salt and pepper to taste

Place the chicken, onion, carrot, celery, basil, Italian seasoning, salt and stock in the slow cooker. Cover and cook on high for 4 hours or on low for 8 hours. Shred the chicken directly in the slow cooker.

Add the cornflour mixture, evaporated milk and gnocchi. Stir and replace cover. Cook for 45 minutes on high until the soup is thick and the gnocchi is soft.

While the soup is thickening, heat oil in a frying pan over medium heat and fry bacon until crispy. Drain on paper towels.

Add garlic to the pan and cook for 1 minute, until fragrant. Add spinach and stir for 2 minutes until it wilts. Remove from heat. Add bacon and spinach to the slow cooker. Stir to combine.

Season with salt and pepper before serving.

SLOW ROAST PORK SHOULDER

1.5kg pork shoulder
1 tbsp olive oil
¼ cup (110g) salt
1 tsp pepper
2 tsps ground coriander
2 tsps dried rosemary, ground or finely chopped
8 cloves garlic, minced
1 cup (250ml) white wine
3 tbsps coriander seeds

Rub the pork roast all over with olive oil, salt, pepper, coriander, rosemary and garlic.

Put the roast and white wine in the slow cooker and cook for 6-8 hours on low. (To retain the firm texture of the meat, don't overcook it. Check at 6 hours. Timing will depend on the width of the cut of meat.)

Pre-heat the grill to medium-high.

Remove meat from slow cooker and place onto a baking tray lined with aluminium foil. Sprinkle with coriander seeds. Set under the grill until meat is nicely browned.

Remove from the grill and cover meat with foil. Allow to rest for 10-15 minutes before serving.

HONEY ROSEMARY CHICKEN

8 chicken drumsticks
4 cloves garlic, minced
½ cup (180g) honey
2 tbsps tomato paste
½ cup (125ml) soy sauce (or tamari)
2 tsps finely chopped rosemary + sprigs for garnish
1 tsp pepper
½ tsp red chilli flakes (optional)

Arrange chicken drumsticks on the bottom of the slow cooker.

In a mixing bowl, combine garlic, honey, tomato paste, soy sauce, rosemary, pepper and chilli flakes, if using, and stir until thoroughly combined.

Pour the sauce over the chicken drumsticks.

Cover and cook on low for 6 hours or on high for 4 hours.

Transfer chicken to a serving plate. Serve on rice, garnished with fresh rosemary sprigs.

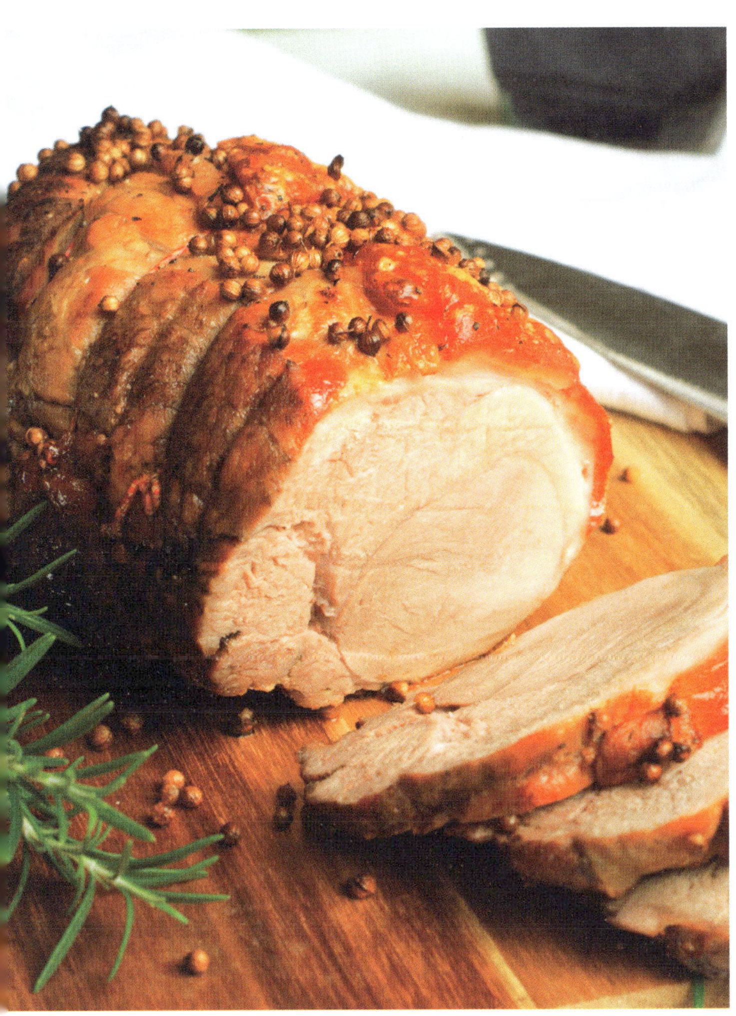

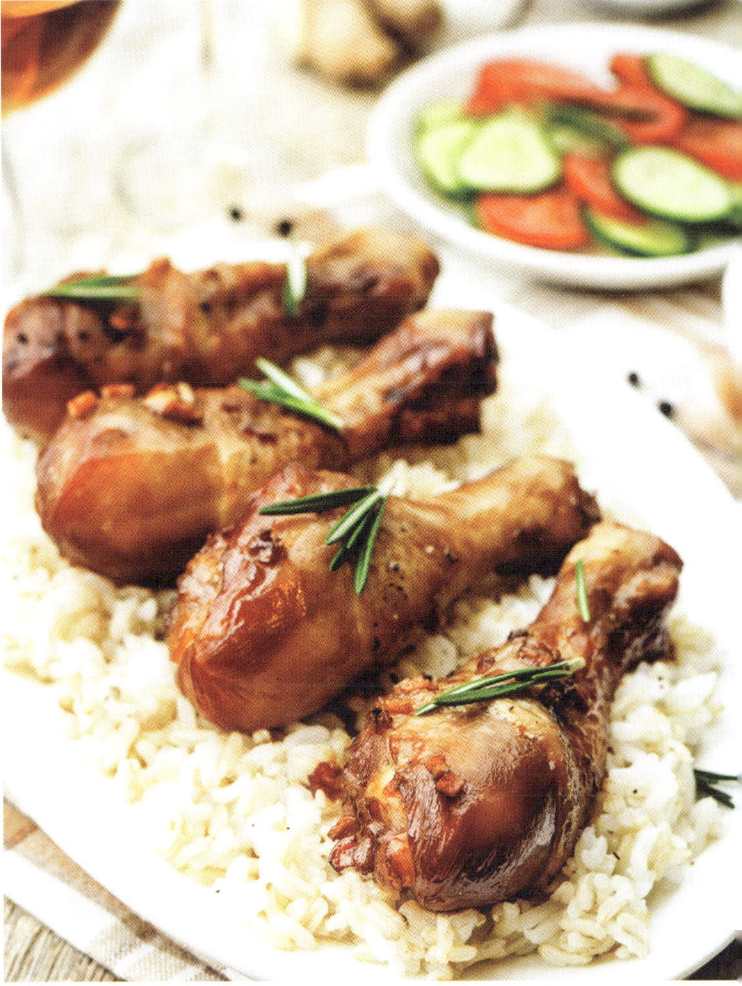

Slow Roast Pork Shoulder

SERVES 6

COOK TIME: LOW 6-8 HRS

GLUTEN FREE • DAIRY FREE

Honey Rosemary Chicken

SERVES 4

COOK TIME: HIGH 4 HRS/LOW 6 HRS

GLUTEN FREE • DAIRY FREE

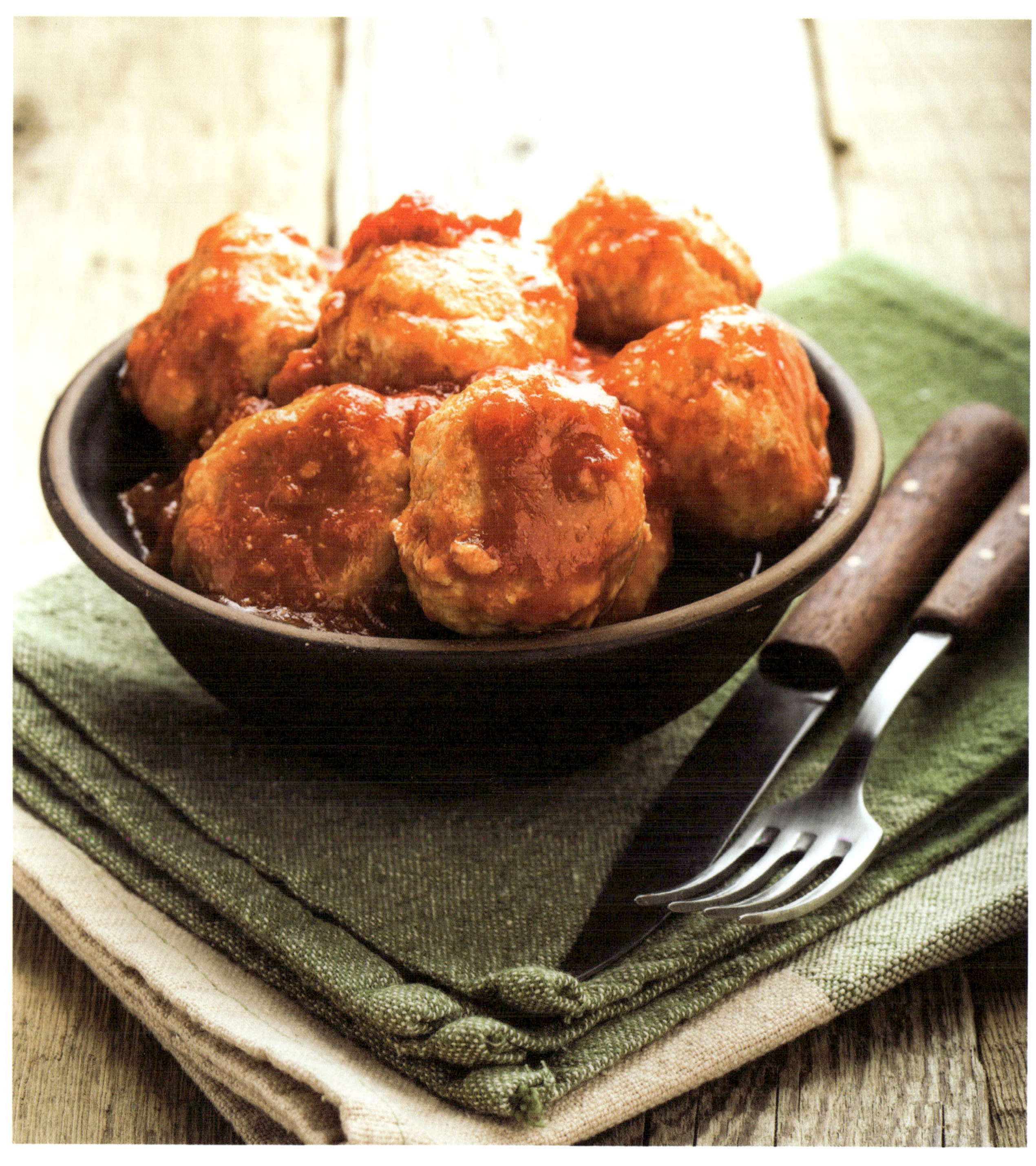

Meatballs with Tomato Sauce

SERVES 8

COOK TIME: HIGH 5 HRS/LOW 8-10 HRS

MEATBALLS WITH TOMATO SAUCE

SAUCE

3 x 400g cans chopped tomatoes
1 onion, finely diced
1 bay leaf
1 tsp sugar
½ tsp dried chilli flakes
½ tsp salt
½ tsp pepper

MEATBALLS

¾ cup (90g) breadcrumbs
½ cup (125ml) milk
4 cloves garlic, minced
¼ cup (10g) chopped fresh parsley
1¾ tsps pepper
1¾ tsps salt
1 tsp dried oregano
½ cup (50g) grated Pecorino
1 large egg
500g beef mince
500g pork mince

Place tomatoes, onion, bay leaf, sugar, chilli flakes, salt and pepper in the slow cooker, stir to combine.

In a medium-sized bowl, combine the breadcrumbs and milk.

To breadcrumbs, add garlic, parsley, pepper, salt, oregano, cheese and egg. Mix it all together with a fork. Add beef and pork mince. Mix together with your hands.

Form into meatballs and place into sauce in slow cooker.

Cover and cook on high for 5 hours or on low for 8-10 hours. Serve with pasta.

SLOW-COOKED PORK RIBS

1 onion, sliced
½ cup (125ml) water
Olive oil, for frying
2kg bone-in pork short ribs, trimmed
¾ cup (260g) plum jam
1 cup (250ml) tomato sauce
¼ cup (40g) brown sugar
2 tbsps red wine vinegar
2 tbsps Worcestershire sauce
2 tbsps Dijon mustard
¼ tsp ground cloves
¼ tsp allspice

Place onion and water in the slow cooker.

Heat oil in a frying pan over a medium-high heat. Add the ribs and brown in batches. Transfer to the slow cooker.

Cover and cook on low for 6 hours until meat is tender.

Place the remaining ingredients in a saucepan over a medium heat. Cook, stirring, until combined and heated through.

Remove ribs from slow cooker. Discard cooking juices.

Return ribs to slow cooker. Pour sauce over top.

Cover and cook on high for 30 minutes or until sticky and well coated.

MIDDLE EASTERN CHICKEN STEW

1kg chicken breast fillets, cut into small chunks
½ tsp salt
2 tbsps tomato paste
2 x 400g cans chopped tomatoes
1 tsp paprika
1 tsp ground coriander
1 tsp ground cinnamon
1 cup (250ml) water
Flat-leaf parsley, to garnish

Place the chicken in the slow cooker and sprinkle with the salt. Add the tomato paste, paprika, coriander and cumin and stir to combine.

Add the chopped tomatoes and water and stir. Cook on high for 4 hours or low for 8 hours, or until the chicken is cooked through and tender.

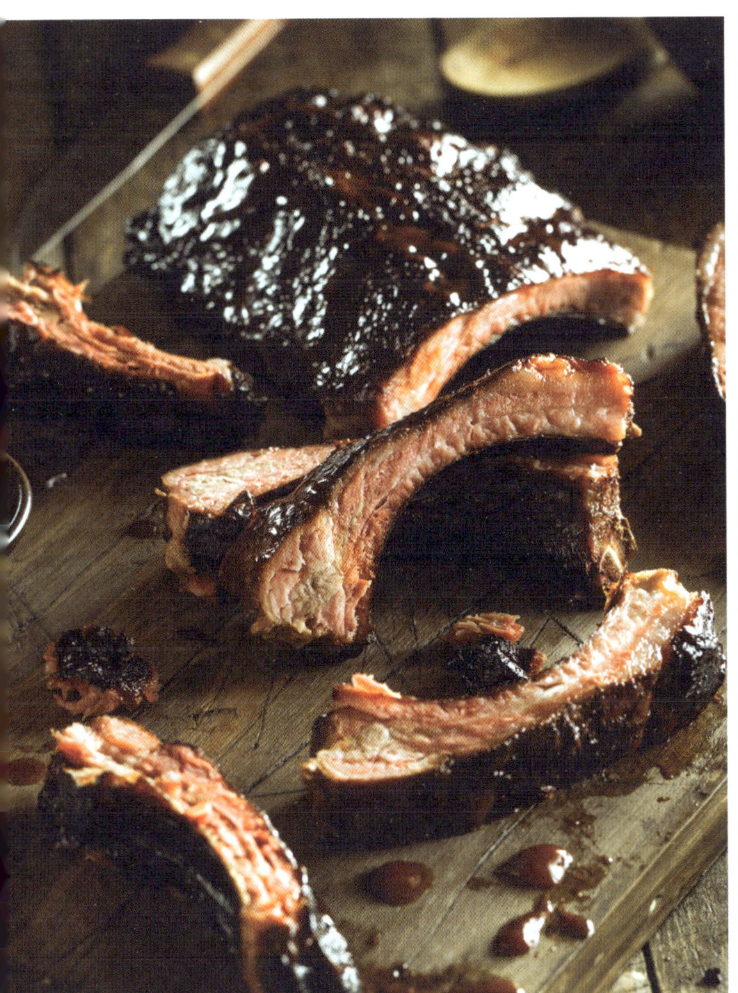

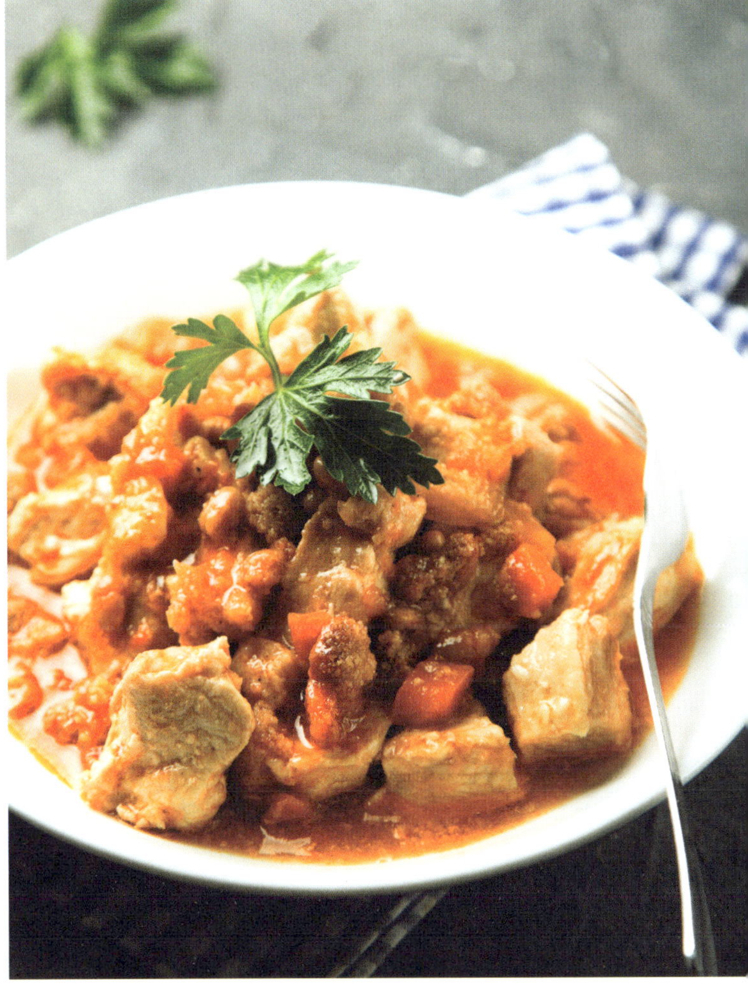

Slow-Cooked Pork Ribs

SERVES 6-8

COOK TIME: LOW 6 HRS + HIGH 30 MINS

GLUTEN FREE • DAIRY FREE

Middle Eastern Chicken Stew

SERVES 4

COOK TIME: HIGH 4 HRS/LOW 8 HRS

GLUTEN FREE • DAIRY FREE

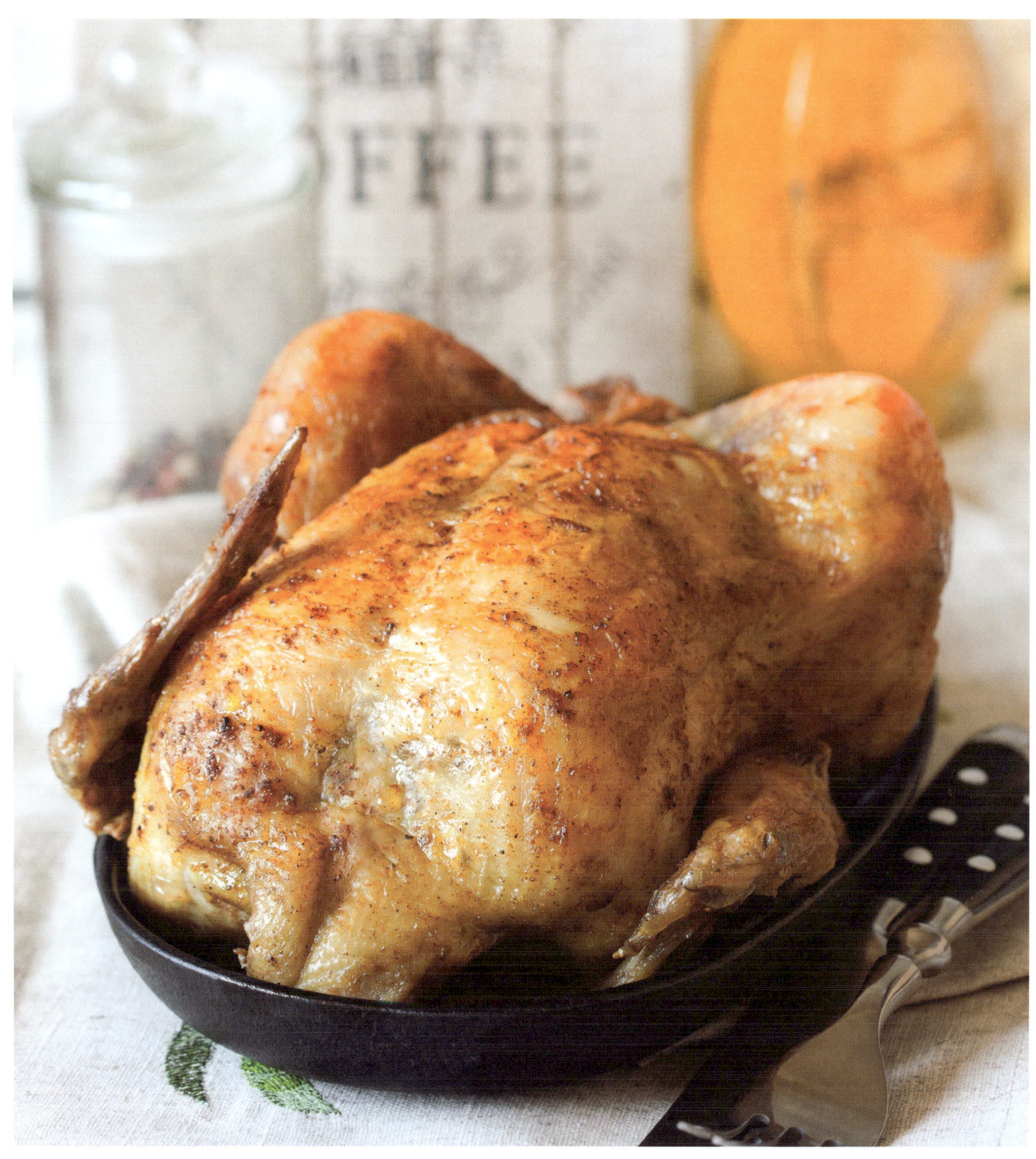

Whole Roast Chicken

SERVES 4

COOK TIME: LOW 8 HRS + 15 MINS IN OVEN

GLUTEN FREE • DAIRY FREE

WHOLE ROAST CHICKEN

2 large onions, ends sliced off and halved
2 medium lemons, washed and halved
1 whole roasting chicken
3 cloves garlic, crushed
2 tbsps olive oil + extra for drizzling
1 tbsp salt
Pepper to taste

Place the onions in the bottom of the slow cooker, with the larger cut end on the bottom.

Stuff three of the lemon halves into the chicken cavity. Squeeze the rest over the chicken.

Rub the chicken all over with the garlic, oil, salt and a couple of good grinds of pepper.

Cover and cook on low 8 hours. In the last 15 minutes of cooking, preheat the oven to 230°C.

Once the chicken is finished cooking in the slow cooker, remove it to a baking dish. Drizzle a small amount of oil over the chicken, then place in the oven for 15 minutes to crisp up.

Remove from oven and serve hot.

THAI PORK CURRY WITH PEANUT BUTTER

Cooking oil spray

1kg pork loin, cut into small chunks

½ cup (125ml) teriyaki sauce

2 tbsps rice wine vinegar

2 cloves garlic, minced

3 tbsps smooth peanut butter

Cooked rice, to serve

Fresh herbs, to garnish

Coat the slow cooker with cooking oil spray. Place the pork in the slow cooker and add the teriyaki sauce, rice wine vinegar and garlic and mix thoroughly.

Cover and cook on low for 9 hours or until the pork is very tender. Remove the pork from the slow cooker and add the peanut butter to the sauce. Stir or whisk thoroughly until the mixture is smooth, return the pork to the slow cooker and cook for another 15 minutes.

Serve with a side of rice and garnish with fresh herbs.

CHICKEN AND SWEETCORN SOUP

2½ cups (450g) frozen corn kernels

½ cup (125ml) warm water

500g chicken thigh fillets

2 leeks, finely sliced (white part only)

Large piece ginger, finely grated

1 tsp sesame oil

4 cups (1L) chicken stock

1 bunch spring onions, thinly sliced, green parts reserved for serving

2 large eggs, lightly beaten

Place half the corn in a food processor with the warm water and process until a coarse puree.

Transfer corn puree to the slow cooker along with chicken thighs, leeks, ginger, sesame oil, stock, remaining corn and white parts of spring onion. Cover and cook on low for 8 hours or until chicken is very tender.

Transfer chicken to a chopping board and shred, using two forks. Return chicken to slow cooker. Increase temperature to high. Slowly pour eggs into soup, stirring constantly until ribbons of cooked egg form. Cover and cook for a further 10 minutes.

Serve soup into bowls and top with reserved spring onion.

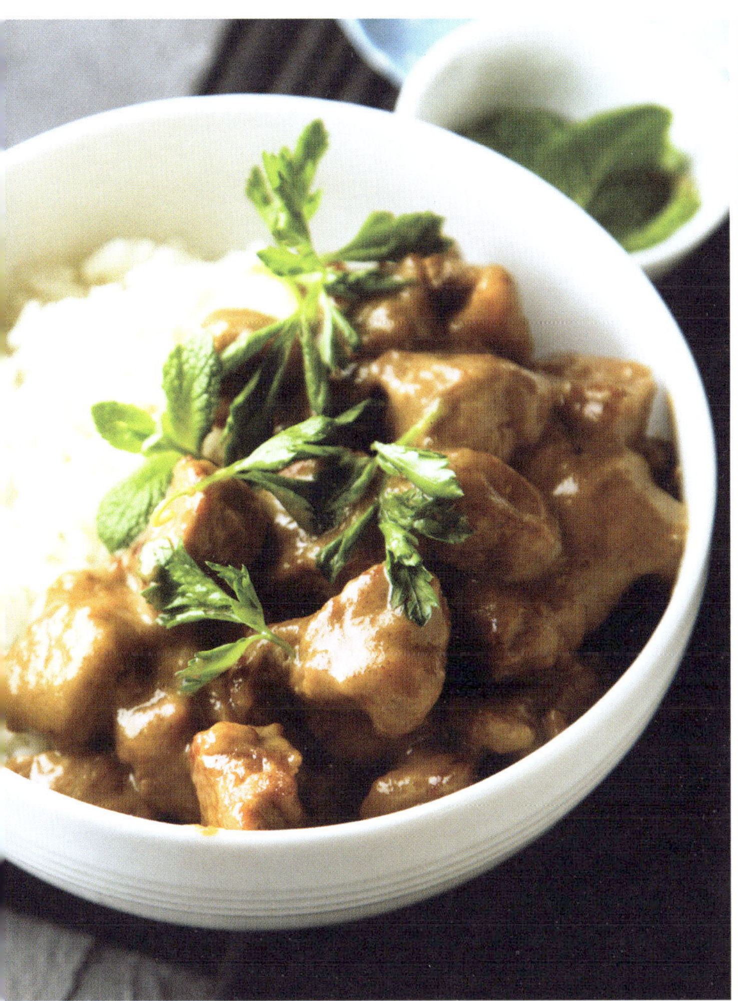

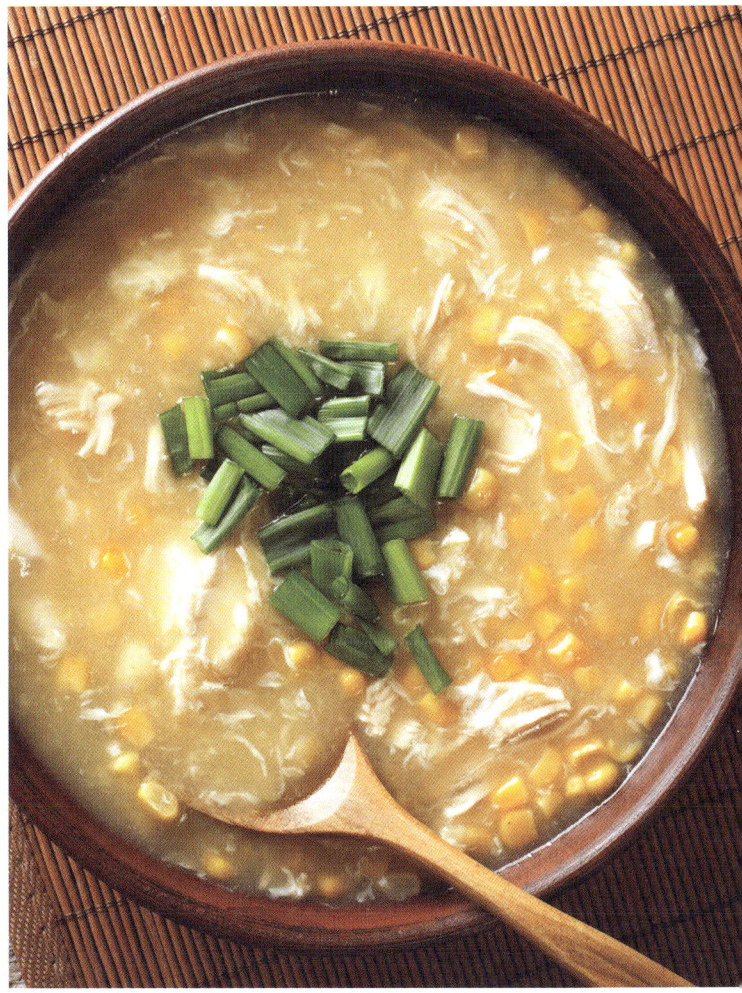

Thai Pork Curry with Peanut Butter

SERVES 4

COOK TIME: LOW 9 HRS

DAIRY FREE

Chicken and Sweetcorn Soup

SERVES 4

COOK TIME: LOW 8 HRS

GLUTEN FREE • DAIRY FREE

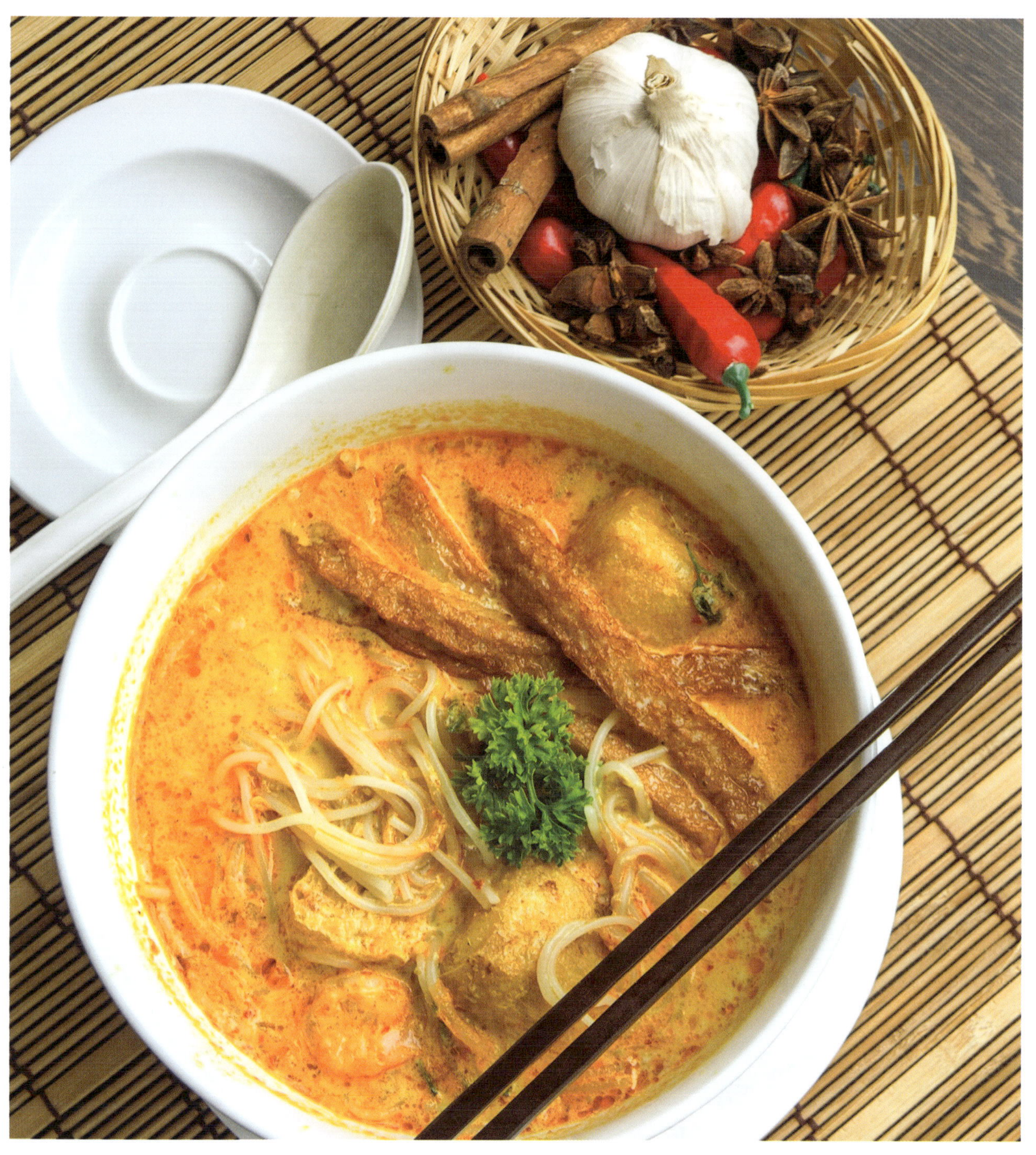

Singapore Chicken Curry

SERVES 4

COOK TIME: HIGH 4 HRS/LOW 8 HRS

GLUTEN FREE • DAIRY FREE

SINGAPORE CHICKEN CURRY

5 cloves garlic, minced

Medium piece ginger, grated

2 tbsps chilli powder

2 tbsps curry powder

1 tbsp ground turmeric

4 tomatoes, grated

4 chicken drumsticks and 4 chicken thighs

4 medium potatoes, peeled and quartered

2 red onions, sliced

1 red chilli, chopped

4 green cardamom pods

2 star anise

12 curry leaves

1 stalk lemongrass, bruised

1 cinnamon stick

2 cups (500ml) water

Salt and pepper to taste

¾-1 cup (200-250ml) coconut milk

2 tbsps soy sauce (or tamari)

400g rice noodles

Combine garlic, ginger, chilli powder, curry powder, turmeric and tomatoes in a large bowl. Add chicken and potatoes and toss to coat. Set aside to marinate for 20 minutes.

Place onions, red chilli, cardamom, star anise, curry leaves, lemongrass and cinnamon into slow cooker. Add the chicken and potato pieces along with marinade. Add the water to the bowl to clean out the last of the marinade and pour into slow cooker. Season with salt and pepper.

Cover and cook on high for 4 hours or low for 8 hours.

In the last hour of cooking, add coconut milk and soy sauce.

Cook the rice noodles according to the directions on the packet. Add to the curry to serve.

SATAY CHICKEN STEW

750g chicken breast fillet, cut into large chunks
4 tbsps soy sauce (or tamari)
3 cloves garlic, crushed
¾ cup (185ml) chicken stock
3 tsps ground cumin
Salt and pepper to taste
¾ cup (185g) smooth peanut butter
Blanched almonds or cashew nuts, to garnish
Fresh coriander, to garnish

Place the chicken pieces in the slow cooker. Pour on 3 tablespoons of soy sauce, garlic, stock, cumin and salt and pepper to taste. Cover then cook on low for 5 hours.

Remove a small amount of liquid for mixing. Add to this the peanut butter and remaining soy sauce. Pour the mixture into the slow cooker and stir well. Cover and cook on high for 30 minutes.

Serve with a garnish of nuts and fresh coriander, if desired.

SPICED CHICKEN WITH PLUMS

2 tbsps butter, melted
1 cup (250ml) plum sauce, store bought
2 tbsps orange juice
1 tsp allspice
1kg chicken breast or thigh, cut into cubes
1 cup (250ml) chicken stock
Salt and pepper to taste
2 large plums, pit removed, cut into quarters
Fresh coriander, to garnish

Place the butter, plum sauce, orange juice and allspice in the slow cooker, stirring to combine.

Add the chicken and stock, and season to taste. Cook on high for 4 hours or on low for 8 hours or until chicken is cooked through and tender. Add the plums to the slow cooker about halfway through on either setting.

Serve with a garnish of fresh coriander leaves.

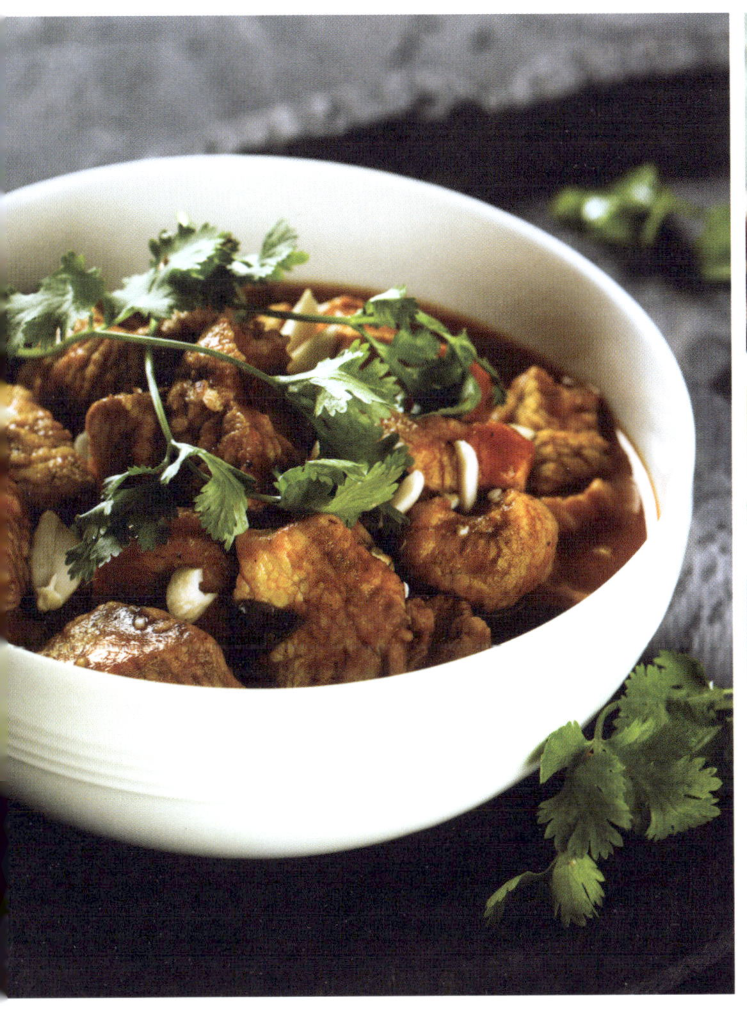

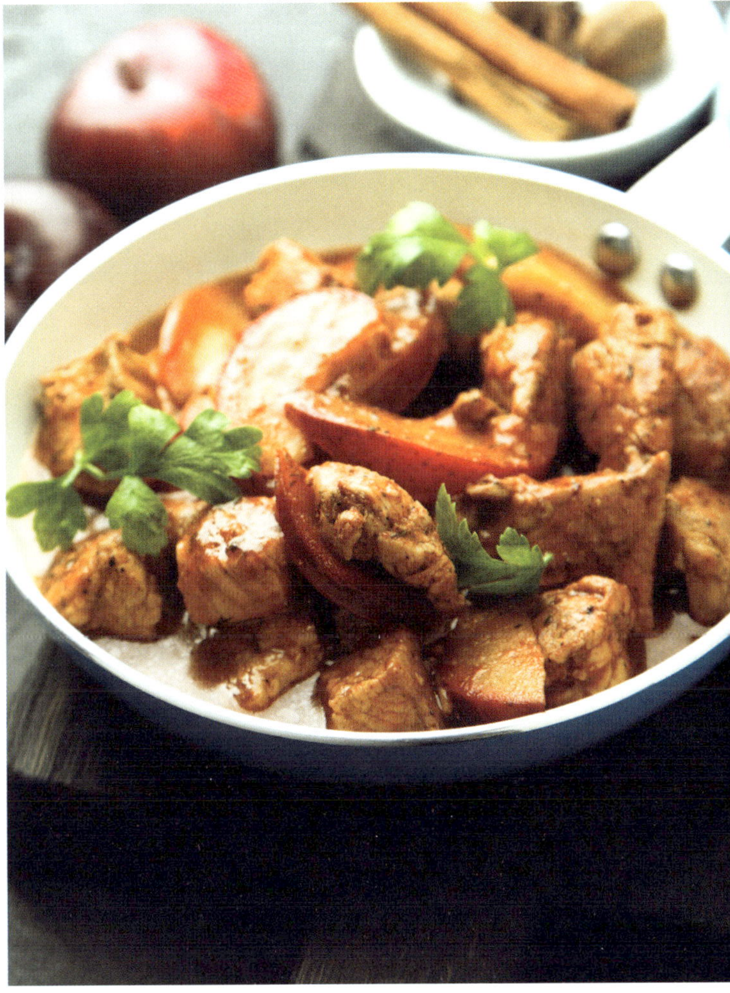

Satay Chicken Stew

SERVES 4

COOK TIME: LOW 5 HRS + HIGH 30 MINS

GLUTEN FREE • DAIRY FREE

Spiced Chicken with Plums

SERVES 4

COOK TIME: HIGH 4 HRS/LOW 8 HRS

GLUTEN FREE

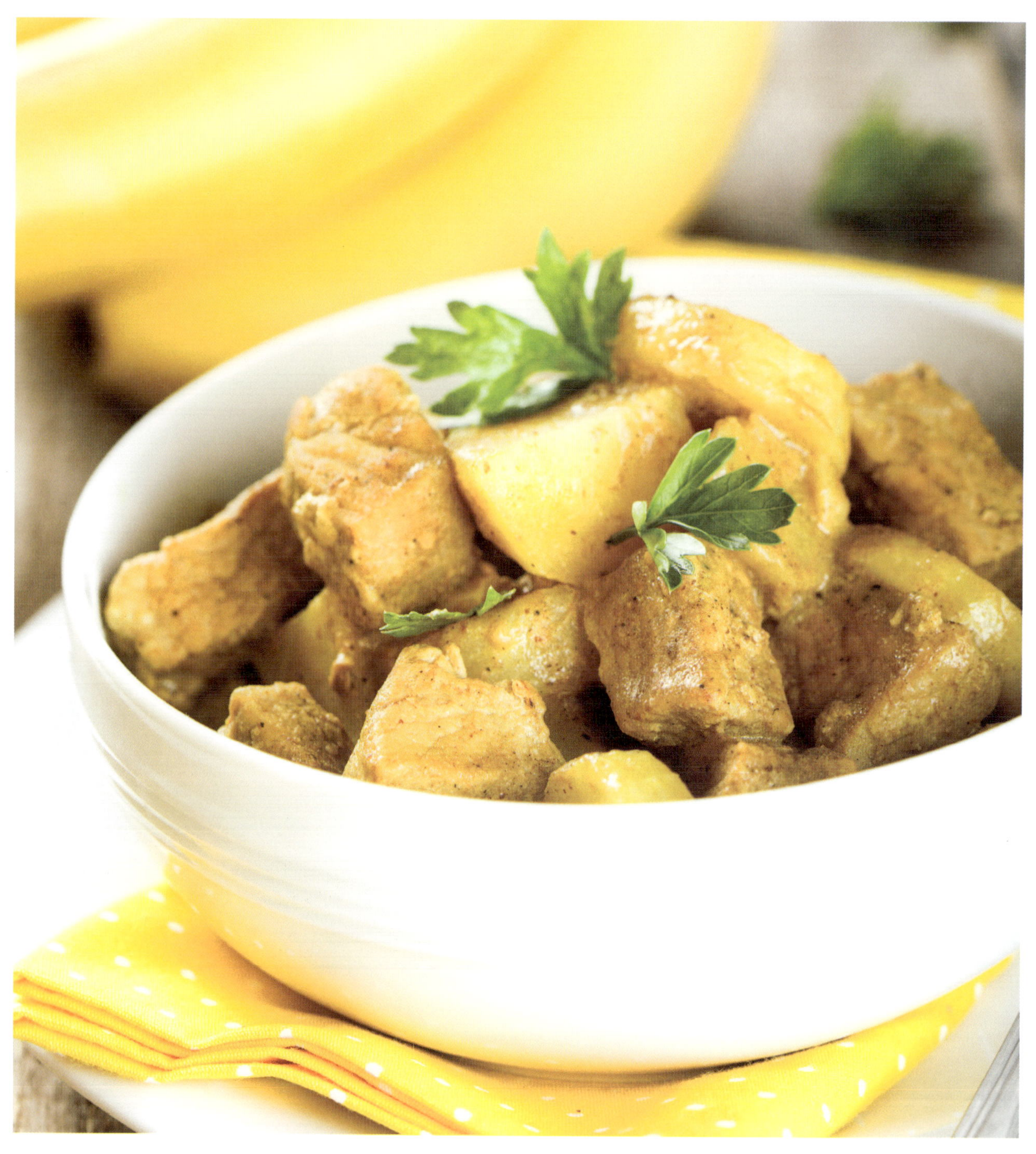

Pork, Potato and Banana Curry

SERVES 4

COOK TIME: HIGH 5 HRS/LOW 6 HRS

GLUTEN FREE • DAIRY FREE

PORK, POTATO AND BANANA CURRY

750g pork loin, cut into small chunks
2 large potatoes, roughly chopped into large chunks
2 tsps curry powder
½ cup (125ml) orange juice
¼ tsp ground cinnamon
Water, to cover
2 tbsps cornflour + 2 tbsps cold water
3 bananas, peeled and sliced into 2cm-thick pieces
Fresh coriander leaves, to garnish

Place the pork, potatoes, curry powder, orange juice and cinnamon in the slow cooker. Add enough water to just cover the meat, if needed. Cover with a lid and cook on low for 6 hours or high for 5 hours, or until the meat is tender.

Increase the heat to high. In a small bowl combine the cornflour and cold water until the mixture is smooth, then stir into the slow cooker.

Add the banana to the slow cooker and cook for 30 minutes, stirring as necessary.

Serve with a garnish of fresh coriander leaves.

Chicken Biriyani

SERVES 3

COOK TIME: LOW 2½-3 HRS

GLUTEN FREE

CHICKEN

2 tbsps ghee or oil
1 large red onion, sliced
2 tsps green chilli paste
5 cloves garlic, minced
Small piece ginger, minced
1 tsp ground turmeric
1 tbsp ground coriander
1 tsp red chilli powder
1½ tbsps garam masala
2 tbsps Greek yoghurt
Salt and pepper to taste
4 chicken drumsticks

RICE

3L + 3 tbsps water
2 tbsps salt
Spice mix: 10 cloves, 5 bay leaves, 1 star anise, 6 green cardamom pods
2¼ cups (450g) basmati rice
¼ cup (30g) cashew nuts

Heat 1 tablespoon ghee or oil in a frying pan over medium heat. Add onion and fry for 5-7 minutes until golden brown.

Take half the fried onion and add to a bowl with chilli paste, garlic, ginger, spices, yoghurt, salt and pepper. Mix to combine. Add chicken and coat well. Cover and transfer to fridge for 2-4 hours.

Heat remaining oil in a frying pan over medium-high heat. Add chicken and brown quickly on all sides. Remove from heat and set aside.

Bring the 3 litres water to the boil, add salt and spice mix. Add rice, bring back up to boil then cook for 4 minutes. Drain immediately and set aside, retaining spices.

Arrange chicken in base of slow cooker. Cover with rice and remaining onion. Sprinkle with 3 tablespoons water and the cashew nuts. Cover cooker with foil, then close lid. Cook on low for 2½-3 hours. Stir the rice and chicken together and serve.

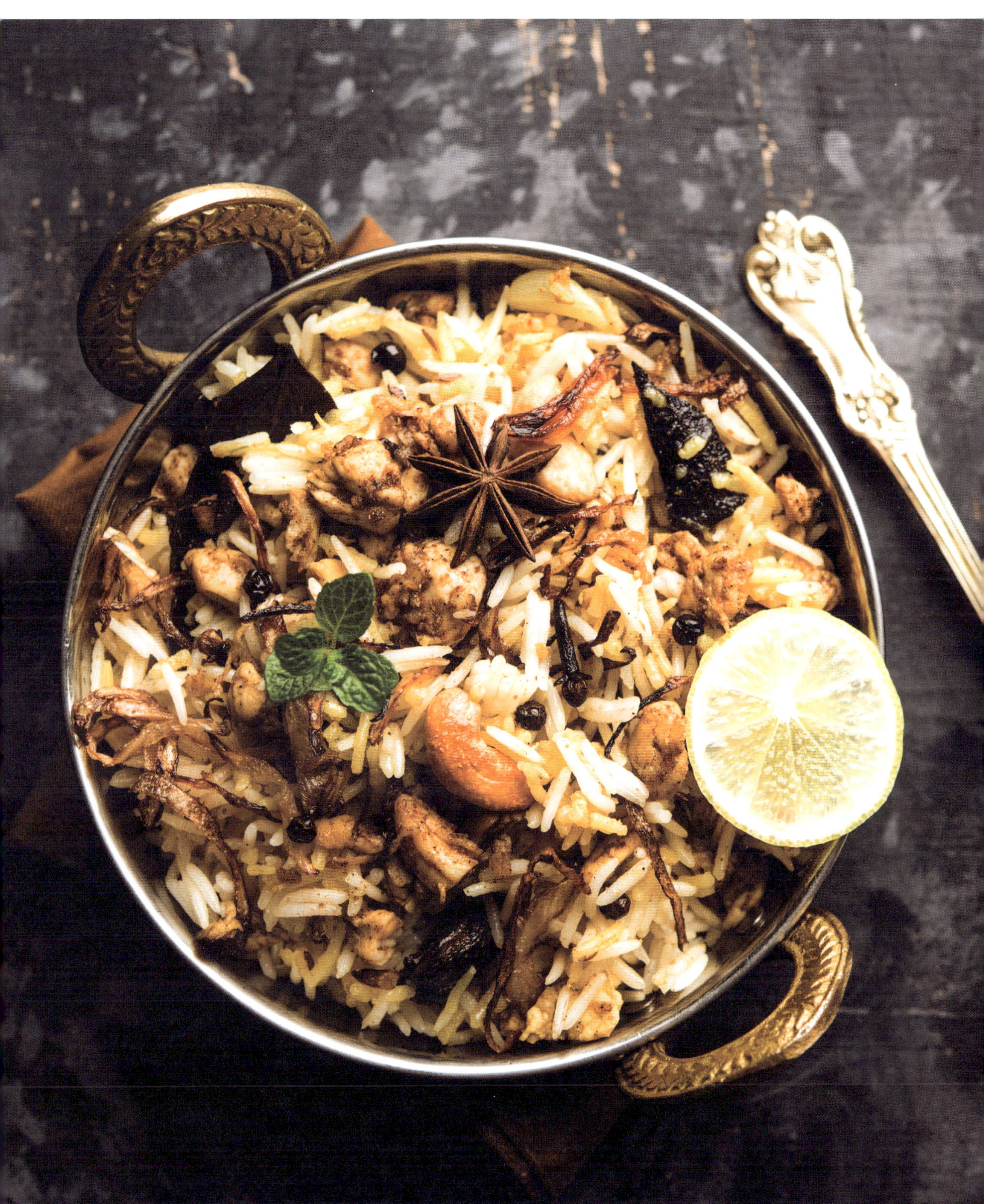

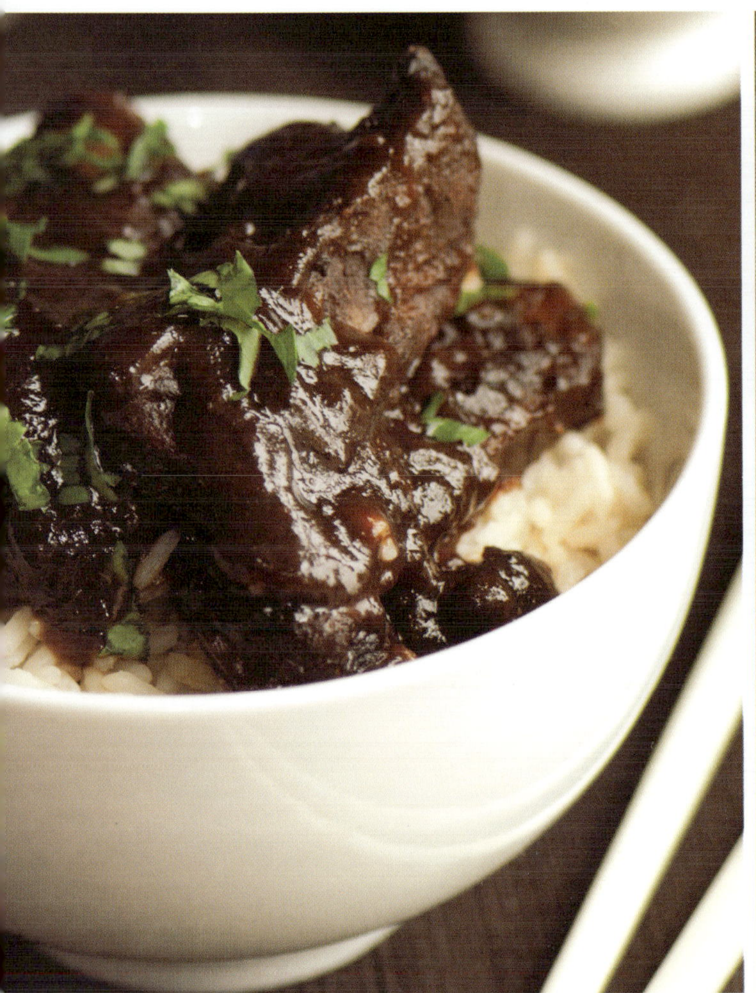

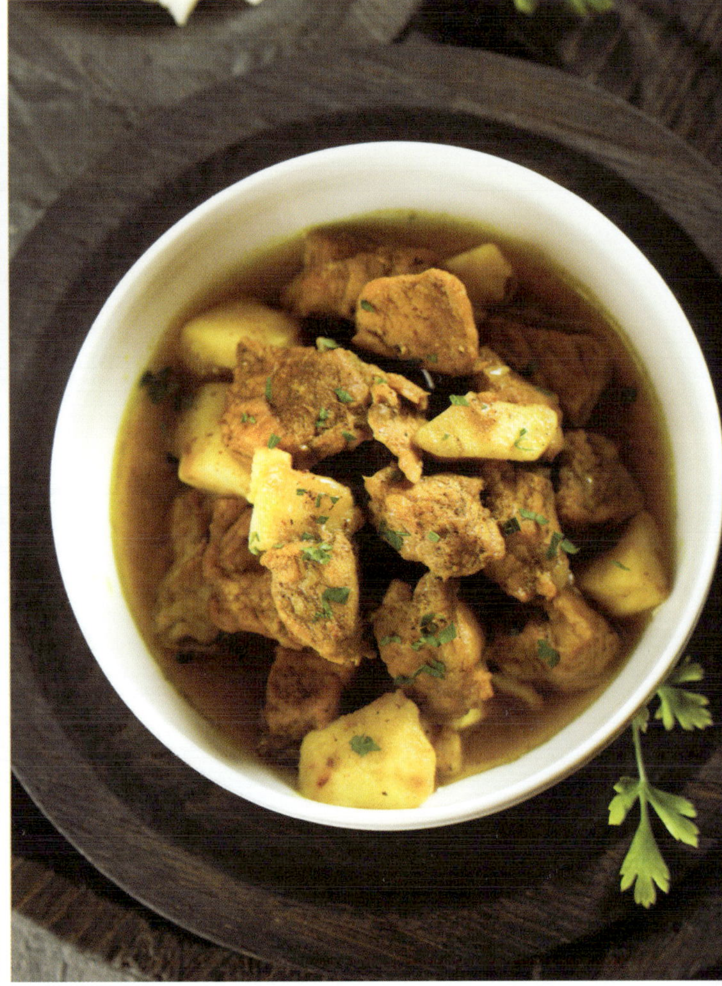

Baby Pork Ribs in Sticky Hoisin Sauce

SERVES 4

COOK TIME: LOW 8 HRS

GLUTEN FREE • DAIRY FREE

Pork and Apple Curry

SERVES 4

COOK TIME: LOW 6 HRS + HIGH 30 MINS

GLUTEN FREE • DAIRY FREE

BABY PORK RIBS IN STICKY HOISIN SAUCE

1kg pork baby back ribs

¾ cup (200ml) hoisin sauce

⅓ cup (100ml) soy sauce (or tamari)

5 cloves garlic, minced

1 tbsp ginger, minced

2 tsps chilli sauce

200g brown sugar

½ cup (125ml) water

2 tsps cornflour

Salt and pepper to taste

Fresh coriander, chopped, to garnish

Cut the racks into individual ribs and place in the slow cooker.

In a large bowl whisk together the hoisin sauce, soy sauce, garlic, ginger, chilli sauce, sugar and water.

Place the ribs in the slow cooker and coat them evenly with the hoisin sauce mixture. Cook on low for 8 hours.

Remove ribs from slow cooker and place on baking sheet. Cover with foil to keep warm.

Skim off the top layer of fat from the liquid in the slow cooker. Pour liquid into a small saucepan and whisk in the cornflour. Bring to a gentle boil and allow to thicken.

Brush thickened sauce over ribs and serve on a bed of rice with chopped coriander as a garnish.

PORK AND APPLE CURRY

1kg pork loin, cut into small chunks

1 large apple, cored, peeled and diced into 3cm pieces

1 tbsp curry powder

½ cup (125ml) orange juice

1 clove garlic, minced

¼ tsp ground cinnamon

2 tbsps cornflour + 2 tbsps cool water

Water, to cover

Fresh coriander, chopped, to garnish

Place the pork, apple, curry powder, orange juice, garlic and cinnamon in the slow cooker. Add enough water to just cover the meat, if needed. Cover with a lid and cook on low for 6 hours or until the meat is tender.

Increase the heat to high. In a small bowl combine the cornflour and 2 tbsps water until the mixture is smooth, then stir into the slow cooker.

Cover and cook for 30 minutes, stirring occasionally.

Serve with a garnish of chopped coriander leaves.

Chicken Fajitas

SERVES 6
COOK TIME: HIGH 2½-3 HRS/LOW 4-6 HRS
DAIRY FREE

1 x 400g can diced tomatoes
3 capsicums (red, green and yellow), sliced
1 large onion, halved and sliced
4 cloves garlic, minced
1 jalapeno chilli, deseeded and chopped
500g boneless, skinless chicken breasts
Salt and pepper to taste
2½ tsps chilli powder
2 tsps ground cumin
1 tsp smoked paprika
1 tsp ground coriander
2 tbsps fresh lime juice
1 tbsp honey
12 large flour tortillas
Chopped spring onion, to serve

Pour half of the tomatoes into the bottom of the slow cooker and spread into an even layer. Top with half of the capsicums and onions. Sprinkle in garlic and jalapeno.

Place chicken breasts in a large bowl. Season with salt and pepper. Add dried spices and toss to coat evenly.

Place chicken in slow cooker.

Top with remaining tomatoes, capsicums and onions.

Cover and cook on low for 4-6 hours or on high for 2½-3 hours, until chicken is cooked and vegetables are tender.

Remove chicken and cut into strips. Ladle out 1 cup of tomato liquid from slow cooker and discard.

In a small bowl whisk together lime juice and honey and add to slow cooker along with chicken and season with additional salt and pepper. Gently toss to combine. Serve warm in warmed tortillas sprinkled with spring onion.

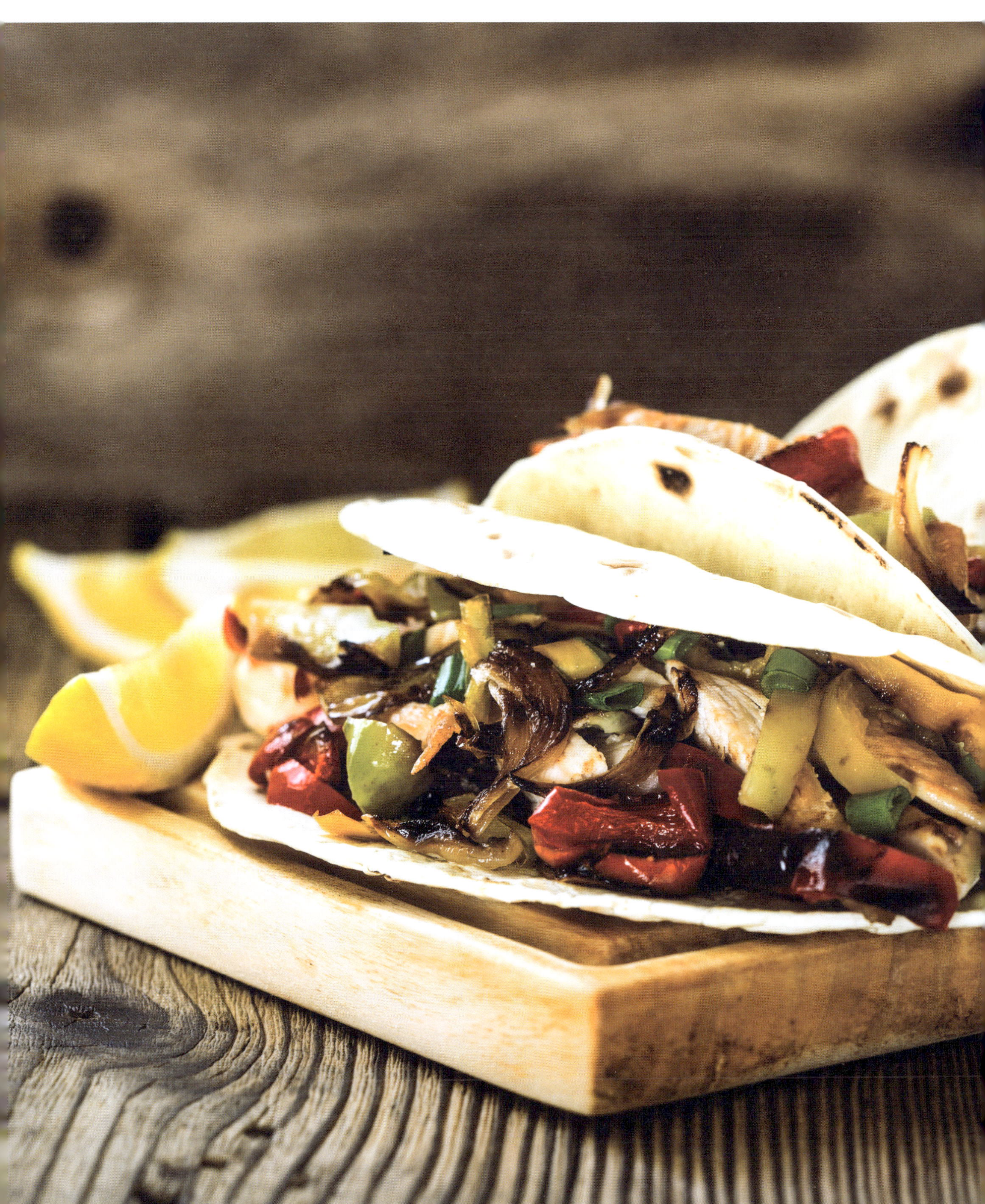

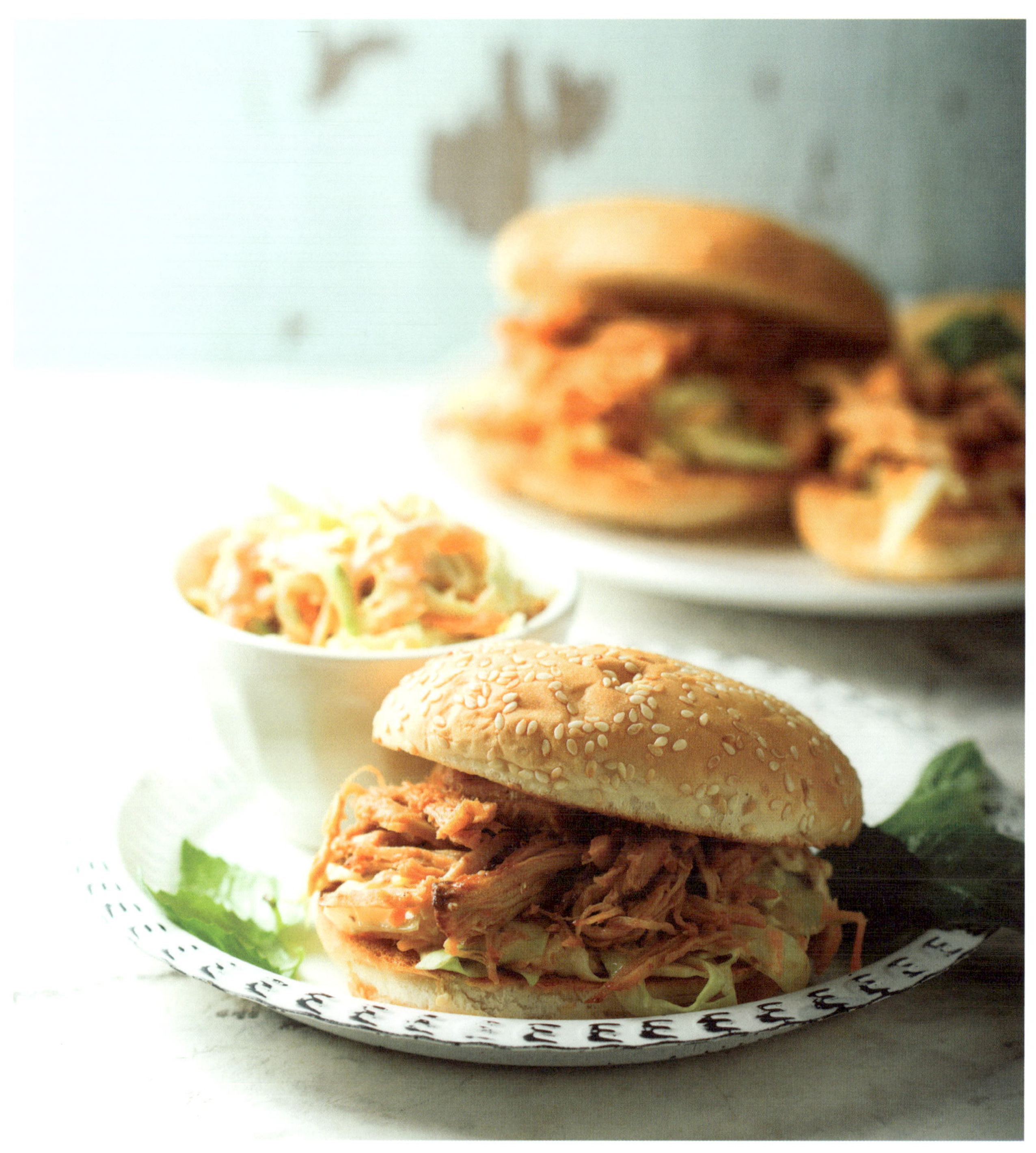

Pulled Pork Burger

SERVES 6

COOK TIME: HIGH 8 HRS/LOW 10 HRS

DAIRY FREE

PULLED PORK BURGER

1.5kg pork shoulder
1 cup (250ml) barbecue sauce
½ cup (125ml) apple cider vinegar
½ cup (125ml) chicken stock
2 cloves garlic, minced
6 sesame-topped burger buns, toasted
Iceberg lettuce, shredded
Coleslaw, to serve

Place the pork in the slow cooker. Pour on the barbecue sauce, vinegar and chicken stock. Add the garlic, cover and cook on low for 10 hours or on high for 8 hours.

Remove the meat from the cooker and place it on a chopping block. Shred the meat using 2 forks, then return the meat to the slow cooker and mix into the juices.

Make up the burgers by placing some meat in the buns with shredded iceberg lettuce and serve with a side dish of coleslaw.

MEATLOAF

2 large eggs, lightly beaten
½ cup (115g) tomato paste
1 carrot, finely grated
1 onion, grated
1 cup (125g) breadcrumbs
Salt and pepper to taste
1kg pork mince
1 cup (250ml) barbecue sauce

Cut four 60cm pieces of foil and fold them over, creating long strips. Place these strips at the bottom of the slow cooker so they stand upright around the sides – these will keep the meatloaf in place and allow you to lift it out of the cooker.

In a large bowl mix together the eggs, tomato paste, carrot, onion and breadcrumbs. Season with salt and pepper. Add the pork mince and using fingers, combine the mixture together.

Scrape the mixture into the foil strips and form a loaf using your hands. Glaze the top with barbecue sauce. Cover and cook for 4 hours on high or 8 hours on low. Lift the meatloaf from the pan using the foil strips and slice to serve.

CHINESE STICKY PORK

1kg boneless pork shoulder, cut into 5cm cubes
2 tbsps honey
4 tbsps soy sauce (or tamari)
4 cloves garlic, minced
2 tbsps rice wine
2 tbsps brown sugar
1 cup (250ml) chicken stock
Chives, chopped, to garnish

Place the pork, honey, soy sauce, garlic, rice wine and sugar in a large bowl and mix thoroughly. Cover and place in the fridge to marinate for at least 4 hours.

Place the pork with marinade mixture and the stock in the slow cooker and mix to combine. Cover and cook on low for 6 hours. Serve with a garnish of chives if desired.

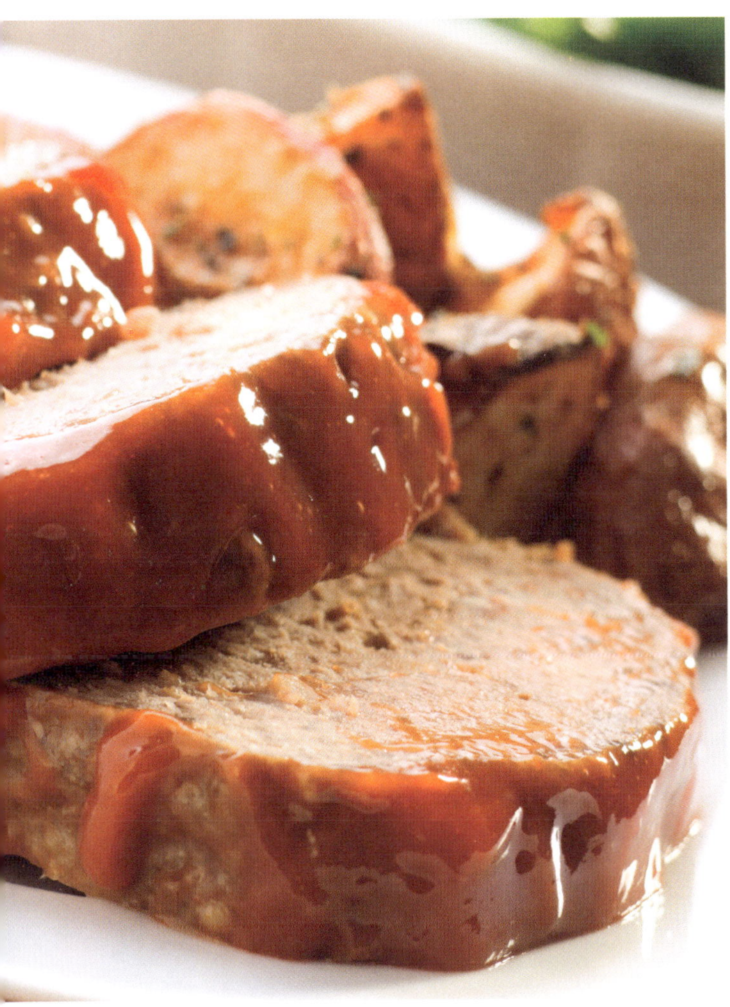

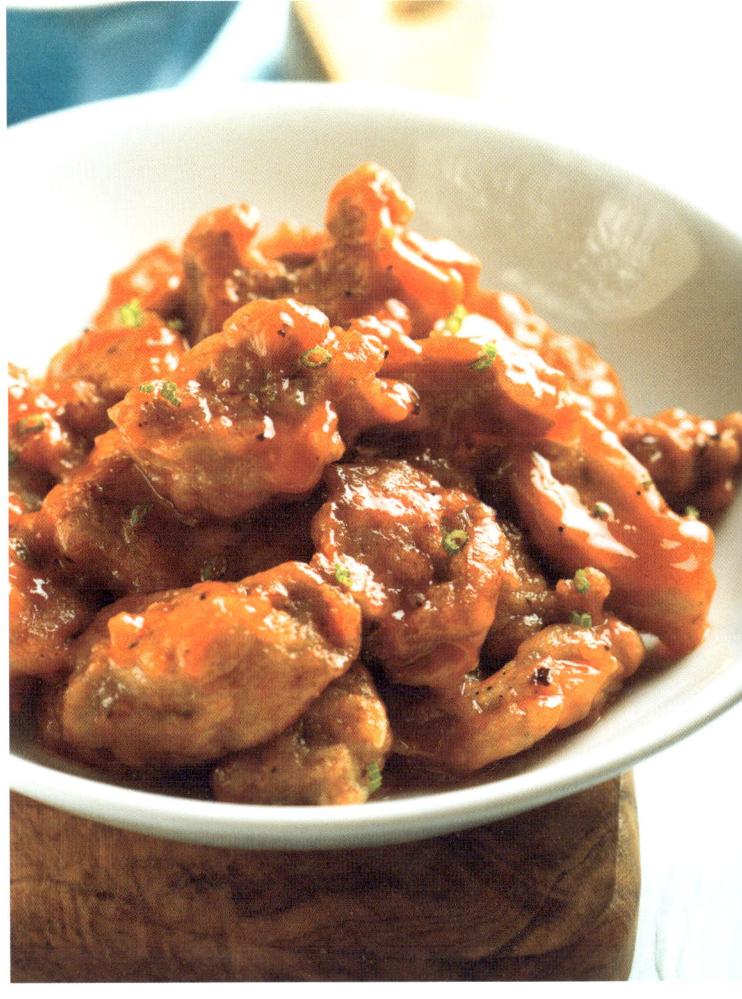

Meatloaf

SERVES 4

COOK TIME: HIGH 4 HRS/LOW 8 HRS

DAIRY FREE

Chinese Sticky Pork

SERVES 4

COOK TIME: LOW 6 HRS

GLUTEN FREE • DAIRY FREE

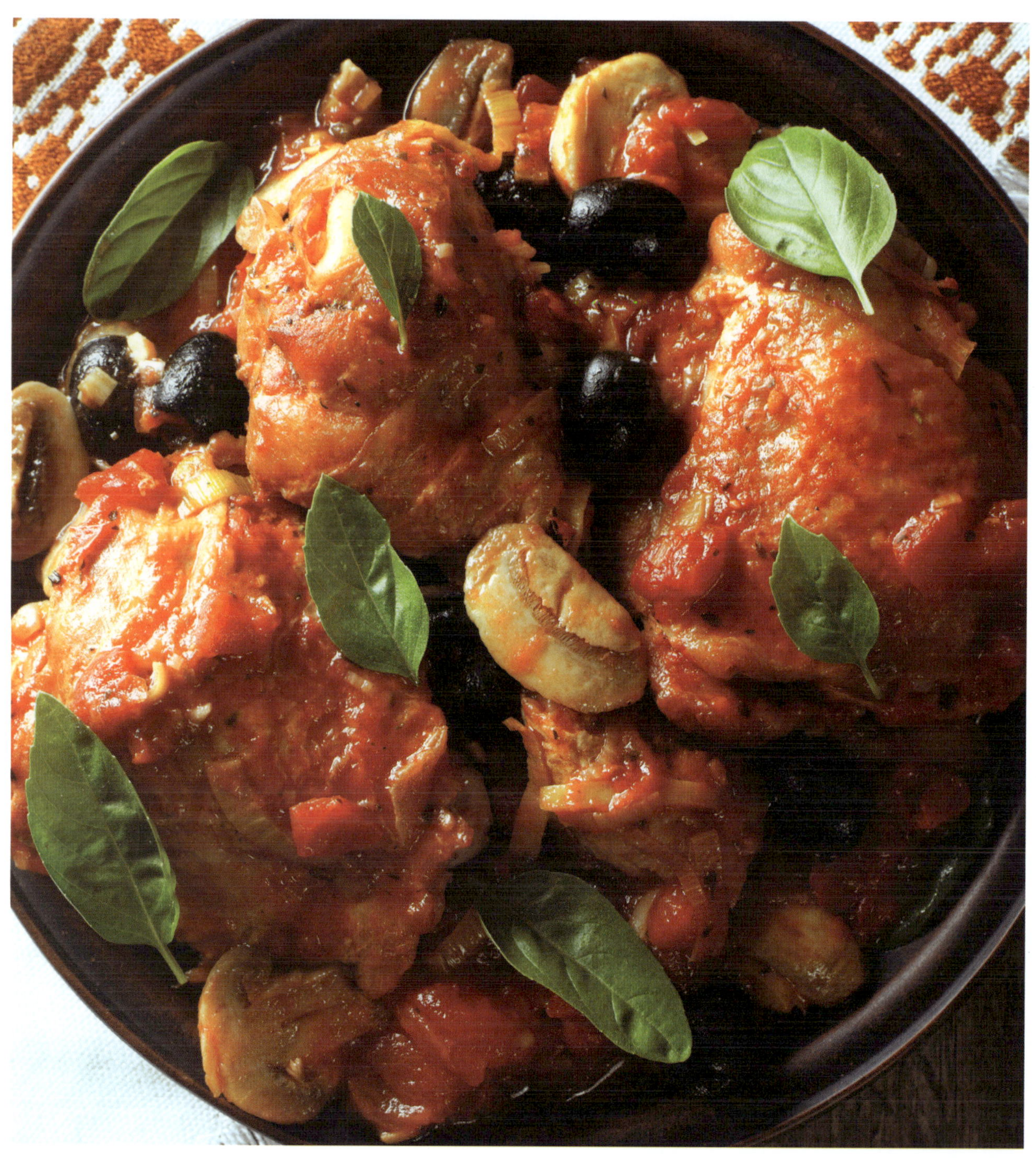

Chicken Cacciatore

SERVES 4

COOK TIME: HIGH 4 HRS/LOW 8 HRS + 1 HR

GLUTEN FREE • DAIRY FREE

CHICKEN CACCIATORE

Olive oil, for frying

6 chicken pieces (leg and thigh), skin on

1 onion, chopped

2 cloves garlic, minced

1 stalk celery, chopped

1 red capsicum, diced

350g button mushrooms, sliced

1 cup (250ml) dry white wine

2 x 400g cans diced tomatoes

½ tsp salt

¼ tsp pepper

¼ tsp chilli flakes

20 Kalamata olives

¼ cup (10g) basil leaves, chopped + extra leaves to garnish

Heat oil in a large frying pan over medium-high heat. Add chicken and cook for 3 minutes on each side, until golden brown. Transfer to the slow cooker.

Place the onion, garlic, celery, capsicum and mushrooms in the slow cooker.

Deglaze the pan with the white wine. Use a spatula to scrape up any brown bits. Pour into the slow cooker.

Add tomatoes, salt, pepper and chilli flakes and stir to mix.

Cover and cook on low for 8 hours or on high for 4 hours.

Add olives and chopped basil and stir. Cook for a further 1 hour, uncovered.

Serve, garnished with basil leaves.

Pork Roulade Stuffed with Apple Sauce

SERVES 4

COOK TIME: LOW 8 HRS

GLUTEN FREE • DAIRY FREE

4 Granny Smith apples, peeled, cored and diced

2 tbsps lemon juice

¼ cup (60ml) water

1.5kg boneless pork loin, chilled

2 tbsps caster sugar

Salt and pepper to taste

Flat-leaf parsley, to garnish

Place the apple, lemon juice and water in a saucepan over a medium-high heat. Bring to the boil then reduce the heat to low. Cook, stirring occasionally, for 15 minutes or until the apple is very soft. Set aside to cool, then stir in the sugar. Place in a blender or food processor and blend until smooth. Cover and allow the sauce to cool completely.

With a long, slender knife, slide the blade through the centre of the loin lengthways, cutting through to the other side. Spoon in the apple sauce until the cavity is entirely filled, pushing it in with the handle of a wooden spoon if necessary.

Season with salt and pepper and place in the slow cooker. Cover and cook on low for 8 hours.

Serve with a garnish of flat-leaf parsley.

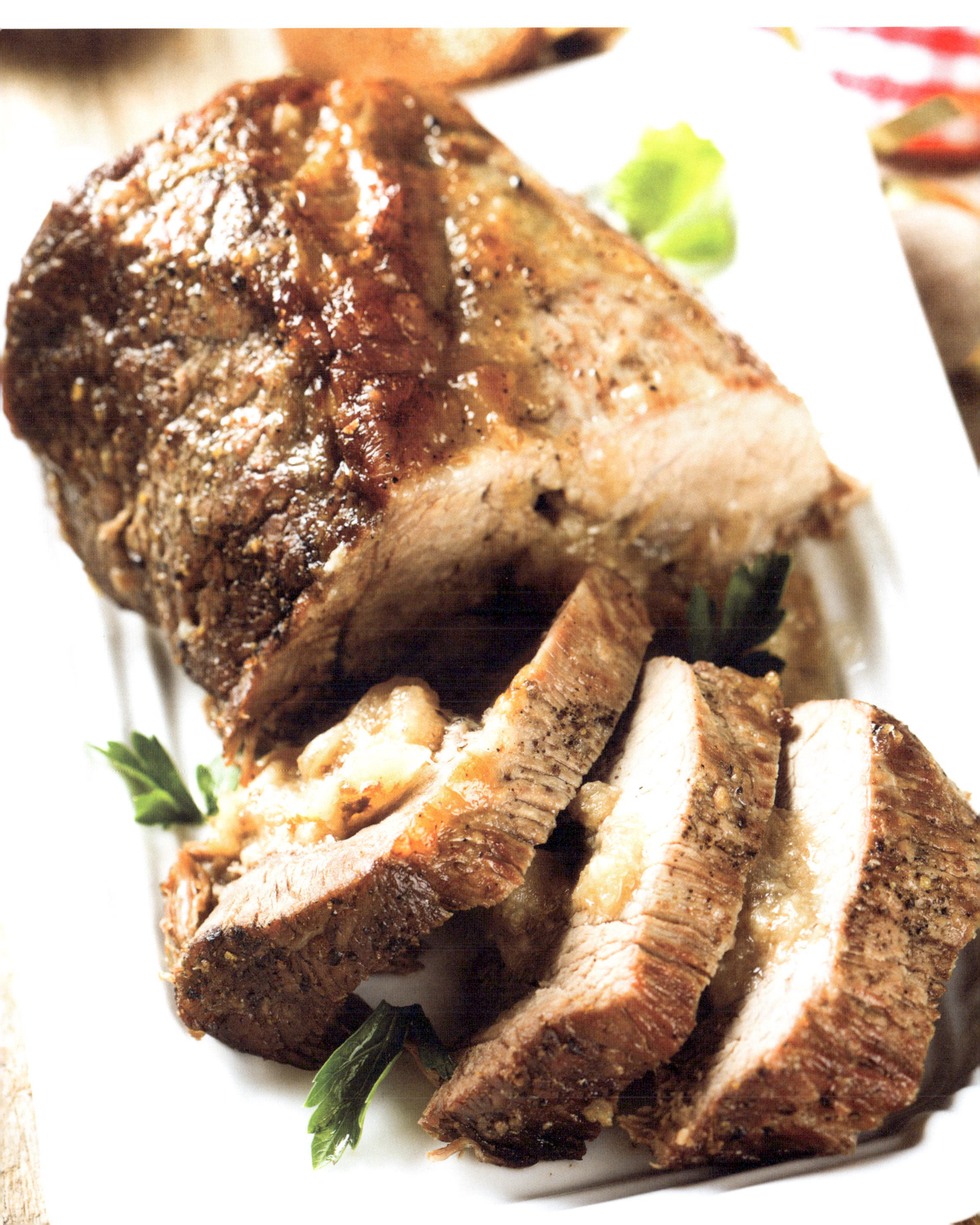

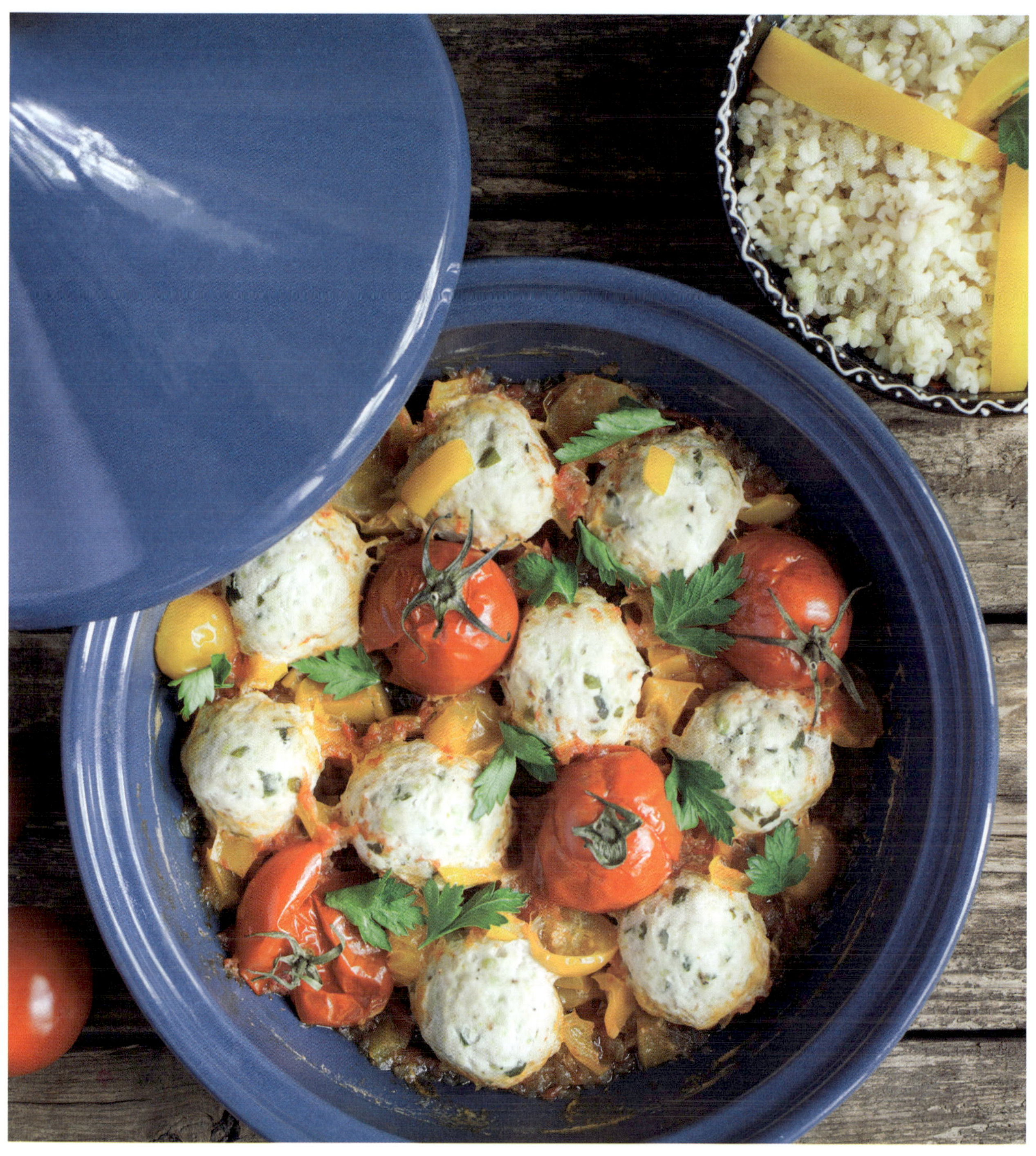

Chicken Kofte Tagine

SERVES 4

COOK TIME: HIGH 3 HRS 30 MINS

DAIRY FREE

CHICKEN KOFTE TAGINE

400g chicken mince

2 red onions, finely chopped

3 cloves garlic, minced

1 tsp cumin

¼ tsp cayenne pepper

1 tsp dried tarragon

1 tbsp ground coriander

1 tsp sweet paprika

2 tbsps breadcrumbs

2 eggs, lightly beaten

¼ cup (10g) roughly chopped parsley + extra to serve

1 tbsp finely chopped fresh coriander

Salt and pepper to taste

4 tbsps olive oil

1 cup (250ml) dry white wine (such as Sauvignon Blanc)

⅓ cup (80g) tomato passata

3 tbsps preserved lemons, finely chopped

1 yellow capsicum, chopped

4 ripe vine tomatoes

Make the meatballs by mixing together the mince, half the onion, two cloves of garlic, ½ teaspoon cumin, cayenne pepper, tarragon, 1 teaspoon ground coriander, paprika, breadcrumbs, eggs, 1 tablespoon chopped parsley, fresh coriander and a good seasoning of salt and pepper.

Form heaped dessertspoons of the mixture into small meatballs using your hands.

Heat 2 tablespoons of olive oil in a large frying pan over medium heat. Cook the meatballs in batches, being careful not to crowd them. Cook them on all sides for 4 minutes until slightly browned. Remove from the pan and set aside.

Use the wine to deglaze the pan, using a spatula to scrape up any brown bits. Pour into the slow cooker.

Add the passata, preserved lemons, capsicum and remaining onion, garlic and spices to the slow cooker. Stir to combine.

Arrange the meatballs and tomatoes in the slow cooker.

Cover and cook on high for about 3½ hours.

Serve sprinkled with fresh parsley and a side of couscous or rice.

Honey-Glazed Ham

SERVES 4

COOK TIME: LOW 6 HRS

GLUTEN FREE • DAIRY FREE

1 tbsp Dijon mustard
½ cup (180g) honey
3 tbsps brown sugar
½ cup (125ml) water
2kg boneless ham, fully cooked

In a large saucepan mix together the mustard, honey, sugar and water. Bring to a simmer over a medium-high heat and cook, while stirring, for 5 minutes.

Spread the glaze on top of the ham. Place the ham in the slow cooker, drizzling any excess glaze over the top.

Cover and cook on low for 6 hours. Slice and serve.

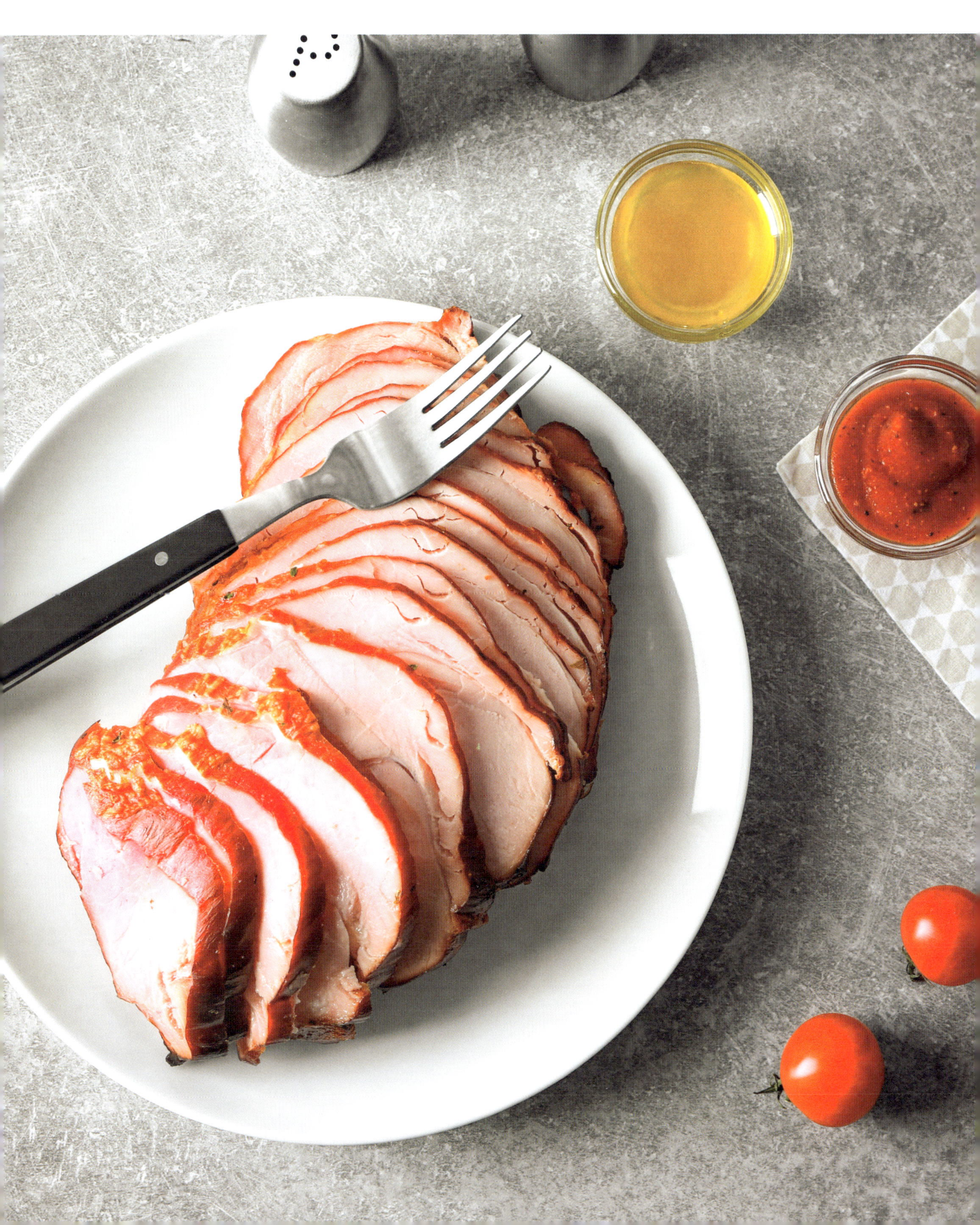

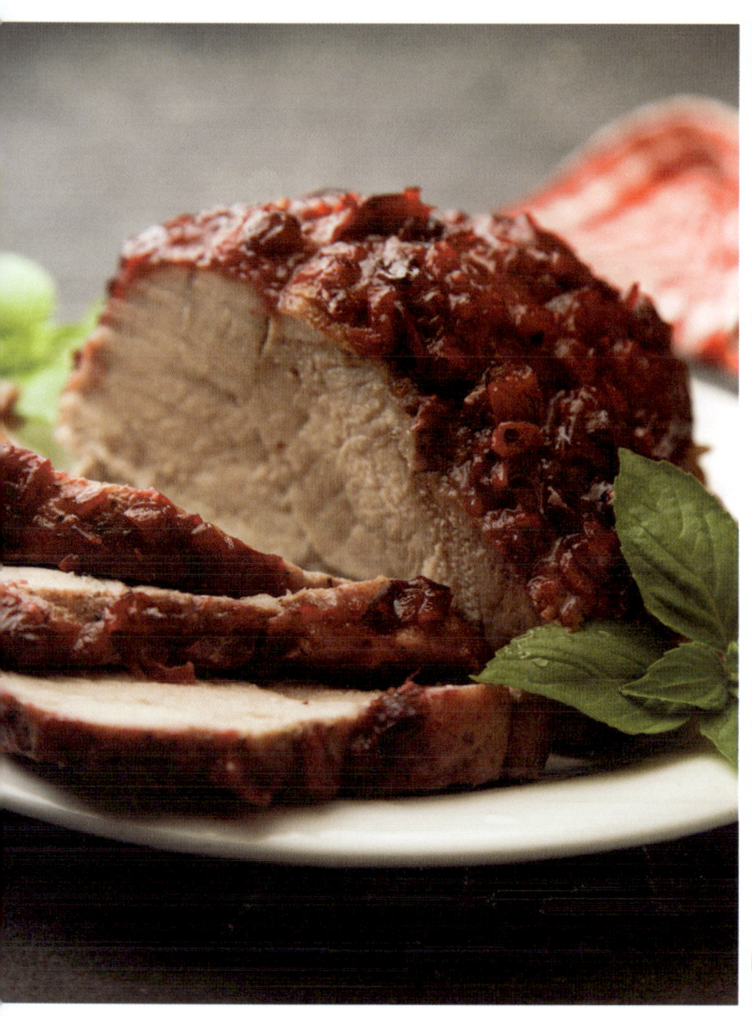

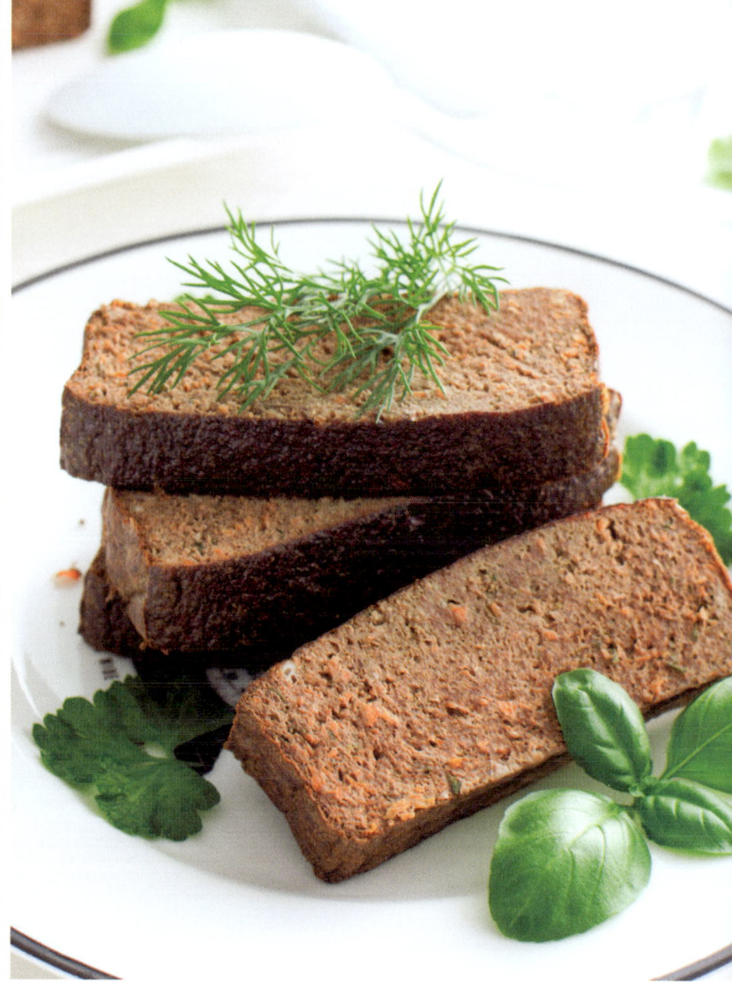

Pork Loin and Cranberry Sauce

SERVES 6

COOK TIME: HIGH 4 HRS/LOW 8 HRS

GLUTEN FREE • DAIRY FREE

Chicken Liver Pate

SERVES 4

COOK TIME: HIGH 1 HR + LOW 8 HRS

GLUTEN FREE

PORK LOIN AND CRANBERRY SAUCE

1 cup (250ml) water
1 cup (220g) sugar
4 cups (400g) fresh or frozen cranberries, rinsed
½ tsp ground cinnamon
1.5kg boneless pork loin
Fresh basil leaves, to garnish

Heat the water and sugar in a saucepan over a medium-high heat. Bring to a boil and stir to dissolve the sugar. Add the cranberries and cook them until they burst. Then lower the heat and simmer for 10 minutes, and mix in the cinnamon. Place in the fridge to cool completely.

Place the pork in the slow cooker and smother the top with the cranberry sauce. Cover and cook on high for 4 hours or low for 8 hours.

Slice and serve with a garnish of fresh basil.

CHICKEN LIVER PATE

600g chicken livers
1 onion, finely chopped
200g butter
2 cloves garlic, grated
2 tbsps brandy
1 tsp sage, chopped
½ tsp salt
1 tsp pepper
Fresh dill, to garnish
Flat-leaf parsley, to garnish

Fry the liver and onions in 15g of butter for 3 minutes in a frying pan over a medium heat. Add the garlic and cook for 2 minutes more.

Stir in the brandy with the remaining butter and the sage. Add salt and pepper. Place in a blender or food processor and blend until the mixture is smooth.

Place the pate in a well-greased terrine mould or loaf tin that will fit the slow cooker, then pour water into the slow cooker to halfway up the tin. Cook on high for 1 hour then low for another 8 hours.

Slice to serve and garnish with fresh dill and parsley.

Sticky BBQ Chicken Legs

SERVES 4

COOK TIME: HIGH 4 HRS/LOW 8 HRS

GLUTEN FREE • DAIRY FREE

2 cloves garlic, minced
1 tsp salt
1 tsp pepper
8 chicken drumsticks (skin on or off)
½ cup (160g) apricot jam
1 cup (250ml) barbecue sauce
2 tsps wholegrain mustard

Rub the garlic, salt and pepper into the chicken flesh or skin. Place chicken in the bottom of the slow cooker, in a single layer if possible.

Cover and cook for 3 hours on high or 6 hours on low.

In a small bowl, mix together the apricot jam, barbecue sauce and mustard. Set aside.

Remove chicken from slow cooker and set aside. Drain juices from slow cooker, then wipe dry with a paper towel. Place chicken back in the cooker. Pour half the sauce over the chicken. Cover and continue cooking on high for 1 hour or low for 2 hours.

Remove chicken from slow cooker and brush with remaining sauce. If desired place under a hot grill for 2-3 minutes to crisp up, or serve as it is.

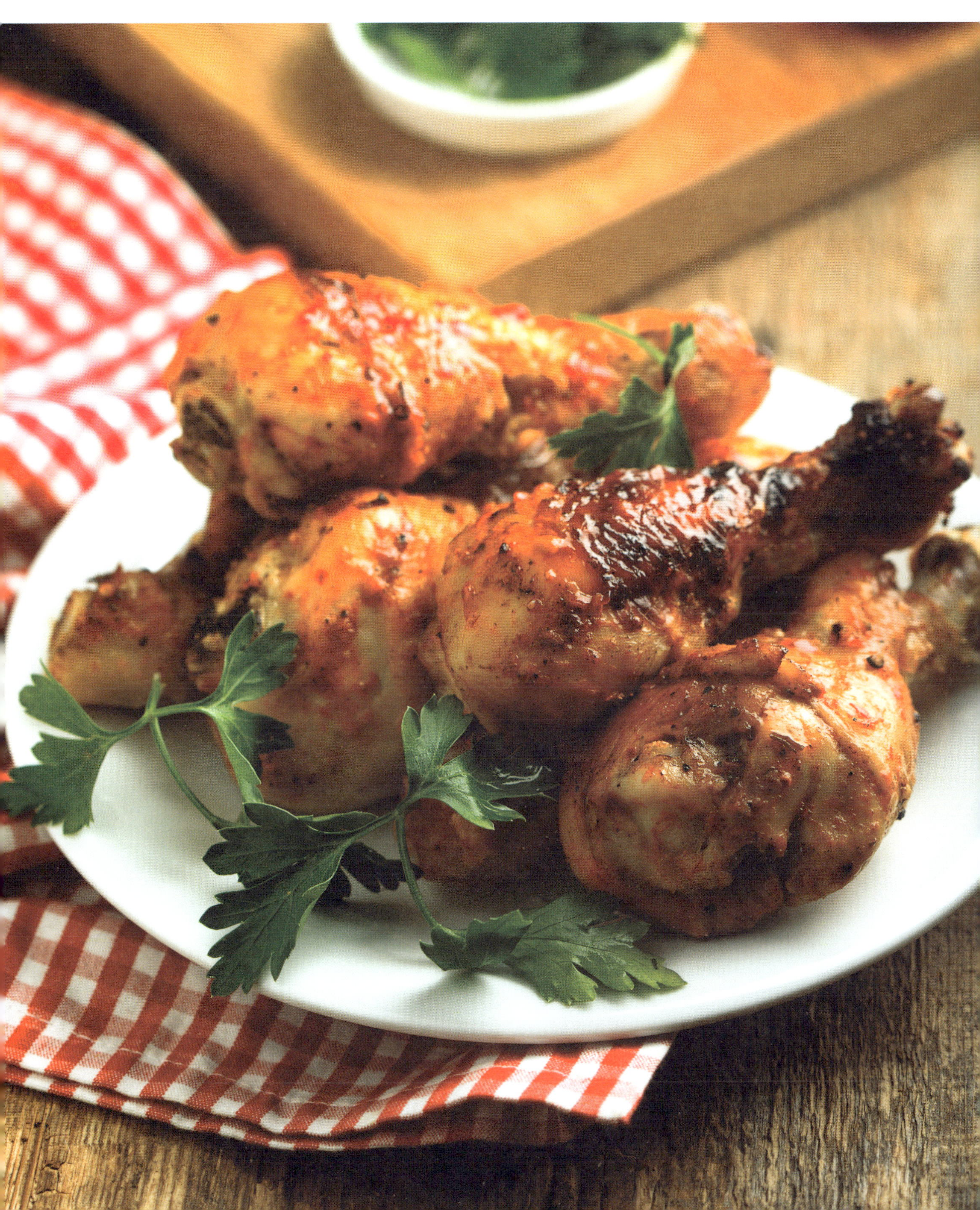

Chapter Three

Fish and Seafood

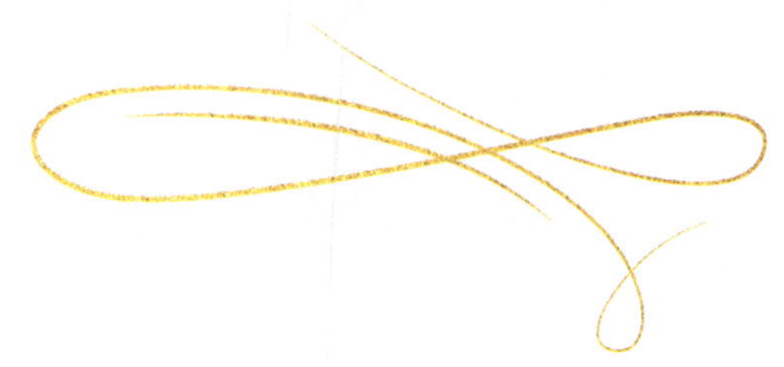

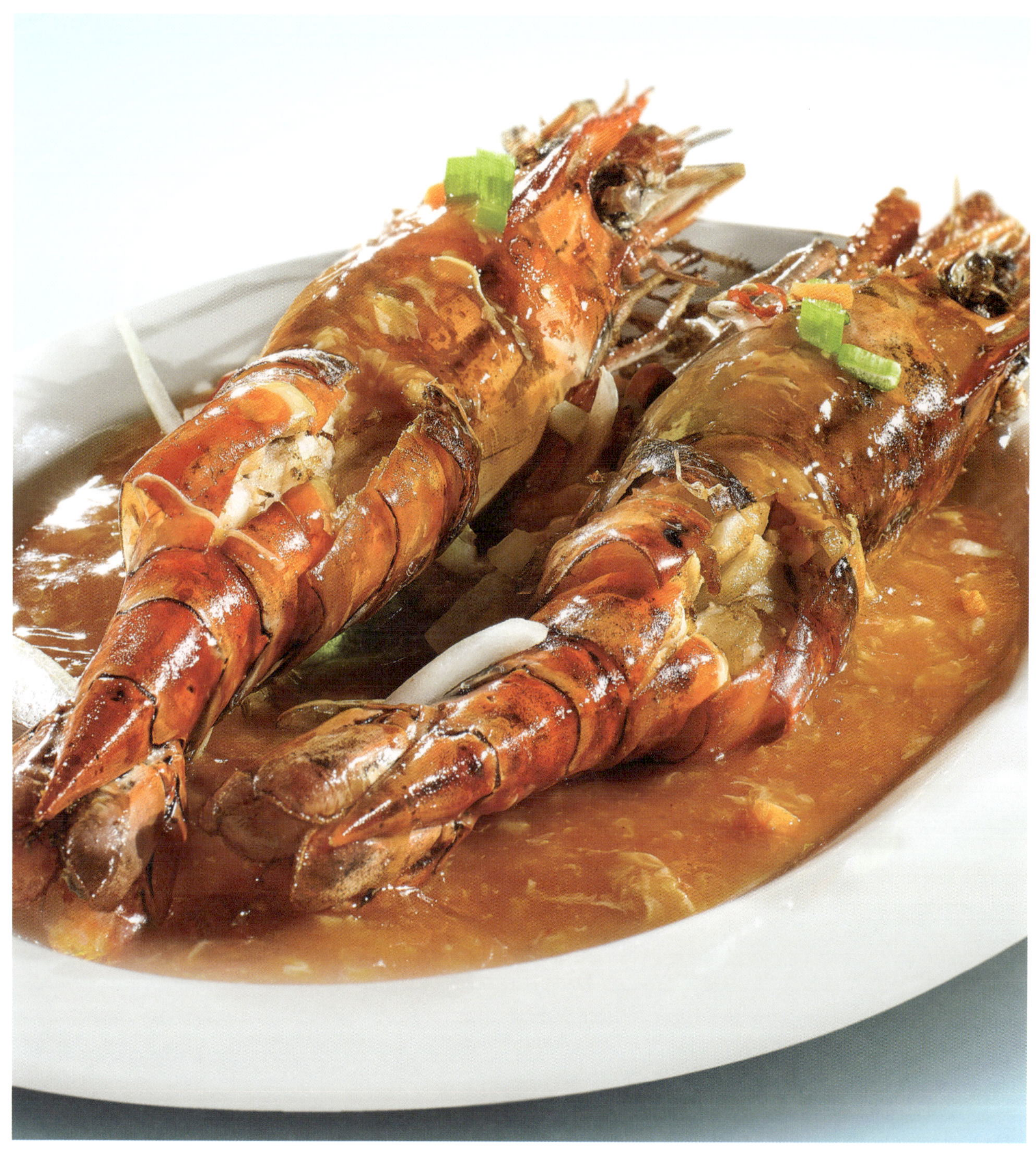

Sweet and Sour Prawns

SERVES 4

COOK TIME: LOW 3-4 HRS + 30 MINS

GLUTEN FREE • DAIRY FREE

SWEET AND SOUR PRAWNS

1 x 400g can crushed pineapple
2 tbsps cornflour
3 tbsps sugar
1 cup (250ml) chicken stock
1 tbsp soy sauce (or tamari)
½ tsp ground ginger
1kg whole jumbo tiger prawns
2 tbsps rice wine vinegar

Drain juice from can of pineapple into a small saucepan. Add cornflour, sugar, chicken stock, soy sauce and ginger. Bring mixture to a boil, stirring. Simmer for 1 minute until thickened.

Transfer to slow cooker with crushed pineapple. Cover and cook on low for 3-4 hours.

Add prawns and continue to cook 30 minutes longer, until prawns are cooked. Add vinegar and stir gently.

Serve immediately.

Fish Chowder

SERVES 4
COOK TIME: HIGH 4 HRS/LOW 8 HRS
GLUTEN FREE

500g white fish fillets (such as Murray cod or Mahi Mahi), chopped into small chunks

2 large potatoes, peeled and diced

2 carrots, peeled and roughly chopped

Salt and pepper to taste

1 x 400g can chopped tomatoes

1 cup (250ml) chicken stock

1 cup (250ml) double cream

3 tbsps butter, melted

2 tbsps cornflour

Place the fish pieces in the slow cooker with the potatoes and carrots. Add salt and pepper to taste and gently mix everything together.

Add the chopped tomatoes and stock and stir to combine. Cover and cook on high for 4 hours or low for 8 hours.

About an hour before the chowder has finished cooking, place the cream, melted butter and cornflour in a blender or food processor and blend so that it is well combined. Stir this into the slow cooker.

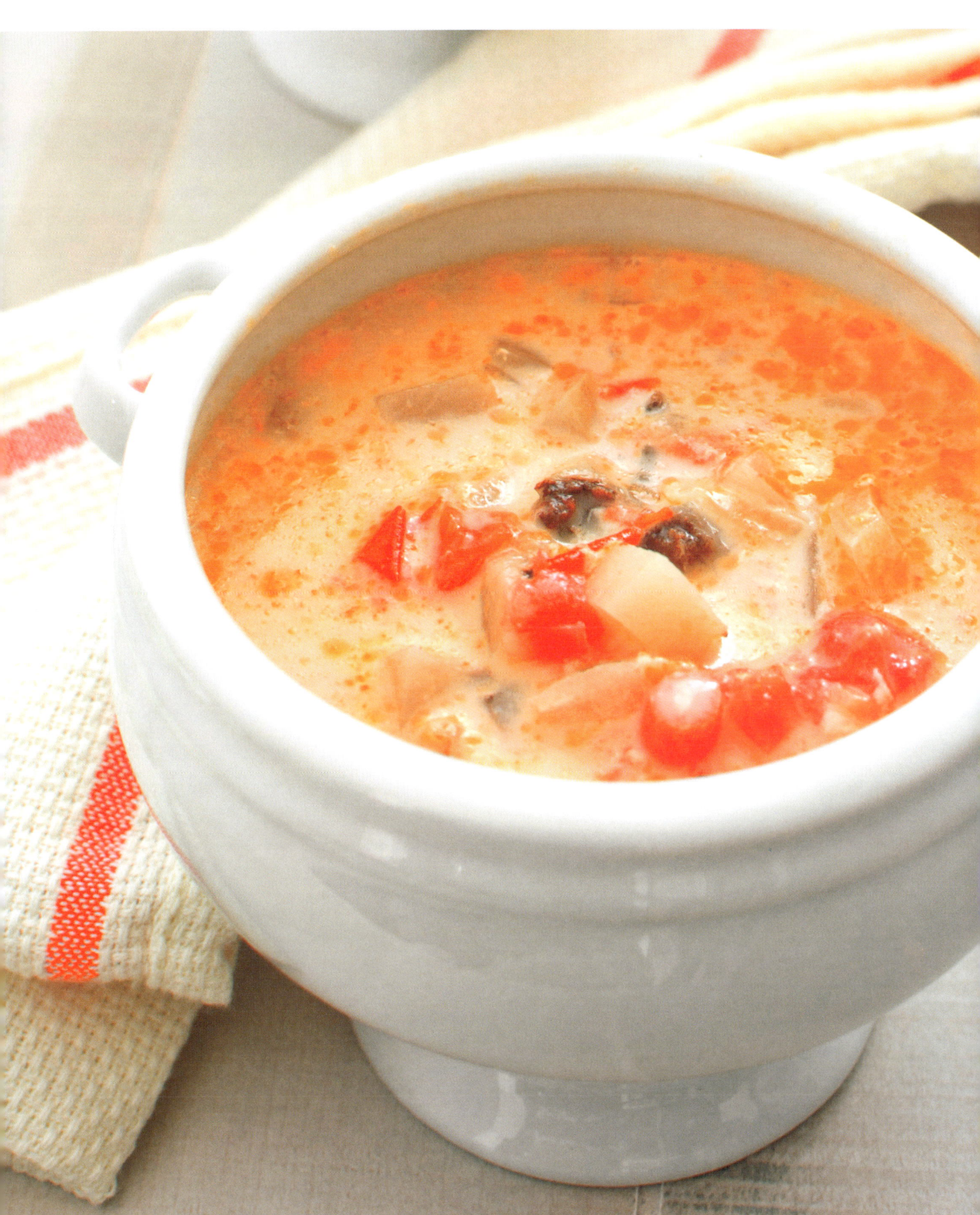

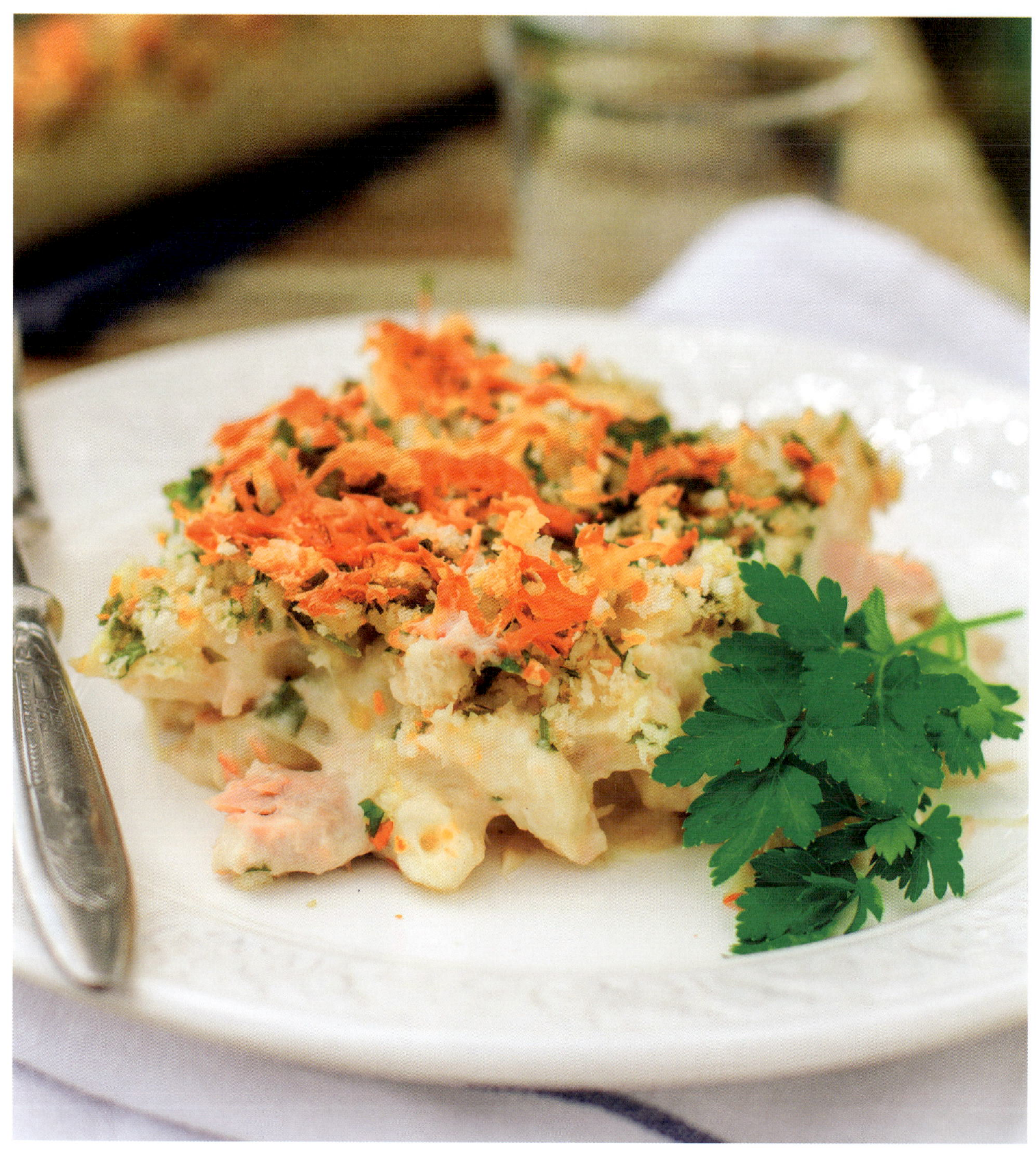

Tuna Mornay

SERVES 4

COOK TIME: LOW 4 HRS + 15 MINS IN OVEN

TUNA MORNAY

3 tbsps butter

3 tbsps plain flour

1½ cups (375ml) milk

Salt and pepper to taste

1 cup (125g) hard cheese (such as Cheddar, Parmesan or Swiss), grated

450g penne or fusilli pasta

3 x 180g cans tuna, drained

2 stems parsley, leaves chopped

½ leek, finely chopped

½ cup (60g) dried breadcrumbs

To make the sauce, melt the butter in a saucepan over a medium high heat. When melted, add the flour and mix thoroughly for 1 minute, making sure the flour doesn't brown. Slowly add the milk while stirring continuously. Bring the sauce to a boil then lower the heat to a simmer and continue to stir for 3-4 minutes. Remove the pan from the heat and season with salt and pepper. Add half of the grated cheese and whisk until the cheese has melted into the sauce.

Add the pasta to the slow cooker then mix in the sauce, tuna, parsley and leek. Cover and cook on low for 4 hours.

Preheat the oven to 200°C. When the pasta is cooked, remove the insert from the slow cooker with the food inside. Sprinkle the rest of the cheese and the breadcrumbs on the top and cook in the oven for 15 minutes or until the cheese is melted and breadcrumbs are crispy.

FISH WITH CREAMY WHITE SAUCE

4 white fish fillets (such as Murray cod or Mahi Mahi), skin removed

2 tbsps plain flour

1 tbsp caster sugar

Salt and pepper to taste

75g butter

½ cup (125ml) thickened cream

1 lemon, juiced

½ cup (125ml) dry white wine

Fresh chives, chopped, to garnish

Pat the fish fillets dry with paper towel and place them in the slow cooker.

In a bowl combine the flour, sugar, a couple of pinches of salt and a good grind of pepper. Melt the butter in a saucepan over a medium heat and stir in the flour mixture. When mixed, add the cream, lemon juice and wine and allow the mixture to simmer, while stirring, for 2 minutes.

Pour the sauce over the fish in the slow cooker, cover, and cook on high for 3 hours. Serve with a garnish of chopped chives.

PRAWN AND SAUSAGE CASSEROLE

300g spicy sausage, chopped into 2cm slices

1 onion, finely chopped

1 x 400g can chopped tomatoes

3 cloves garlic, minced

2 cups (500ml) chicken stock

½ cup (60g) plain flour

300g prawns, deveined and tails removed

2 tbsps olive oil

Cooked rice, to serve

Spring onions, sliced, to garnish

Place the sausage in the slow cooker with the onion, tomatoes and garlic.

In a large bowl, whisk the stock with the flour until no lumps remain. Pour into the slow cooker, cover, and cook on high for 5 hours.

After 5 hours, stir in the prawns. Re-cover and cook for a further 30 minutes.

Serve with rice, garnished with spring onions.

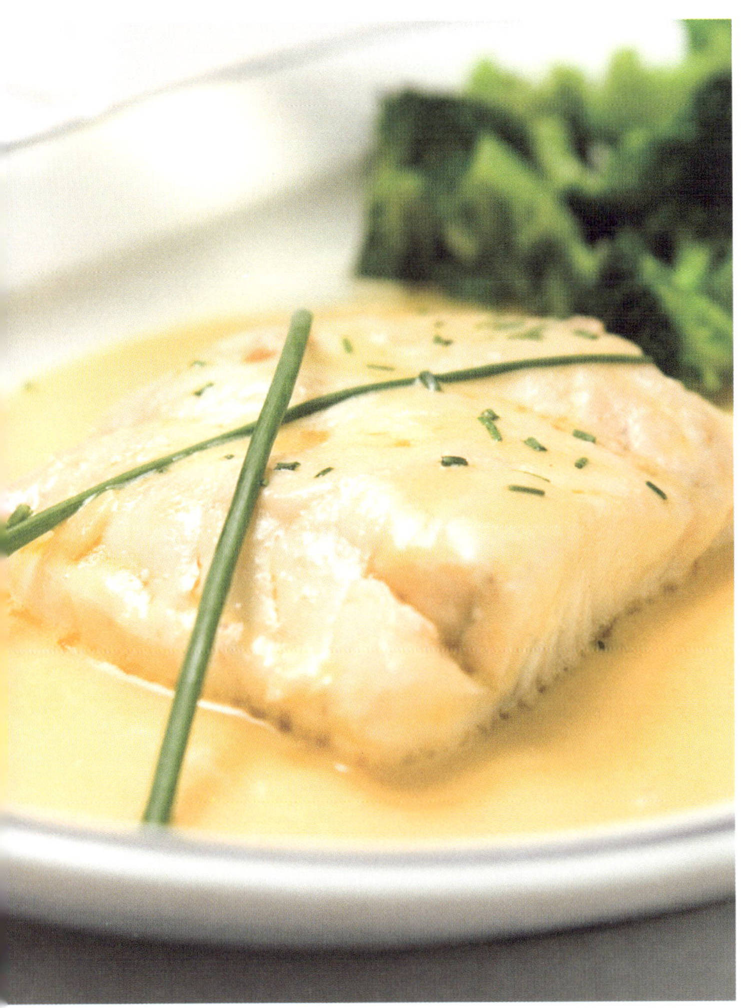

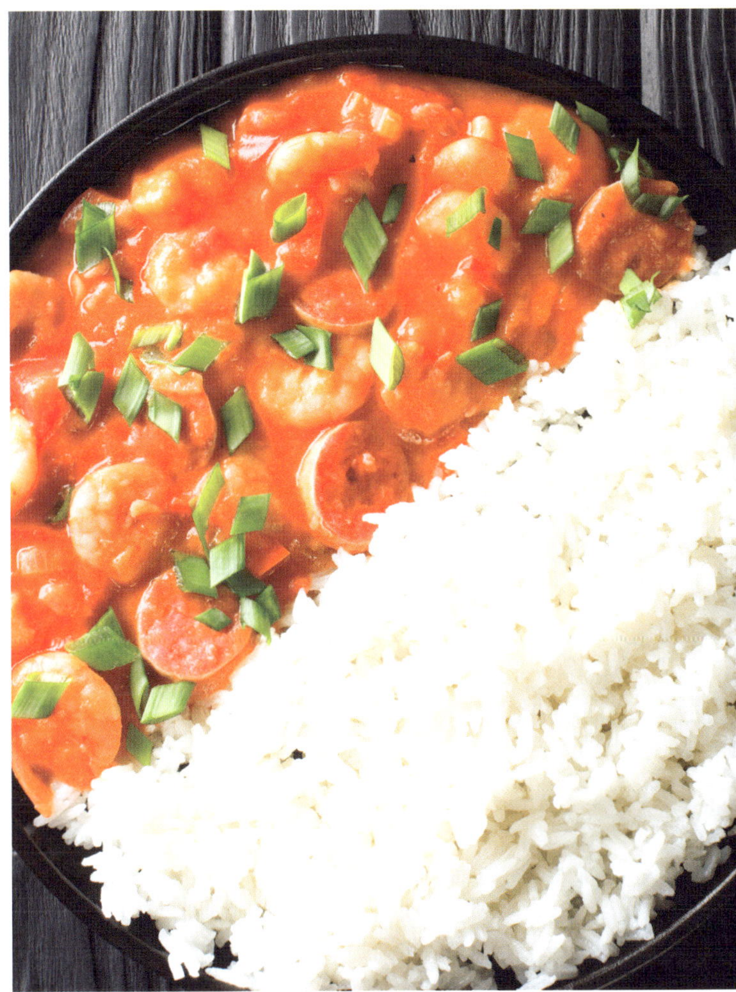

Fish with Creamy White Sauce

SERVES 4

COOK TIME: HIGH 3 HRS

Prawn and Sausage Gumbo

SERVES 4

COOK TIME: HIGH 5 HRS 30 MINS

DAIRY FREE

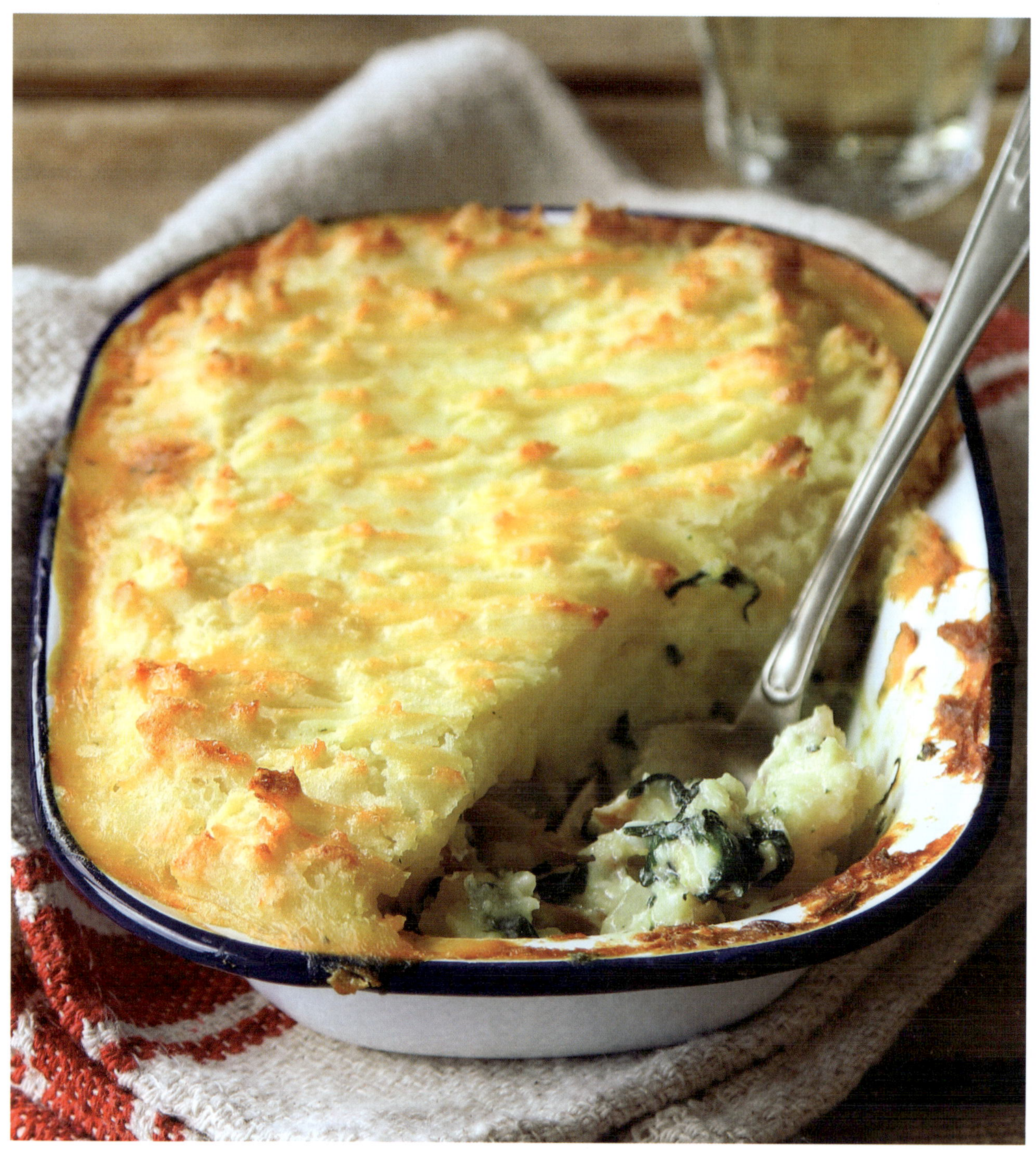

Fish and Spinach Pie

SERVES 4

COOK TIME: HIGH 8 HRS + LOW 3 HRS

GLUTEN FREE

FISH AND SPINACH PIE

3 potatoes, peeled and roughly chopped

40g butter

¼ cup (60ml) milk

600g fish (barramundi, snapper, salmon or a combination), cut into 3cm chunks

150g baby spinach

1 lemon, juiced

Salt and pepper to taste

Place the potatoes in a large saucepan and cover with salted water. Boil for 20 minutes until potatoes are tender. Drain then return the potatoes to the pan and mash with a potato masher. Add the butter and milk and continue to mash until the potato is fluffy. Set aside to cool completely.

Place the fish, spinach and lemon juice in the slow cooker and season with salt and pepper. Cook on high for 1 hour. Stir thoroughly then spread the cold potato mash on top and cook on low for 3 hours.

Place under a hot grill to finish if desired.

Fish Balls in Tomato Sauce

SERVES 4

COOK TIME: HIGH 2 HRS + LOW 2 HRS

DAIRY FREE

2 x 400g cans chopped tomatoes

1 red capsicum, finely chopped

1 cup (250ml) vegetable stock

Salt and pepper to taste

500g white fish fillets (such as Murray cod or Mahi Mahi), roughly chopped into large chunks

½ cup (60g) dried breadcrumbs

1 tsp dried oregano

1 egg, beaten

2 tbsps olive oil

Pour the tomatoes into the slow cooker with the capsicum and stock and season well with salt and pepper. Cook on high for 2 hours.

In the meantime, place the fish in a food processor or blender. Pulse the fish on its own before adding the breadcrumbs, oregano, egg and further seasoning and blending until the mixture is fine, but not a mush.

Place the mixture in a bowl and using wet hands, roll it into fish balls. Set aside until about 30 minutes before the 2 hours is up.

Heat the olive oil in a large frying pan over a medium-high heat. Cook the fish balls in batches until slightly browned, then add to the slow cooker. Reduce to low and cook for a further 2 hours.

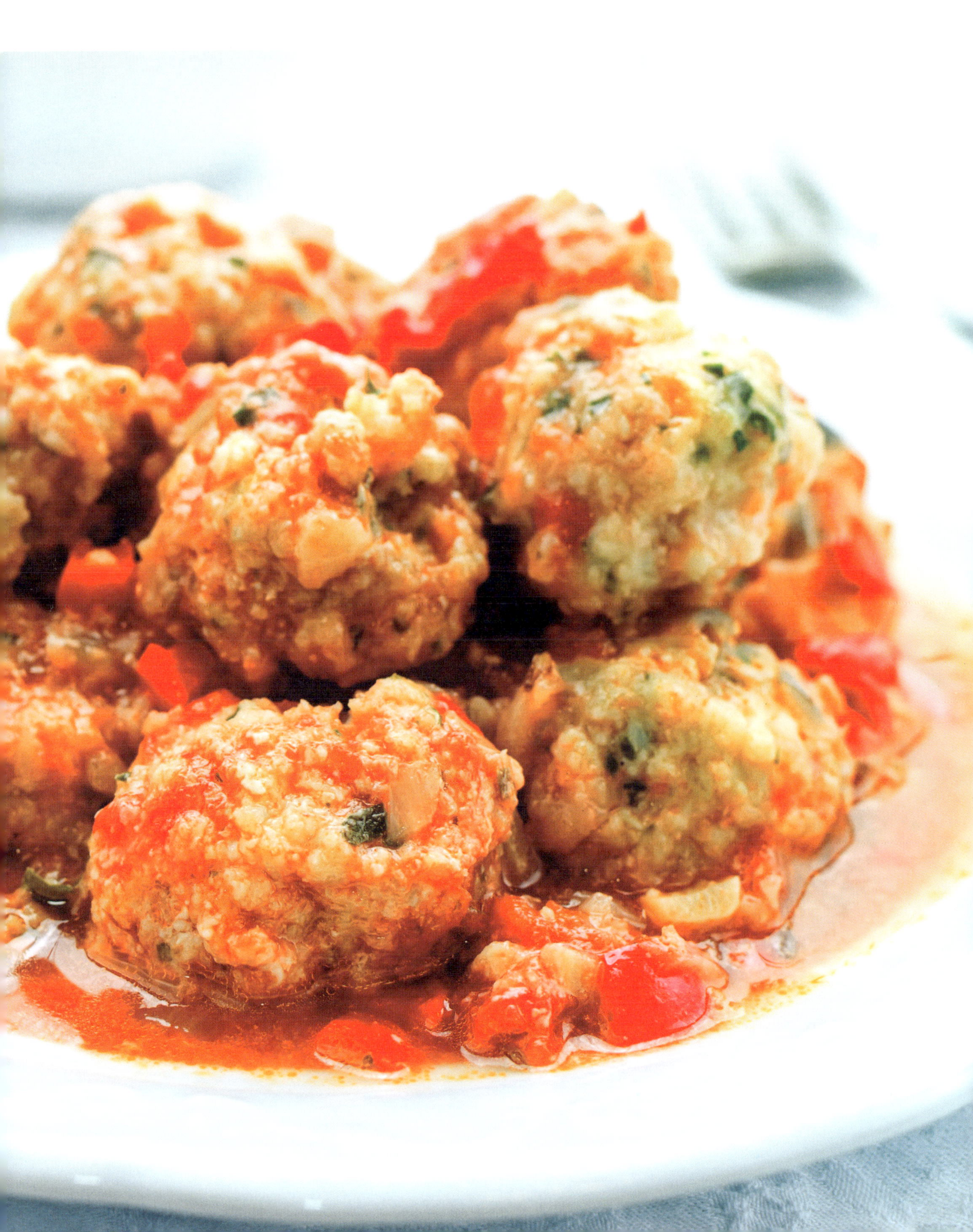

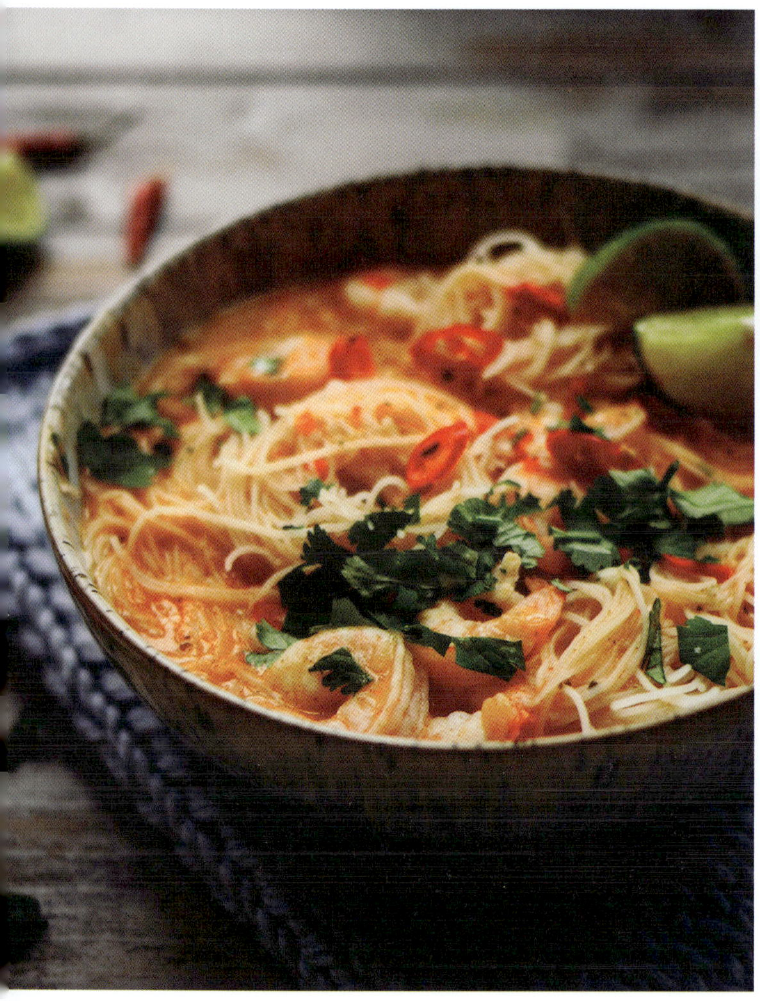

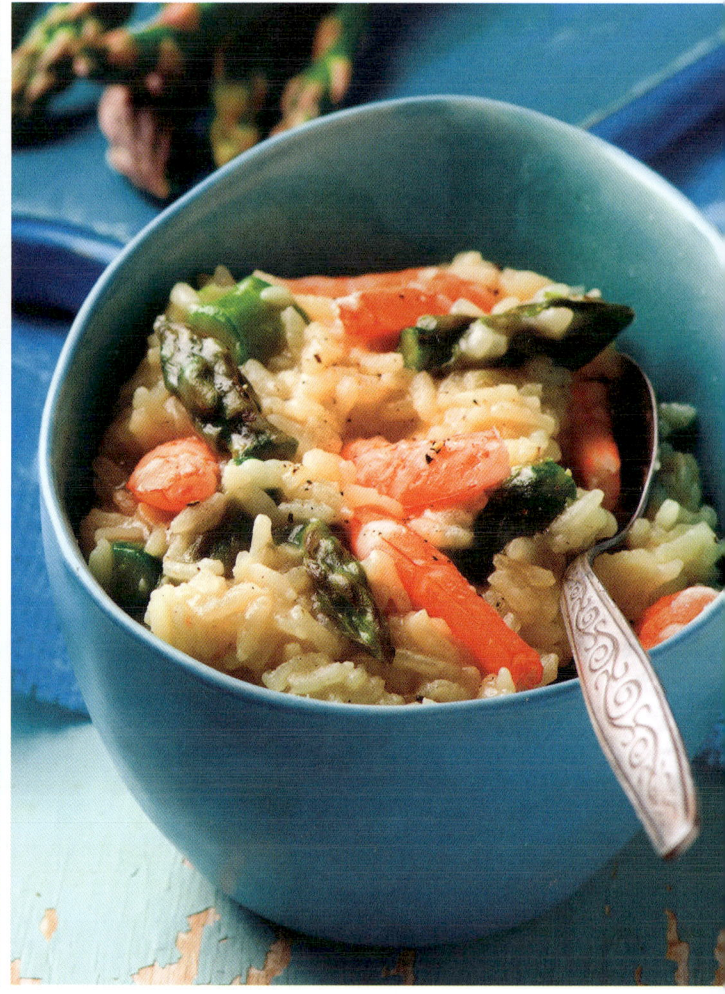

Easy Prawn Laksa

SERVES 4

COOK TIME: HIGH 1 HR

GLUTEN FREE • DAIRY FREE

Prawn and Asparagus Risotto

SERVES 4

COOK TIME: HIGH 1 HR + LOW 1 HR 30 MINS

GLUTEN FREE

EASY PRAWN LAKSA

1 x 400ml can coconut milk
3 tbsps laksa paste
2 cups (500ml) vegetable stock
2 tbsps fish sauce
200g rice vermicelli noodles
Fresh coriander, chopped, to garnish
Red chillies, chopped, to garnish
400g prawns, deveined, tails removed

Place all the ingredients except for the prawns in the slow cooker and cook on high for 30 minutes. Stir after 20 minutes when the noodles start to soften.

Add the prawns and vermicelli and cook for a further 30 minutes.

Serve with garnishes of fresh coriander and red chillies.

PRAWN AND ASPARAGUS RISOTTO

1½ cups (235g) Arborio rice
3 cloves garlic, minced
2 cups (500ml) chicken stock
450g prawns, deveined and tails removed
1 bunch asparagus, ends trimmed and finely chopped
1 cup (100g) Parmesan cheese, grated

Place the Arborio rice, garlic and chicken stock in the slow cooker. Cover and cook on high for 1 hour.

Turn the cooker to low, add the prawns and asparagus and cook for 1 hour.

Add half of the cheese and cook for another 30 minutes. Stir through the rest of the cheese just prior to serving.

Sardines in Tomato Sauce

SERVES 4

COOK TIME: HIGH 6 HRS

GLUTEN FREE • DAIRY FREE

1kg sardine fillets

2 x 400g cans chopped tomatoes

2 tbsps tomato paste

3 cloves garlic, minced

½ cup (125ml) water

1 tsp salt

2 tbsps white wine vinegar

1 lemon, sliced into wedges, to garnish

Fresh parsley, to garnish

Place the sardines in the bottom of the slow cooker. Add the tomatoes, tomato paste, garlic, water, salt and vinegar and cook on high for 6 hours.

Serve with lemon wedges and parsley.

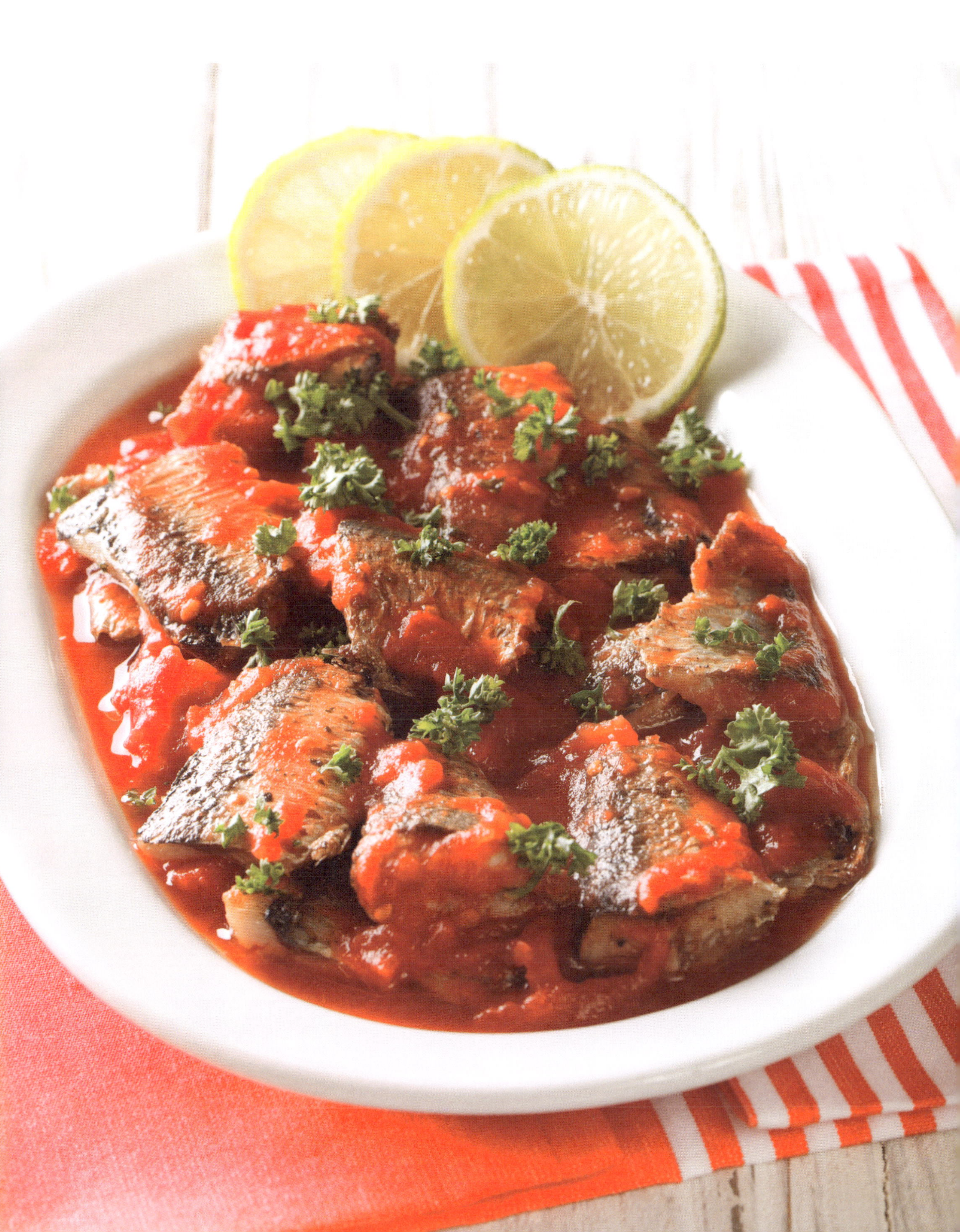

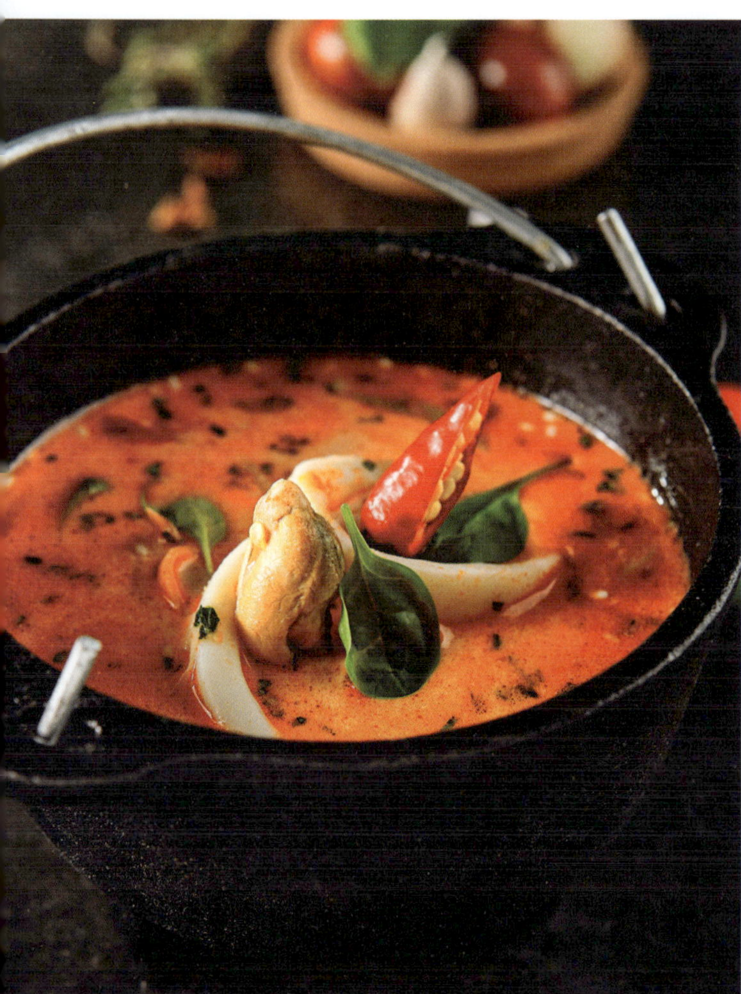

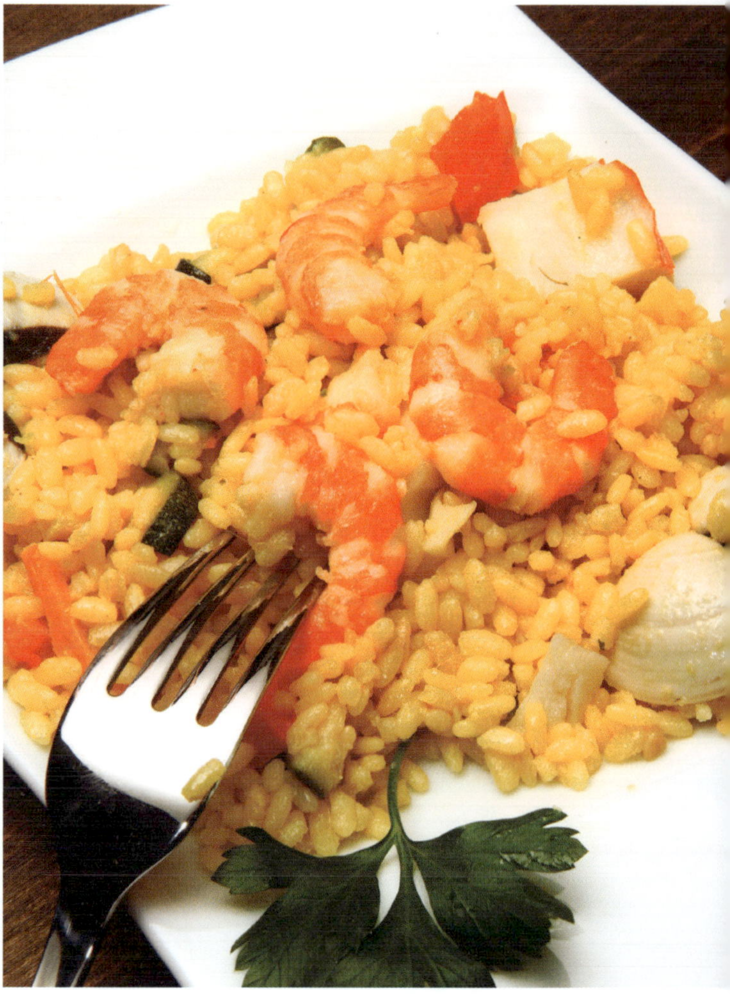

Hot and Sour Squid Soup

SERVES 4

COOK TIME: HIGH 3 HRS/LOW 6 HRS

GLUTEN FREE • DAIRY FREE

Saffron Seafood Paella

SERVES 4

COOK TIME: LOW 5 HRS

GLUTEN FREE • DAIRY FREE

HOT AND SOUR SQUID SOUP

4 cups (1L) chicken stock

⅓ cup (80ml) soy sauce (or tamari)

⅓ cup (80ml) rice wine vinegar

1 tbsp Srirarcha or other hot chilli sauce

1 tsp sugar

2 tsps tomato paste

500g squid, cleaned and cut into 4cm strips

¼ cup (10g fresh coriander, finely chopped

Pour the chicken stock into the slow cooker and stir in the soy sauce, rice wine vinegar, Sriracha and sugar. If you prefer your soup to have more tomato flavours, add tomato paste too. Add the squid pieces and cook on high for 3 hours, or low for 6 hours.

Stir in the chopped coriander just before serving.

SAFFRON SEAFOOD PAELLA

1½ cups (235g) Arborio or other short-grain white rice

2 tbsps olive oil

½ tsp crushed saffron

1 x 400g can chopped tomatoes

2 cups (500ml) water

Salt to taste

200g clams or mussels, fresh or frozen, shucked and cleaned

100g crab sticks, roughly chopped

250g prawns, deveined, tails left on

Place the rice and oil in the slow cooker and mix. Stir in the saffron, tomatoes, water and salt to taste then add the clams and crab sticks.

Cover and cook on low for 5 hours. About 30 minutes before serving, add the prawns and increase the slow cooker to high.

Millet Soup with Salmon and Cabbage

SERVES 4

COOK TIME: HIGH 1 HR + LOW 1 HR

GLUTEN FREE • DAIRY FREE

500g salmon fillet, skin removed, cut into bite-size chunks

Salt and pepper to taste

4 cups (1L) chicken stock

¾ cup (150g) millet

3 cups (300g) white cabbage, shredded

2 eggs, hard-boiled, peeled and quartered, to garnish

Season the salmon with salt and pepper then place in the slow cooker with half the stock. Cover and cook on high for 1 hour.

Reduce to low, mix in the millet and the rest of the stock and cook for another 30 minutes.

Add the cabbage and cook for 30 minutes more, ensuring the salmon is flaky and cooked through before serving.

Serve with quartered hard-boiled eggs.

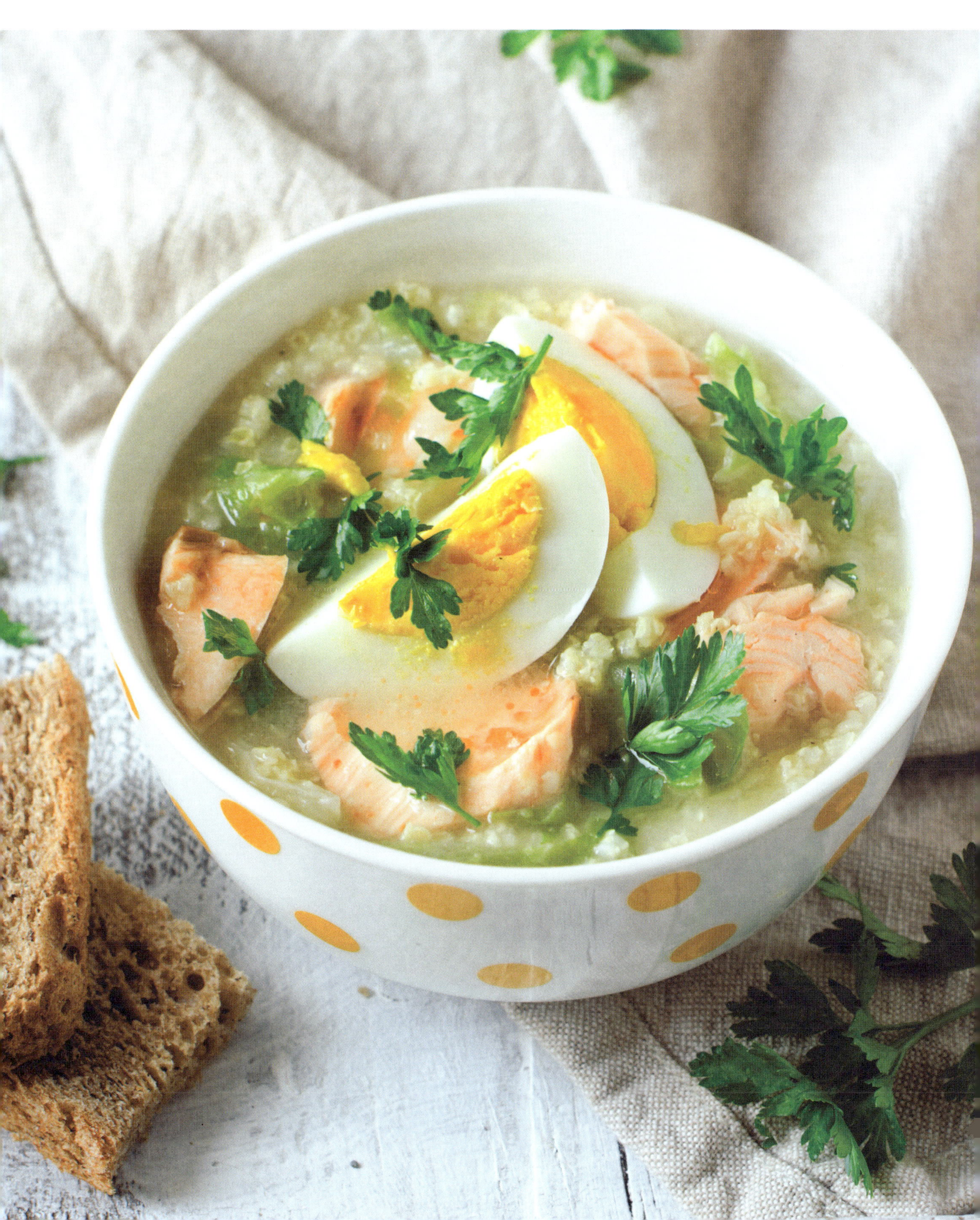

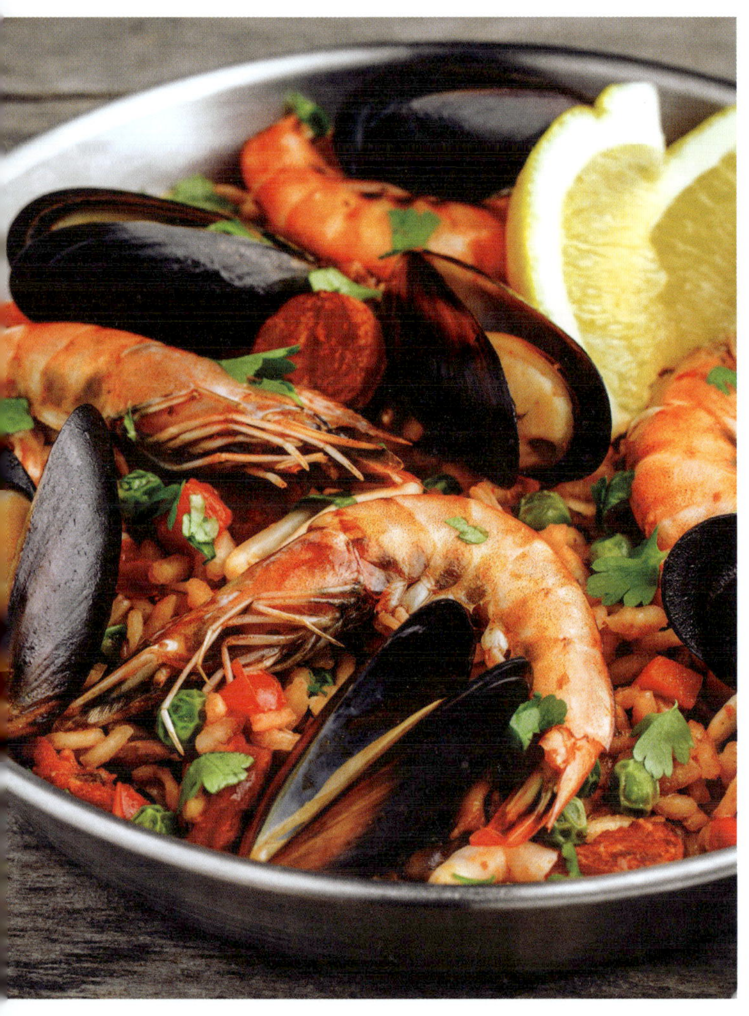

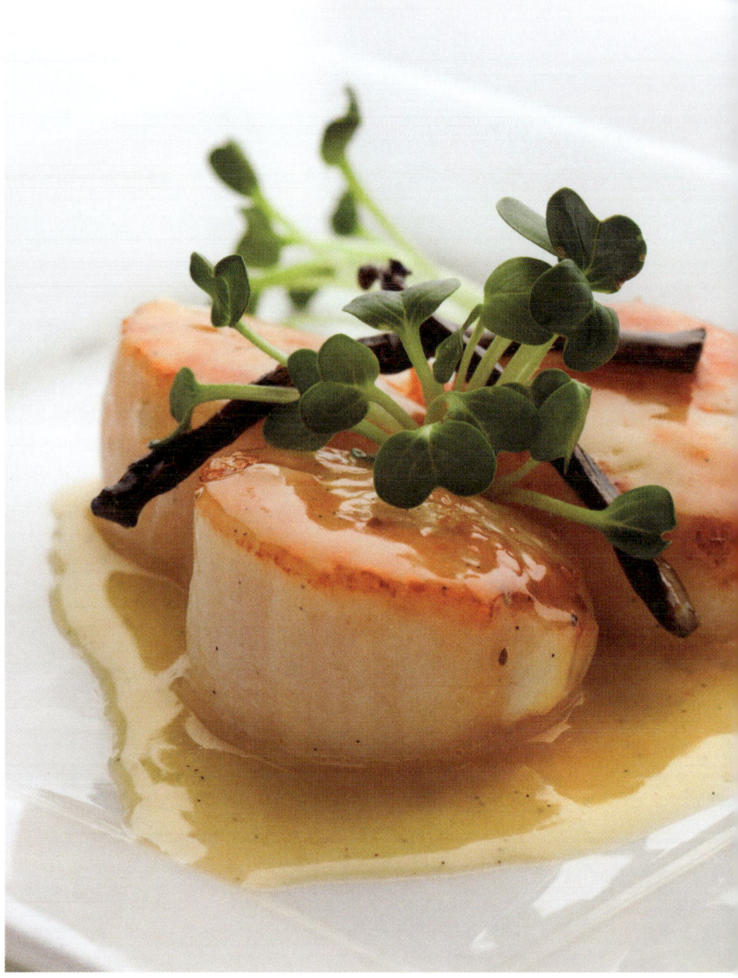

Paella

SERVES 4
COOK TIME: HIGH 4 HRS
GLUTEN FREE • DAIRY FREE

Scallops in Vanilla Butter Sauce

SERVES 4
COOK TIME: HIGH 1 HR 30 MINS/LOW 3 HRS
GLUTEN FREE

PAELLA

2 tbsps olive oil
200g chorizo, sliced
1½ cups (235g) short-grain rice
1 medium onion, chopped
3 cloves garlic, minced
1 red capsicum, chopped
1 x 400g chopped tomatoes
1½ cups (375ml) chicken stock
Salt to taste
Pinch of saffron threads
½ tsp ground paprika
500g whole, shell-on prawns
500g mussels, scrubbed and debearded
½ cup (125ml) white wine
Lemon wedges and parsley leaves, to serve

Heat 1 tablespoon olive oil in a frying pan over medium-high heat. Add chorizo and cook for 3-5 minutes until browned.

Add to the slow cooker with rice, onion, garlic, capsicum, tomatoes, stock, salt and spices. Mix to combine.

Cook on high for 4 hours.

Heat remaining oil in a large saucepan or stock pot. Add seafood and wine and cover. Cook for 5 minutes until mussels are open and prawns are pink.

Spoon paella into a serving dish. Top with seafood, lemon wedges and chopped parsley to serve.

SCALLOPS IN VANILLA BUTTER SAUCE

250g butter
½ cup (125ml) thickened cream
½ vanilla bean, split and scraped
1½ tsps salt
12 jumbo scallops, cleaned

Melt the butter in a large saucepan over a medium heat. Add the cream and simmer for 5 minutes. Add the scraped vanilla and salt and simmer for 1 minute more.

Place the scallops in the slow cooker and pour the vanilla and cream sauce over them.

Cook on high for 1 hour 30 minutes or low for 3 hours.

Seafood Stew

SERVES 6
COOK TIME: HIGH 4 HRS + LOW 30 MINS
GLUTEN FREE

1 onion, roughly chopped
2 x 400g cans chopped tomatoes
½ cup (125ml) dry white wine
2 tbsps tomato paste
1 tbsp red wine vinegar
½ tsp sugar
½ cup (125ml) water
Salt and pepper to taste
500g white fish, cut into 3cm pieces
400g mussels, fresh or frozen, shucked and cleaned
Fresh coriander, chopped
Feta cheese, crumbled (optional)

Place the onion, tomatoes, wine, tomato paste, vinegar, sugar, water and salt and pepper in the slow cooker.

Cover and cook on high for 4 hours. Stir in the fish and mussels. Reduce the slow cooker to low and cook for a further 30 minutes, or until the fish is flaky and tender.

Add chopped coriander as a garnish, and if desired sprinkle crumbled feta over the top.

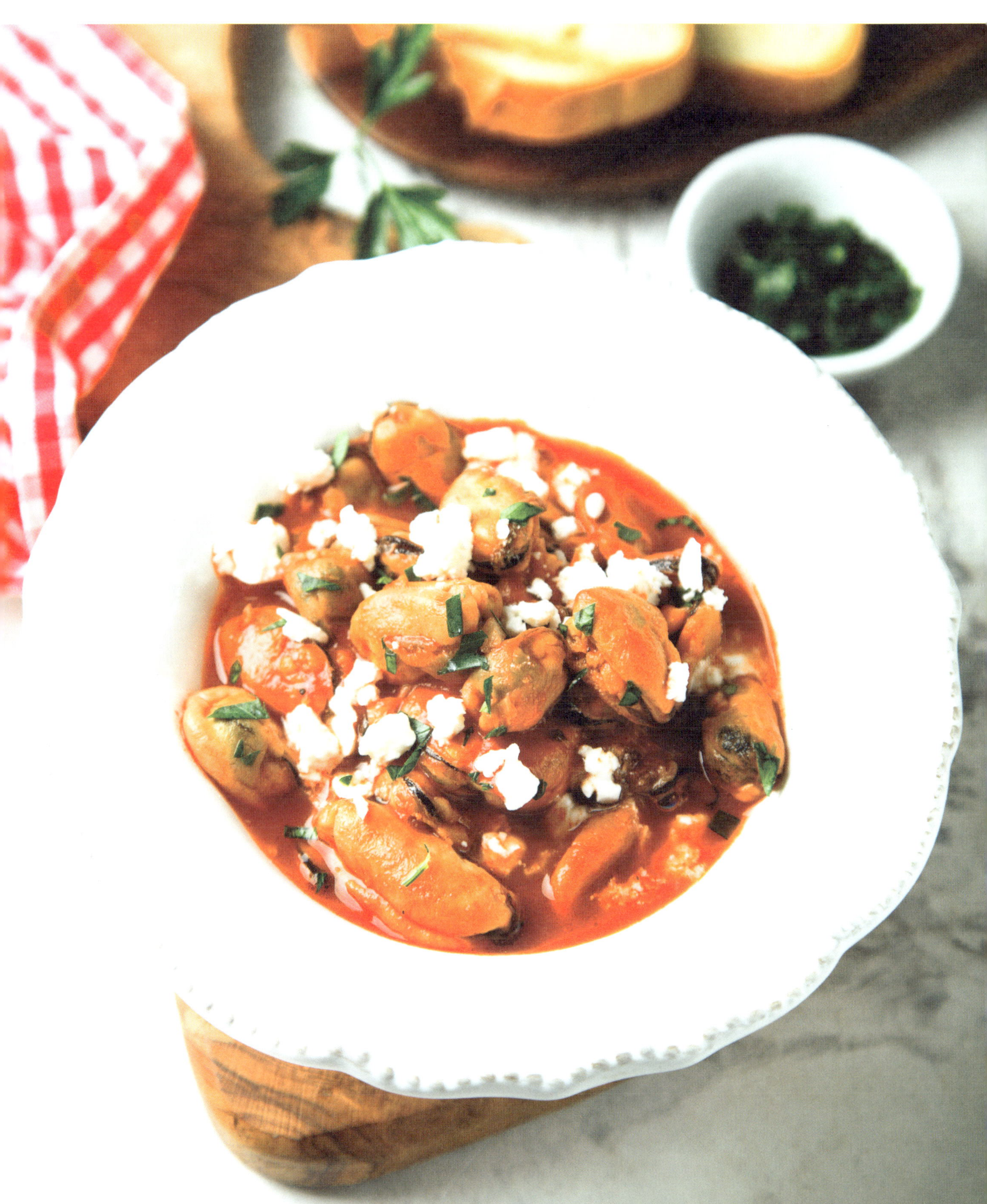

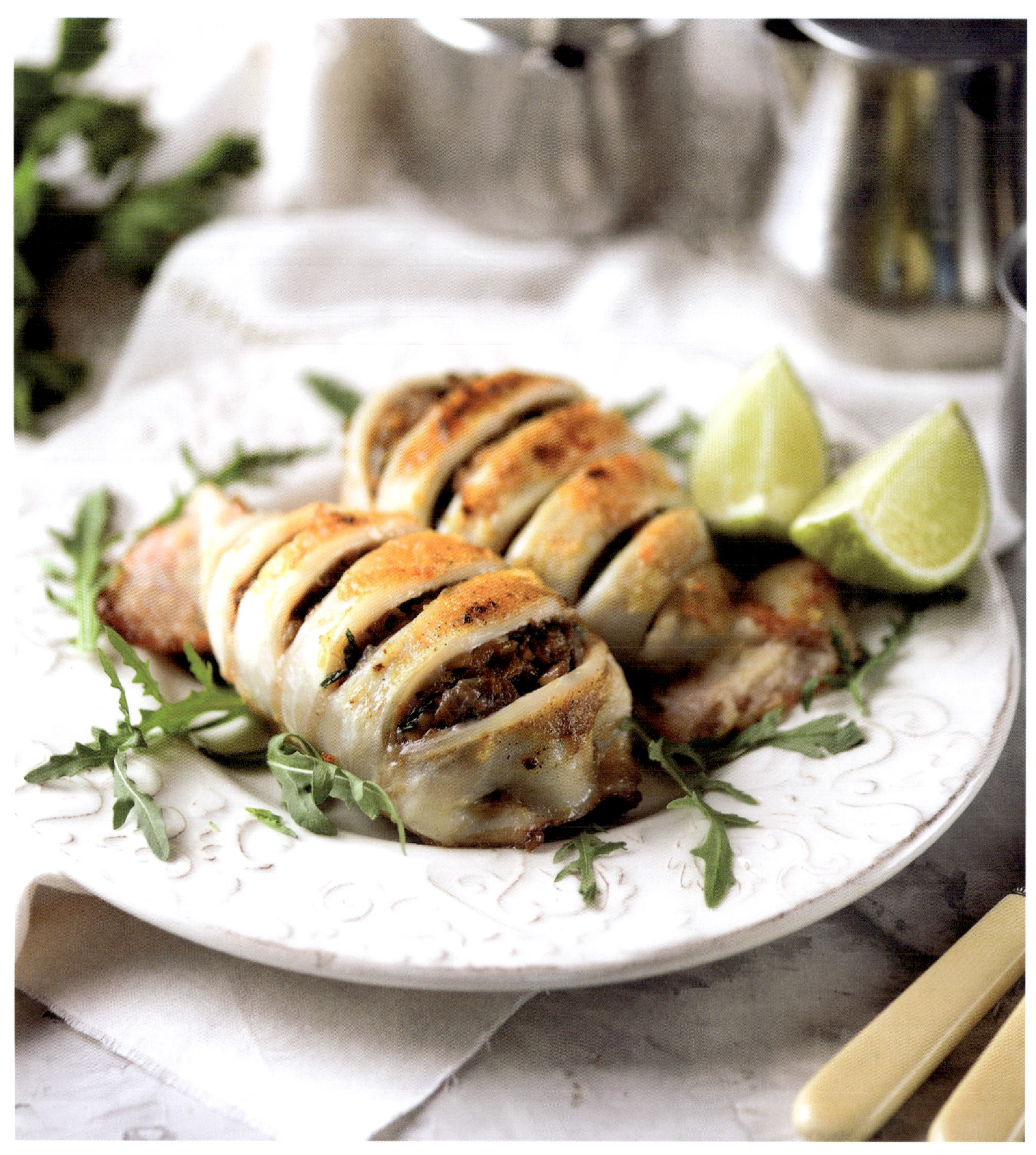

Squid Stuffed with Bacon and Mushrooms

SERVES 4

COOK TIME: LOW 2 HRS 30 MINS

DAIRY FREE

SQUID STUFFED WITH BACON AND MUSHROOMS

4 squid, cleaned
1 tbsp olive oil
2 onions, finely diced
2 cloves garlic, minced
4 rashers bacon, finely chopped
500g mushrooms, finely chopped
1 cup (250ml) white wine
Salt and pepper to taste
2 tbsps chopped fresh parsley leaves
½ cup (60g) breadcrumbs
1 cup (250ml) water
1 tsp paprika

Cut off the squid tentacles and chop finely.

Heat oil in a large frying pan over medium-high heat. Add onion and cook for 3-5 minutes until soft and translucent. Add garlic and cook for 1 minute until fragrant. Add bacon, mushrooms and the chopped tentacles. Cook for a further 5 minutes until mushrooms are soft.

Add half the wine to the pan. Allow the wine to bubble and reduce by half then remove from the heat. Season with salt and pepper. Add parsley and breadcrumbs and stir through.

Fill the squid tubes with the stuffing. Thread the top with one or more toothpicks to close. Use a sharp knife to cut three or four slits on top of the tubes and place in the slow cooker.

Add water and remaining wine to slow cooker. Sprinkle squid with paprika. Cover and cook on low for 2½ hours.

HONEY SOY SALMON

4 salmon fillets
2 tbsps soy sauce (or tamari)
2 tbsps honey
2 tbsps lemon juice
2 tsps sesame seeds
2 tsps grated ginger

Line the base and sides of the slow cooker inset with aluminium foil, allowing it to cover about halfway up the sides.

Place fish on the aluminium foil in one layer and drizzle with soy sauce, honey and lemon juice.

Cover with another piece of foil, tucking in on all sides.

Cook on low for 2 hours.

Use a fish slice to remove fillets from slow cooker and a spoon to scoop out the juices.

To serve, spoon juices over the fish, sprinkle with sesame seeds and top with a little fresh ginger.

FISH IN CREAMY MUSHROOM SAUCE

4 white fish fillets, such as snapper
Salt and pepper to taste
400g mushrooms (such as button), roughly chopped
¼ cup (60ml) chicken stock
1¼ cups (300ml) cream
2 tbsps cornflour

Season the fillets with salt and pepper and place in the slow cooker, followed by the mushrooms.

Whisk the stock into the cream in a large mixing bowl and pour over the fish and mushrooms. Add more seasoning if desired.

Cover and cook on low for 4 hours, or until the fish is flaky and cooked through. For a thicker sauce, stir in the cornflour with 1 hour left of cooking.

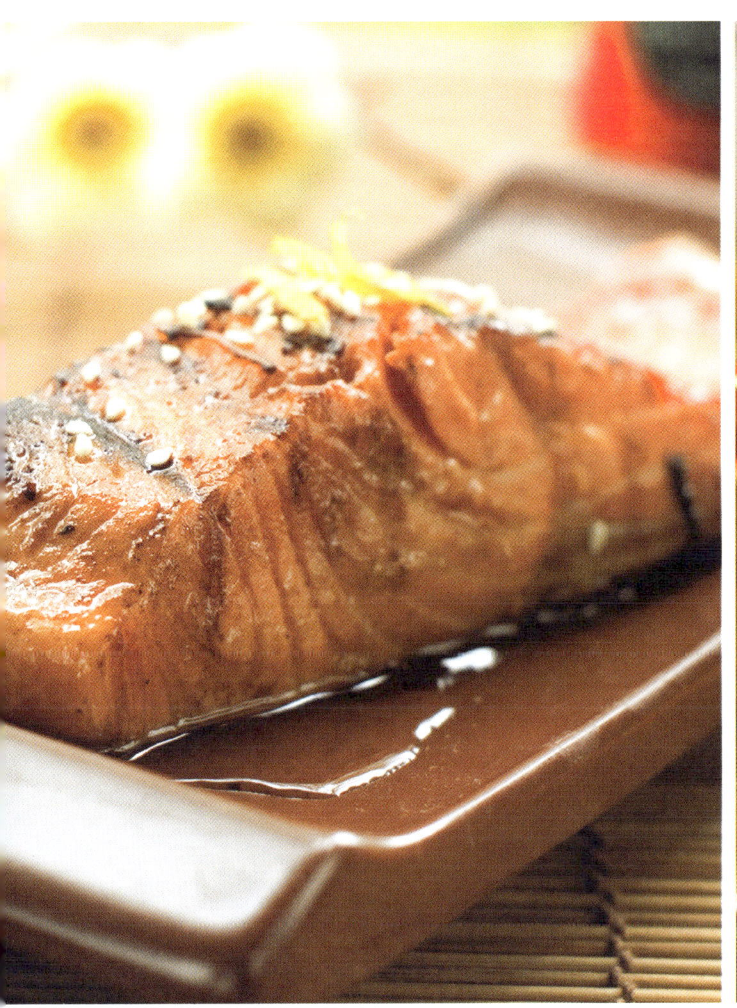

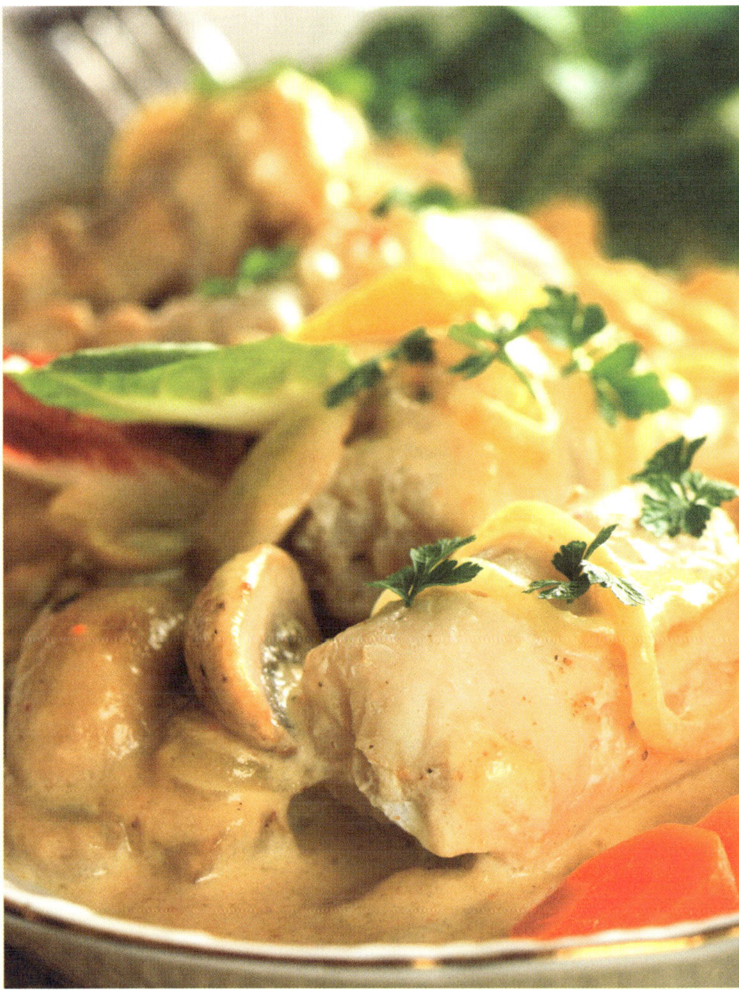

Honey Soy Salmon

SERVES 4

COOK TIME: LOW 2 HRS

GLUTEN FREE • DAIRY FREE

Fish in Creamy Mushroom Sauce

SERVES 4

COOK TIME: 4 HRS

GLUTEN FREE

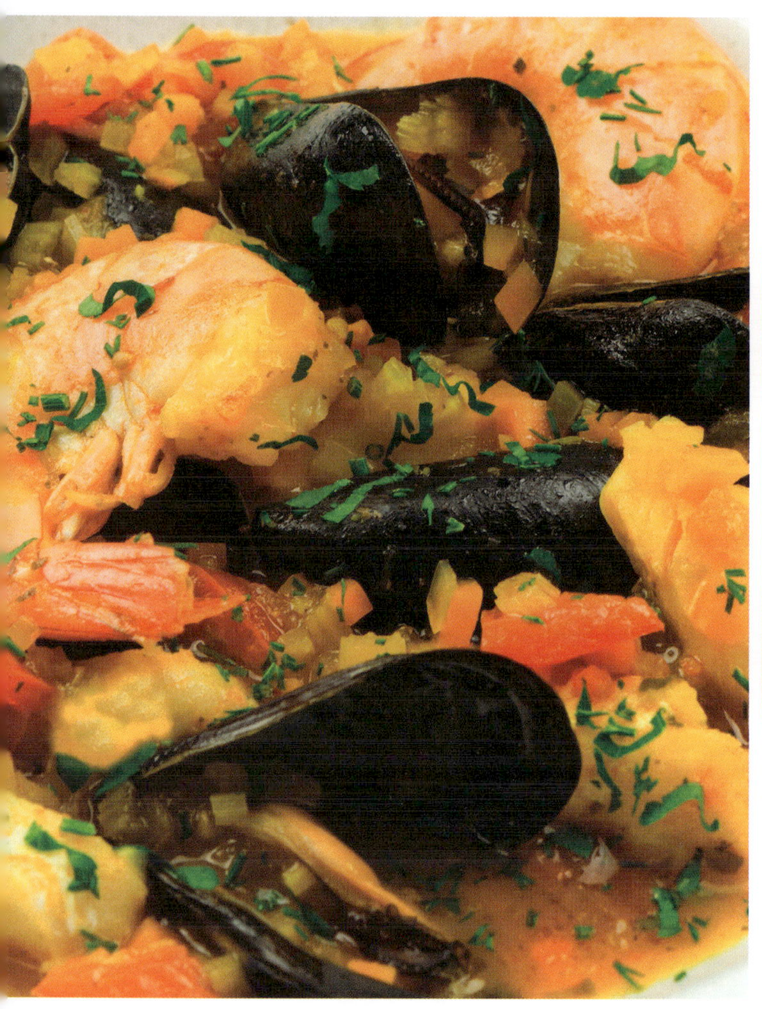

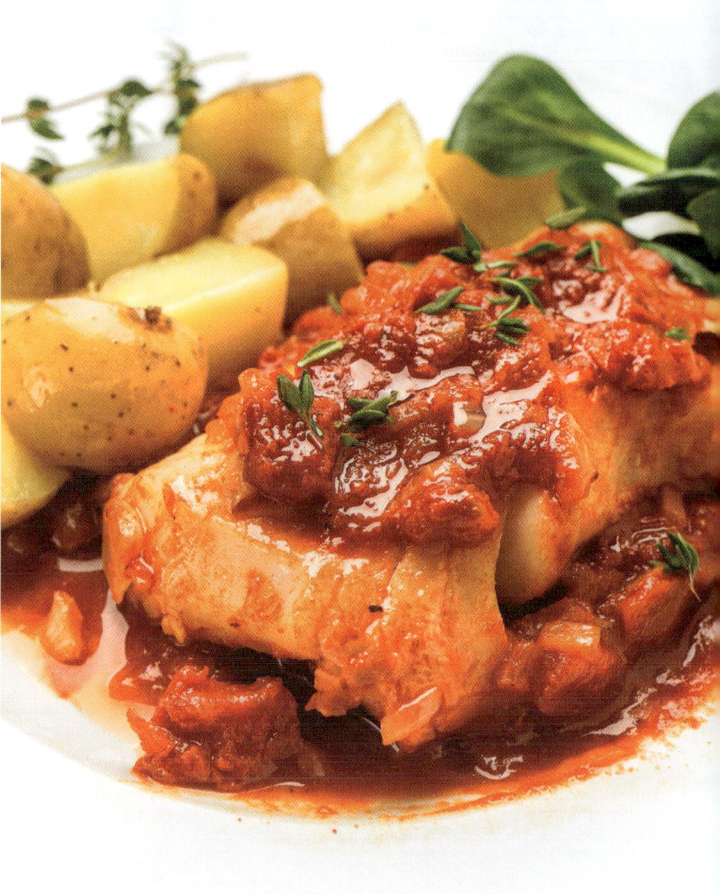

Seafood Cioppino

SERVES 4

COOK TIME: LOW 9 HRS

GLUTEN FREE • DAIRY FREE

Braised Cod in Tomato and Thyme Sauce

SERVES 4

COOK TIME: HIGH 1 HR/LOW 3 HRS

GLUTEN FREE • DAIRY FREE

SEAFOOD CIOPPINO

300g white fish, such as flathead or snapper, cut into bite-size pieces

1 stalk celery, finely diced

1 cup (250g) canned diced tomatoes

1 tsp dried oregano

1 cup (250ml) water

Salt and pepper to taste

250g prawns, deveined, tails left on

250g mussels, shells on

Fresh coriander, chopped, to garnish

Combine the fish, celery, tomato, oregano and water in the slow cooker. Season well with salt and pepper.

Cover and cook on low for 9 hours. With 1 hour left to cook, add the prawns and mussels and turn to high.

Serve with chopped coriander as a garnish.

BRAISED COD IN TOMATO AND THYME SAUCE

2 tbsps olive oil

1 large onion, finely chopped

2 cloves garlic, minced

4 Murray cod fillets (or use Mahi Mahi)

1 x 400g can chopped tomatoes

½ cup (125ml) dry white wine

1 sprig fresh thyme, leaves stripped, plus extra to garnish

½ cup (125ml) water

Salt and pepper to taste

Boiled potatoes, to serve

Green salad, to serve

Heat the olive oil in a frying pan over a medium heat. Saute the onion and garlic until softened and fragrant.

Add the cod fillets to the pan and sear for 2 minutes on each side, then place the fish, onion and garlic in the slow cooker.

Add in the tomatoes, wine, thyme, water and salt and pepper and cook on high for 1 hour 30 minutes or low for 3 hours, or until the fish is tender and flaky.

Serve with potatoes and green salad.

Coconut and Lime Fish Stew

SERVES 4

COOK TIME: HIGH 2 HRS/LOW 4 HRS

GLUTEN FREE • DAIRY FREE

1kg white fish (such as Murray cod or Mahi Mahi), skinned, boned and cut into large chunks

4 tbsps lime juice

Salt and pepper to taste

1 x 400ml can coconut milk

1 x 400g can chopped tomatoes

1½ tbsps paprika

1 yellow or green capsicum, finely chopped

Fresh parsley, to garnish

Place the fish pieces in a large bowl, and add the lime juice. Mix well until the fish is coated, then season with salt and pepper and set aside for at least 30 minutes.

Place the coconut milk, tomatoes, paprika and capsicum in the slow cooker. Add the fish with the lime juice. Cook on high for 2 hours or low for 4 hours.

Serve garnished with parsley.

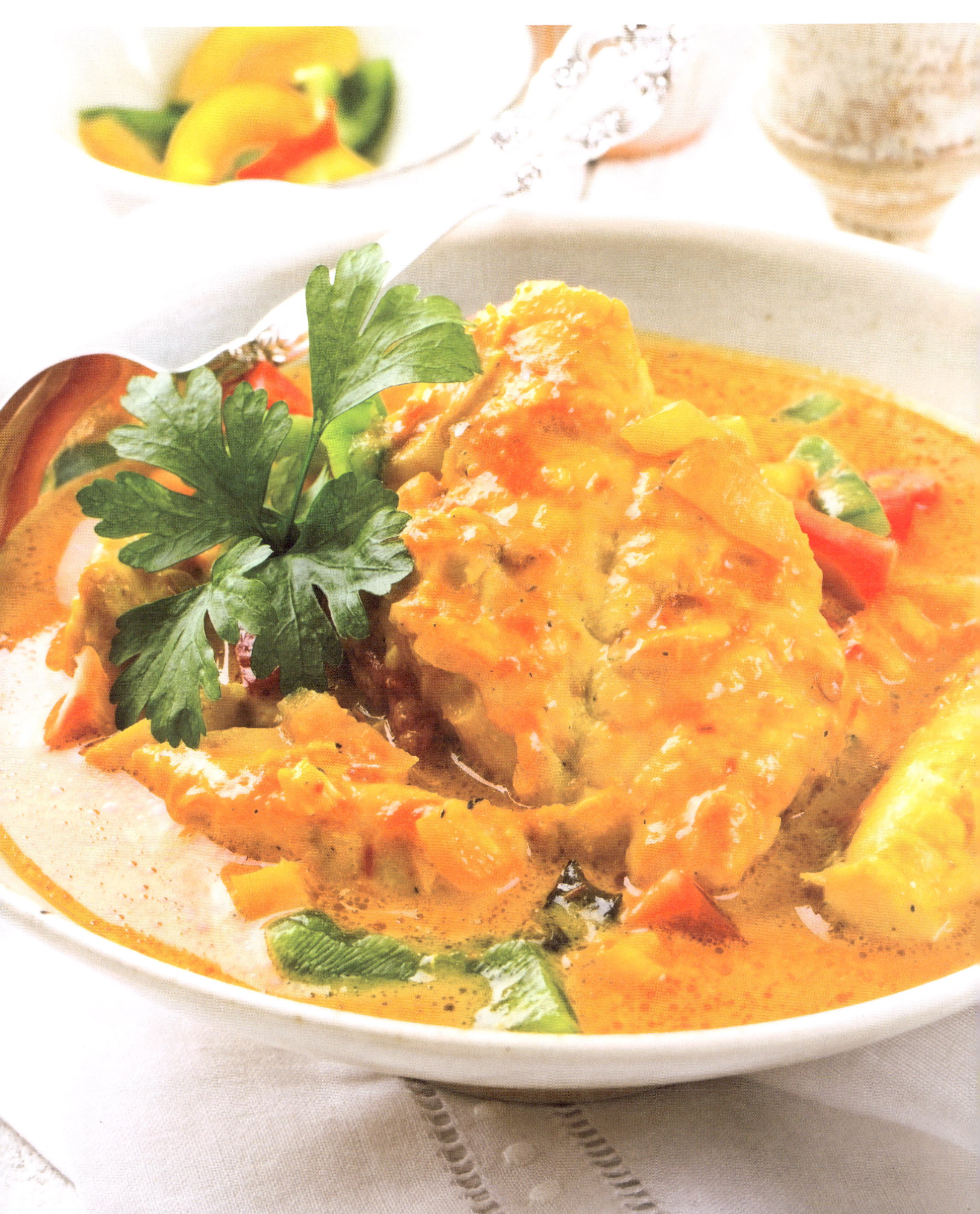

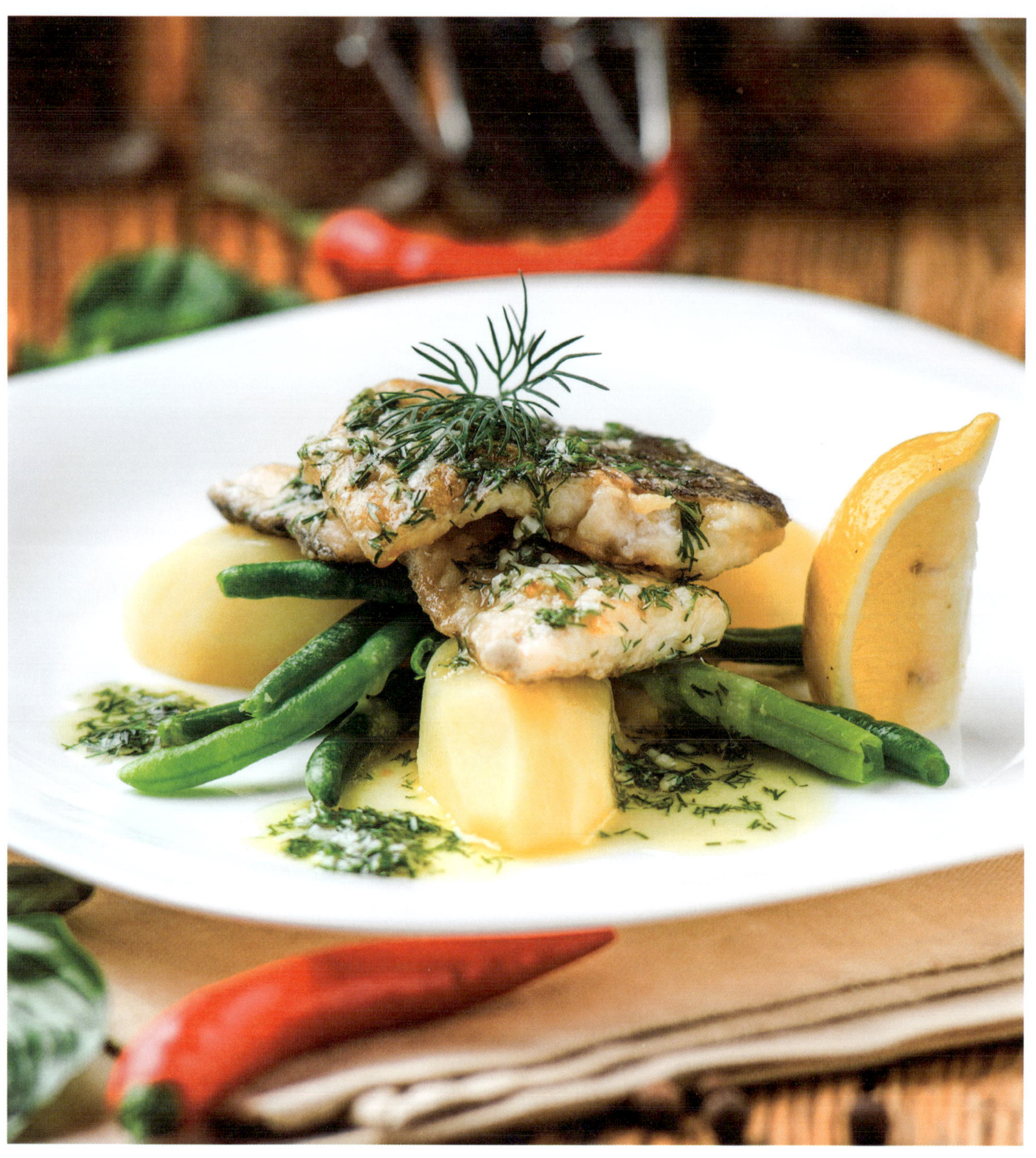

Dill Baked Fish

SERVES 6

COOK TIME: HIGH 2 HRS

GLUTEN FREE

DILL BAKED FISH

6 white fish fillets
¼ cup (60ml) dry white wine
2 tbsps butter, melted + 25g butter, room temperature
1 tbsp olive oil
½ lemon, juiced
2 cloves garlic, minced
¼ cup (10g) dill, finely chopped
¼ tsp salt
¼ tsp pepper
Boiled potatoes and green beans, to serve

Line the base and sides of the slow cooker inset with aluminium foil, allowing it to cover about halfway up the sides. Place fish on the aluminium foil in one layer and drizzle with white wine, melted butter, olive oil and lemon juice.

Sprinkle garlic, dill and salt and pepper over the fish. Finish with a knob of butter on each fillet. Cover with another piece of foil, tucking in on all sides.

Cook on high for 2 hours. Use a fish slice to remove fillets from slow cooker and a spoon to scoop out the juices. Spoon juices over the fish and serve with boiled potatoes and green beans.

Bouillabaisse

SERVES 4
COOK TIME: LOW 4 HRS
GLUTEN FREE • DAIRY FREE

½ tsp saffron strands
1 cup (250ml) white wine
1 orange, juiced and zested
1 tbsps olive oil
1 onion, diced
1 bulb fennel, trimmed, cored and thinly sliced
2 cloves garlic, minced
1 tsp dried mixed herbs
½ tsp salt
¼ tsp pepper
4 cups (1L) fish stock
1 medium tomato, diced
1 bay leaf
500g snapper fillets, cut into bite-size pieces
350g mussels, cleaned and scrubbed
350g large whole king prawns
¼ bunch parsley, chopped

Soak the saffron strands in a small bowl with the wine and orange juice. Set aside.

Heat the oil in a large saucepan over a medium-high heat. Add the onion and fennel and fry, stirring, for 5 minutes until soft. Add the garlic, mixed herbs, salt and pepper and fry for 30 seconds until aromatic.

Add the saffron-wine mixture and bring to a gentle boil. Add the fish stock, orange zest, tomato and bay leaf and stir to combine. Transfer the mixture to the slow cooker.

Cover and cook on low for 4 hours.

Turn the cooker to high. After 15 minutes, add the fish, mussels and prawns and cook for a further 15 minutes.

Discard the bay leaf.

Scatter with parsley to serve.

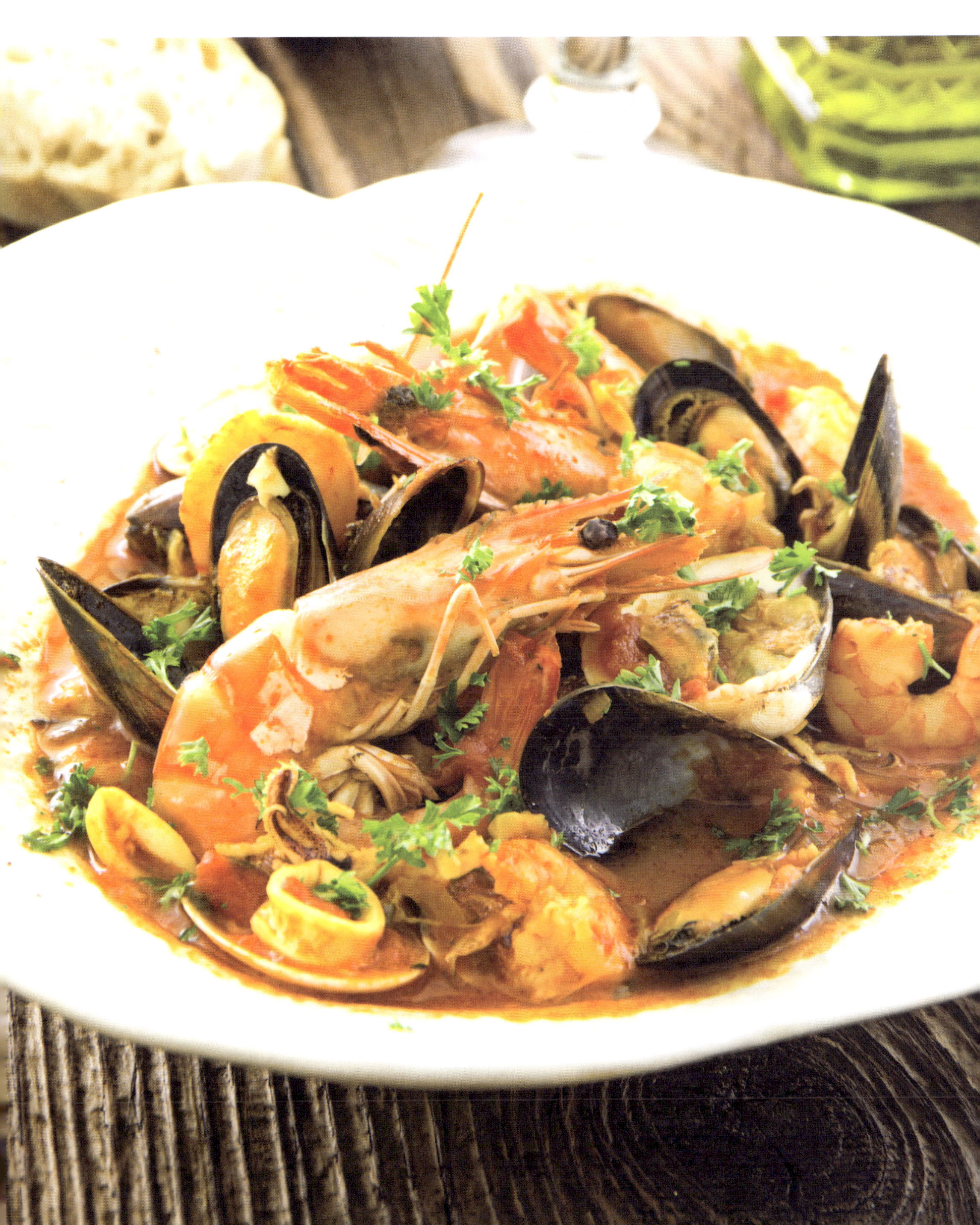

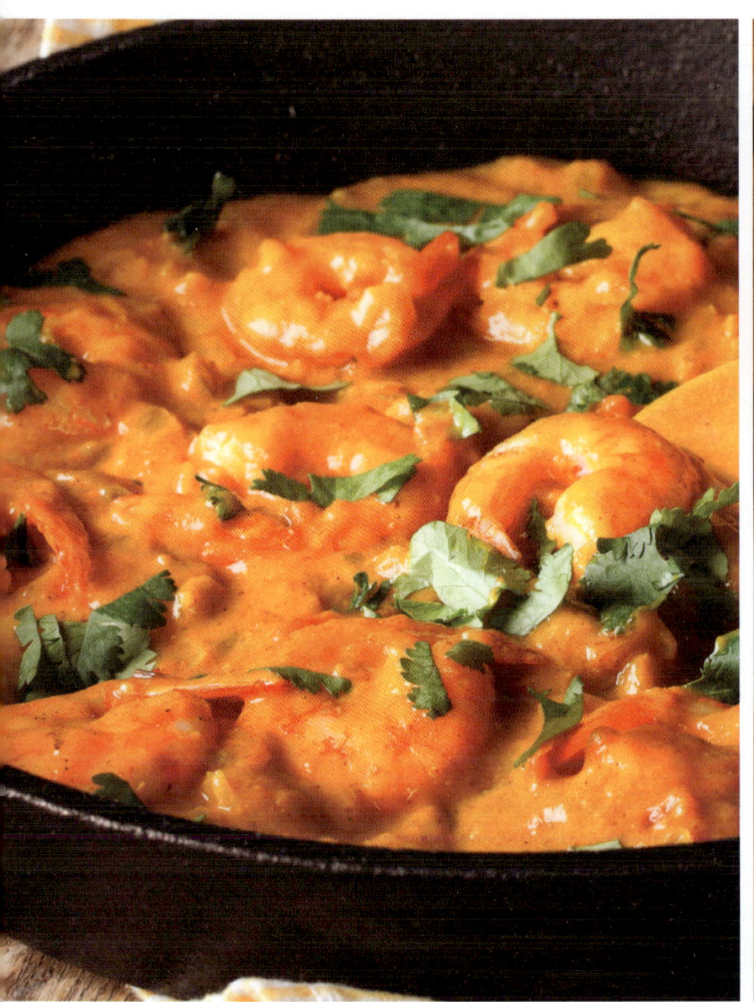

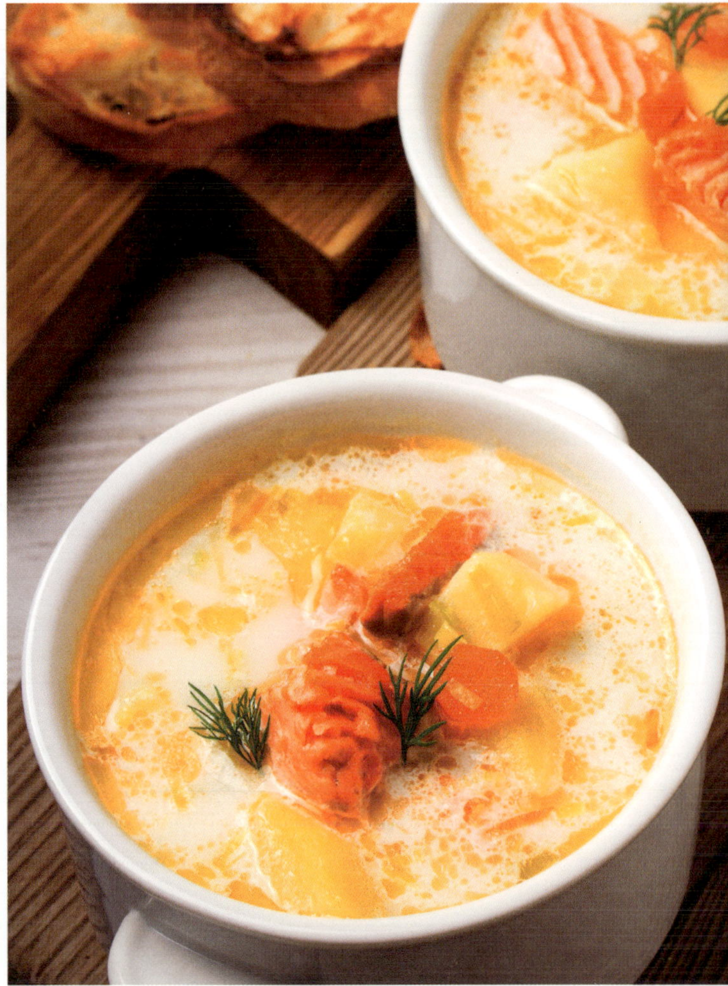

Prawn Curry

SERVES 4

COOK TIME: LOW 2 HRS + HIGH 1 HR

GLUTEN FREE

Creamy Salmon Soup

SERVES 4

COOK TIME: HIGH 4 HRS

GLUTEN FREE

PRAWN CURRY

1 x 400g can chopped tomatoes

2 tbsps korma paste

1 tsp ground cinnamon

2 tsps ground cumin

750g prawns, deveined and tails removed

⅔ cup (150ml) cream

Fresh coriander, chopped, to garnish

Place the tomatoes, korma paste, cinnamon and cumin in the slow cooker and mix well to combine. Cook on low for 2 hours.

Add the prawns with the cream and stir thoroughly. Increase the heat and cook on high for 1 hour.

Serve with a garnish of fresh coriander.

CREAMY SALMON SOUP

2 potatoes, peeled and diced

600g salmon fillet, skinned and chopped into bite-size chunks

⅓ cup (100ml) thickened cream

2 cups (500ml) chicken stock

1 large carrot, peeled and roughly chopped

1 tsp paprika

2 tbsps cornflour

Place the potatoes at the bottom of the slow cooker. Add the fish, cream, stock, carrots and paprika and stir thoroughly to combine the ingredients.

Cover and cook on low for 4 hours. About 30 minutes before serving, stir in the cornflour until the soup has reached a thicker consistency.

PRAWN AND CHORIZO GUMBO

2 tbsps olive oil
350g chorizo, sliced
2 stalks celery, sliced
1 onion, diced
1 red capsicum, diced
1 clove garlic, minced
1 tbsp cornflour
1 cup (250ml) water
1¼ cups (310ml) chicken stock
1 x 400g can diced tomatoes
1 tbsp thyme leaves
2 tsps smoked paprika
455g prawns, deveined and peeled, tails intact
1 tbsp chopped parsley, to garnish

Heat half the oil in large frying pan over a medium-high heat. Add chorizo and cook, stirring, for 3-4 minutes until browned. Drain and set aside. Wipe pan clean with paper towel and heat remaining oil.

Add celery, onion and capsicum and cook for 4-5 minutes until almost soft. Add garlic and cook for a further 1 minute until fragrant.

Combine cornflour and water in a small mixing bowl to create a slurry, stirring to combine well.

Place chorizo and celery-onion mixture in the slow cooker. Pour over the stock and tomatoes. Add thyme and smoked paprika and stir in the cornflour slurry.

Cover and cook on low for 3½ hours.

Add prawns and cook for a further 1 hour.

Serve gumbo over rice, garnished with parsley.

SEAFOOD MARINARA

1 x 400g can diced tomatoes
⅔ cup (150ml) passata
2 tbsps chopped fresh parsley
3 cloves garlic, minced
½ tsp dried basil
1 tsp dried oregano
Salt and pepper to taste
1kg mussels, scrubbed and debearded
500g spaghetti

Combine canned tomatoes, passata, parsley, garlic, basil, oregano, salt and pepper in the slow cooker. Mix well.

Cover and cook on low for 2-3 hours.

Add mussels and cook on high for 15-20 minutes or until the mussels are open.

Meanwhile place spaghetti in a pan of boiling salted water. Cook according to the packet directions, until al dente. Drain well and combine with marinara sauce.

Spoon onto plates to serve.

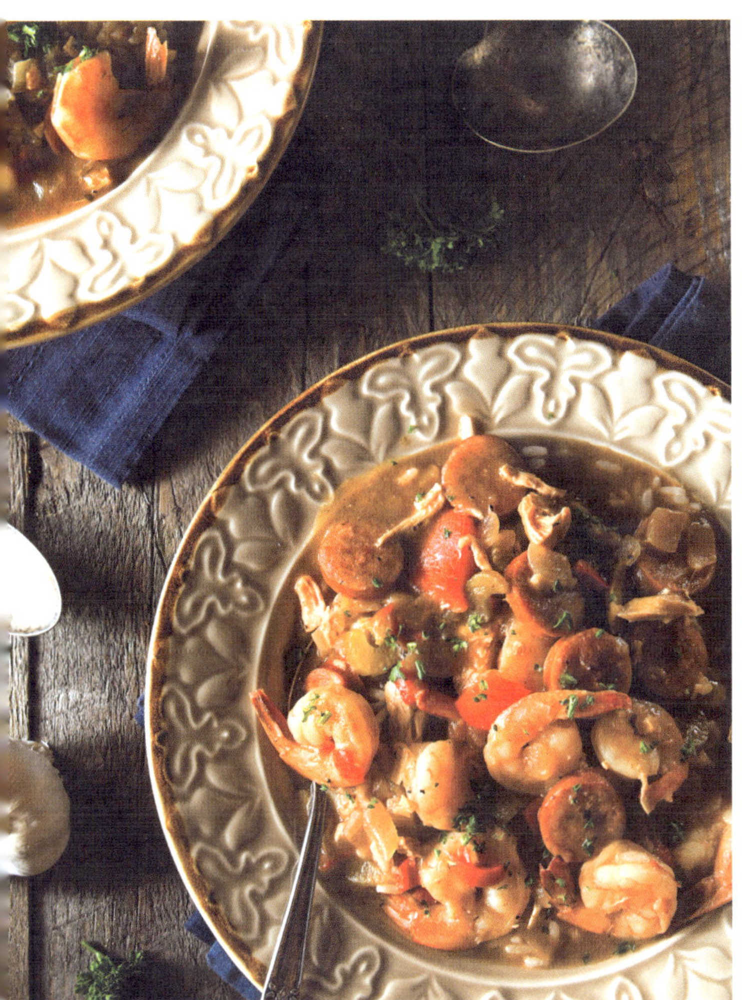

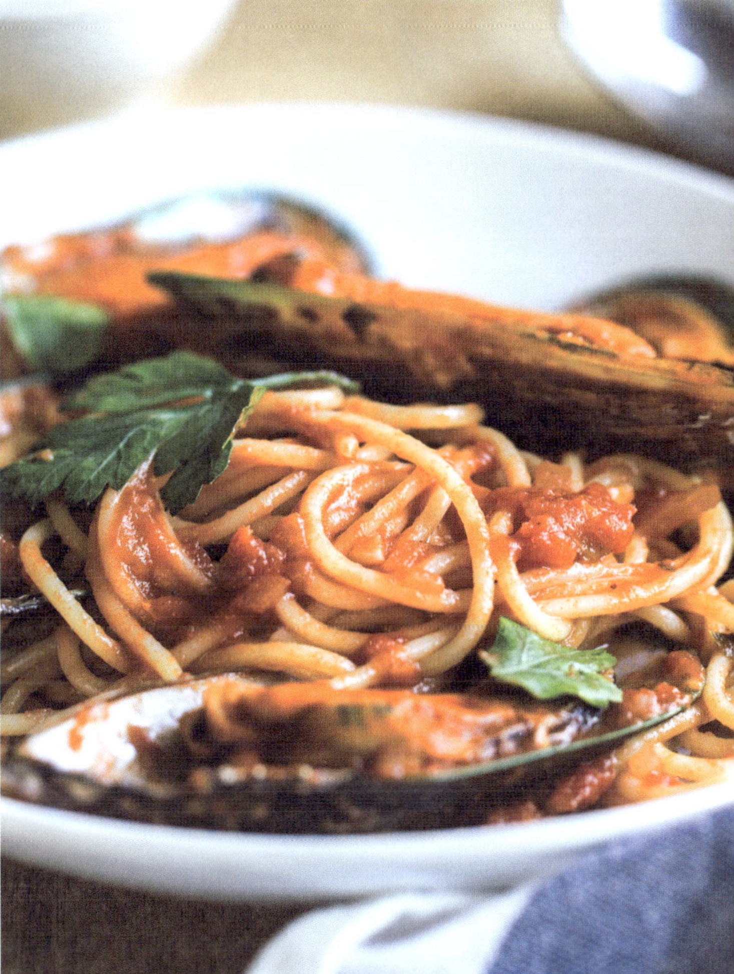

Prawn and Chorizo Gumbo

SERVES 4

COOK TIME: LOW 3 HRS 30 MINS + 1 HR

GLUTEN FREE • DAIRY FREE

Seafood Marinara

SERVES 4

COOK TIME: LOW 2-3 HRS + HIGH 15-20 MINS

DAIRY FREE

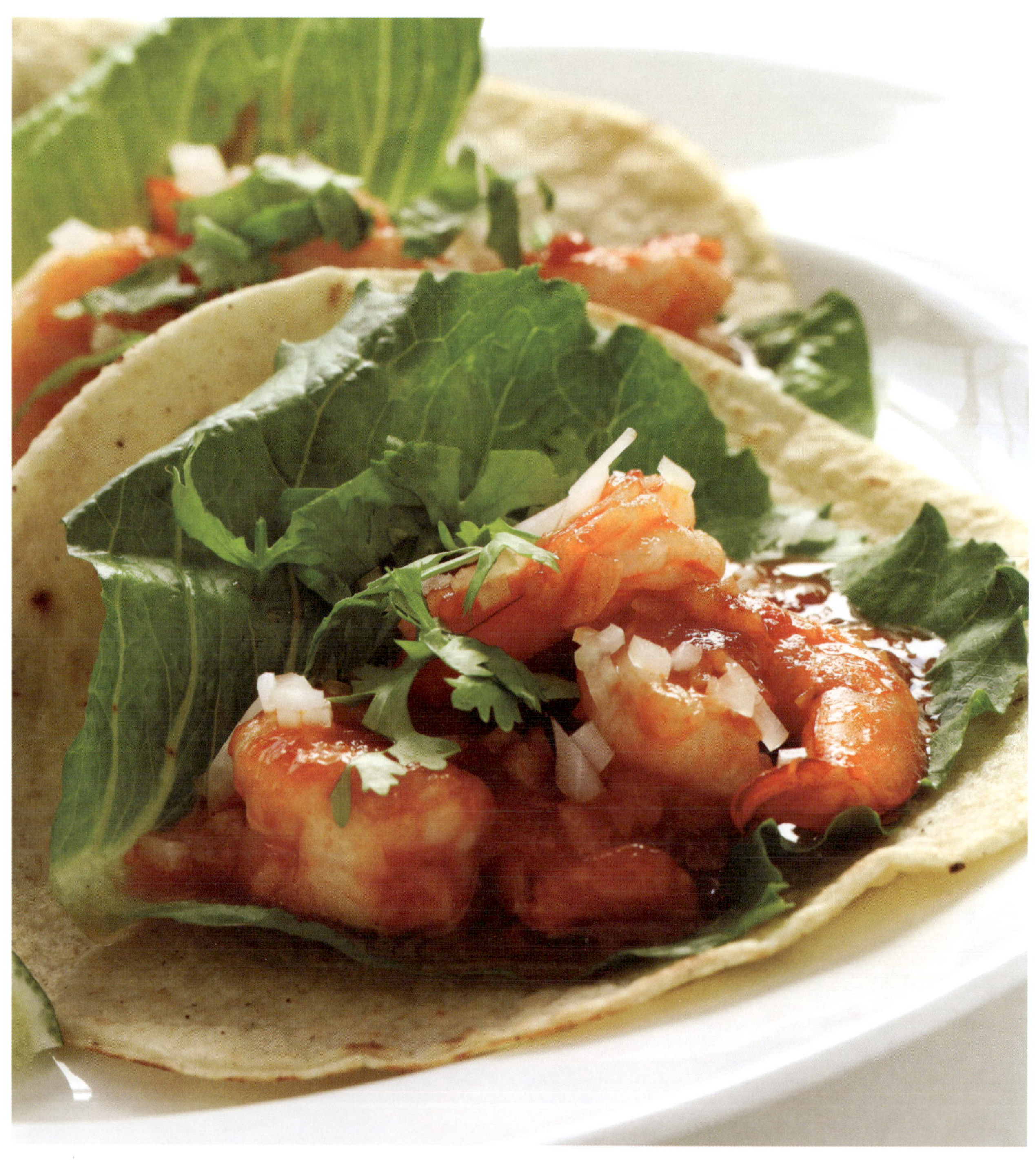

Prawn Tacos

SERVES 4

COOK TIME: HIGH 1 HR 30 MINS/LOW 2 HRS

DAIRY FREE

PRAWN TACOS

500g prawns, peeled, tails off
1 tbsp olive oil
1 red onion, finely chopped
1 tsp minced garlic
1¾ cups (400g) cherry tomatoes, diced
1 red capsicum, chopped
½ cup (135g) chunky salsa + more to serve
½ tsp cumin
½ tsp chilli powder
½ tsp smoked paprika
⅛ tsp cayenne pepper
Salt and pepper to taste
12 corn tortillas, warmed
12 lettuce leaves
½ white onion, finely diced
3-4 tbsps chopped coriander

Place prawns in slow cooker. Drizzle with olive oil. Add red onion, garlic, tomatoes, capsicum, salsa and spices. Season with salt and pepper. Mix together.

Place slow cooker on low for 2 hours or on high for 90 minutes.

Serve the prawns in warmed corn tortillas on a lettuce leaf. Add extra salsa as required and sprinkle with white onion and coriander to serve.

Kedgeree

SERVES 4
COOK TIME: HIGH 3 HRS
GLUTEN FREE

- 1 tbsp olive oil
- 1 onion, diced
- ¼ tsp ground mace
- ½ tsp ground turmeric
- ½ tsp ground cumin
- ½ tsp ground coriander
- 2 cups (310g) basmati or long-grain white rice
- 1 bay leaf
- Zest of 1 lemon + 2 tbsps juice
- 6 cups (1.5L) vegetable stock
- 40g butter
- 300g smoked haddock fillets or other hot-smoked fish
- 2 tbsps chopped fresh parsley
- 1 tbsp chopped chives
- 4 eggs, hard-boiled and quartered

Heat the olive oil in a frying pan over a medium-high heat. Add the onion and fry, stirring, for 3 minutes until soft. Add the spices and stir for 1 minute or until fragrant. Add rice and fry, stirring, for 2-3 minutes until grains are lightly toasted.

Place the rice mixture into the slow cooker, add the bay leaf, lemon zest and juice, stock and butter. Stir gently.

Lay fish fillets skin-side down on top of the rice mixture. Cook on high for 3 hours.

Lift out fish fillets onto a plate and remove the skin. Flake the fish and add back to the rice along with chopped parsley and chives. Stir well to combine.

Add the eggs and serve.

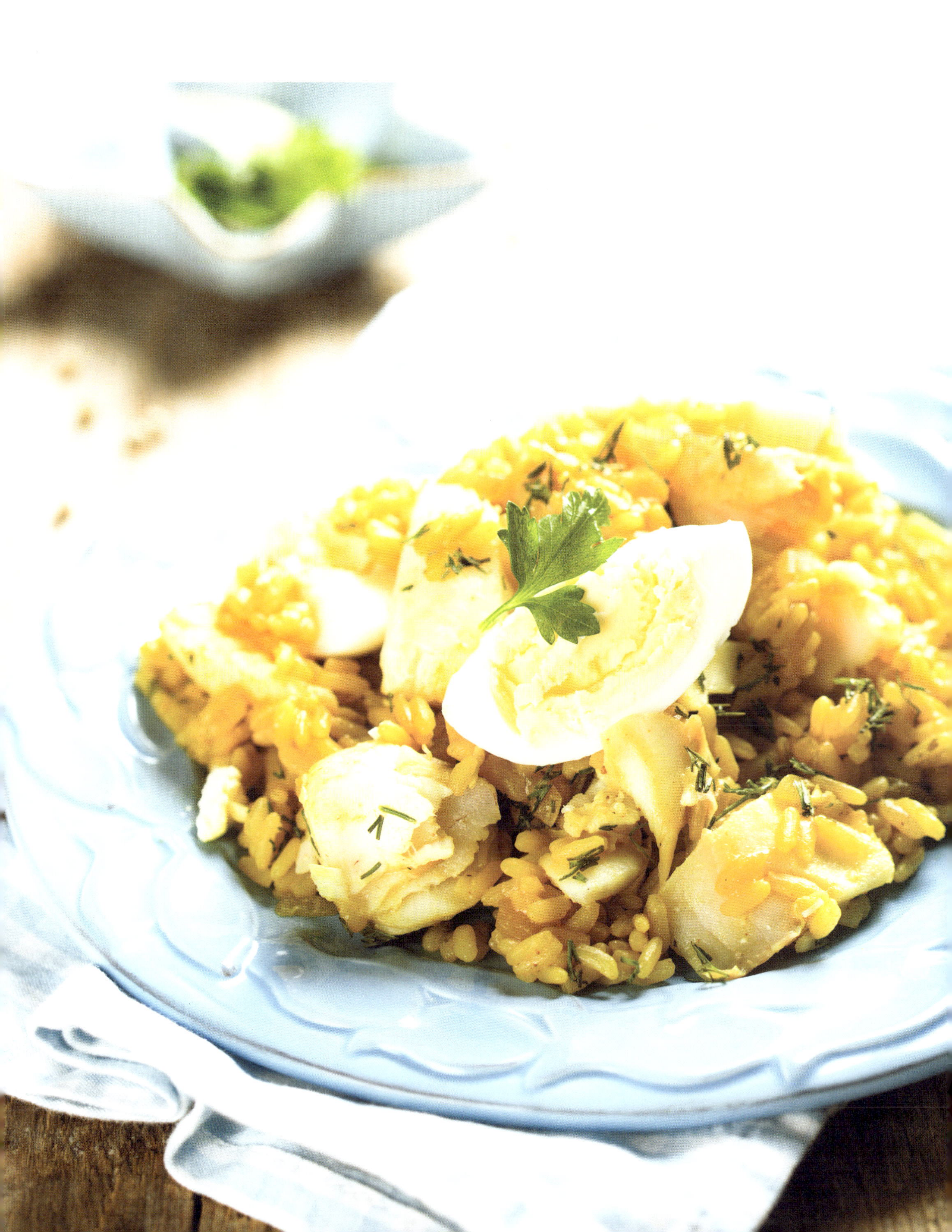

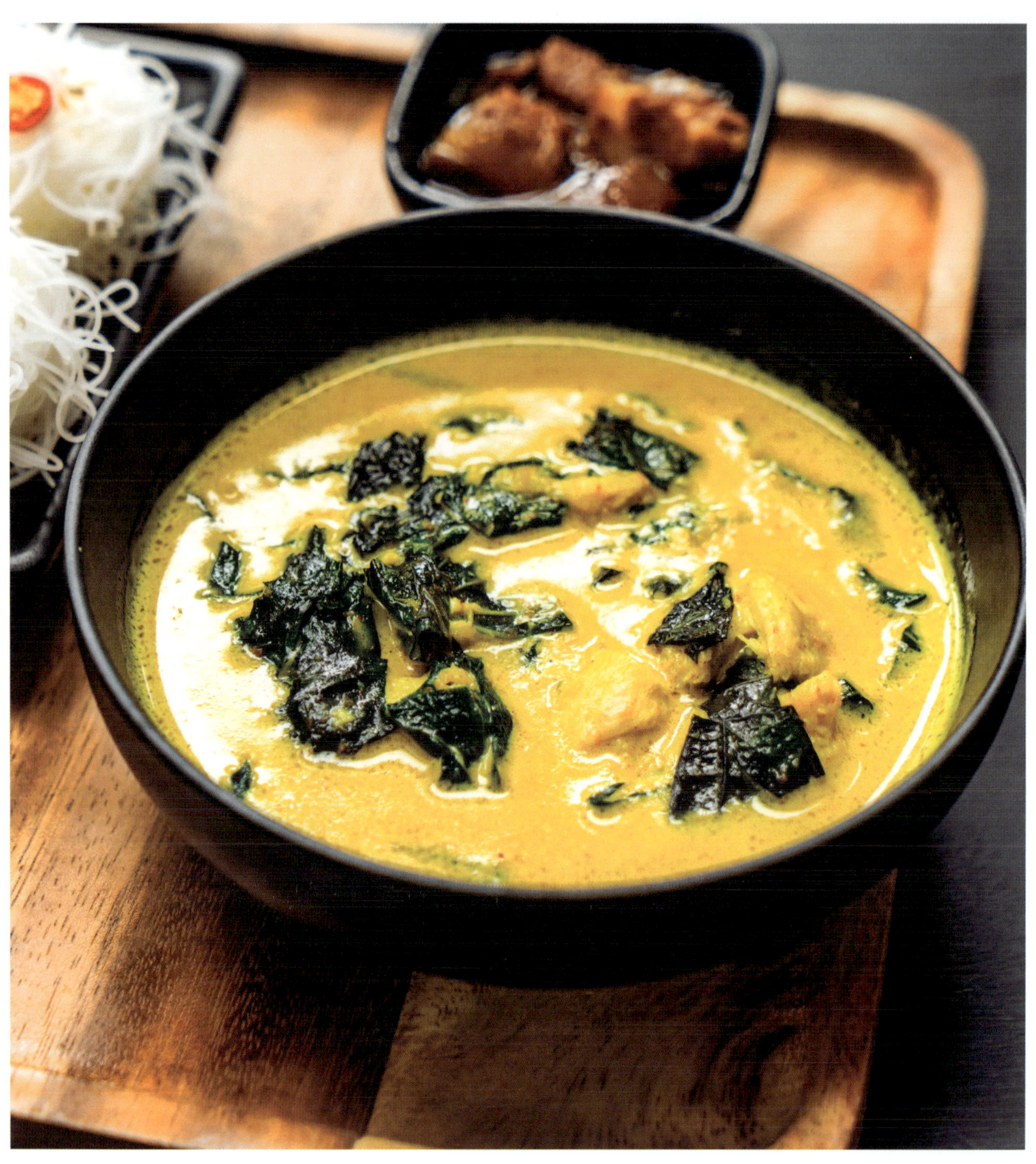

Thai Coconut Curry Soup with Crab

SERVES 4

COOK TIME: HIGH 3 HRS/LOW 6 HRS

GLUTEN FREE • DAIRY FREE

THAI COCONUT CURRY SOUP WITH CRAB

2 tbsps Thai green curry paste
2 cups (500ml) chicken stock
1 x 400ml can coconut milk
400g crab meat
½ cup (15g) baby spinach leaves
1 tbsp lime juice

In a large bowl mix the curry paste, stock and coconut milk. Add to the slow cooker with the crab meat and cook on high for 3 hours or low for 6 hours.

Mix in the spinach with 30 minutes of cooking to go, and stir through the lime juice just before serving.

MUSSELS IN WHITE WINE

2 tbsps melted butter
4 cloves garlic, thinly sliced
½ red chilli, finely chopped
¼ tsp salt
1 sprig thyme
1 sprig rosemary
1 bay leaf
1.5kg mussels, scrubbed and debearded
½ cup (125ml) dry white wine

Set the slow cooker to high. Add butter, garlic, chilli, salt and herbs. Cover and cook for 5 minutes.

Add mussels and wine. Cover and cook for 15-20 minutes on high until mussels open.

Spoon into bowls and serve with crusty bread.

LEMON HERB SALMON

4 x 200g salmon fillets
1 lemon; ½ juiced and ½ sliced
2 tsps cracked pepper
2 tsps dried thyme
2 tsps dried parsley
2 sprigs fresh dill, to garnish

Lay out a piece of foil twice as big as one salmon fillet. Place a single fillet on the foil. Repeat with the other three salmon fillets. Top the fillets with lemon juice, pepper, herbs and a couple of lemon slices each. Fold the foil over and crimp edges together, creating an airtight parcel for the fish.

Place the foil parcels in the slow cooker, stacked on top of one another if space requires.

Cover and cook on low for 2 hours.

Remove foil parcels from the slow cooker and carefully open over a plate to catch the juices. Serve garnished with fresh dill.

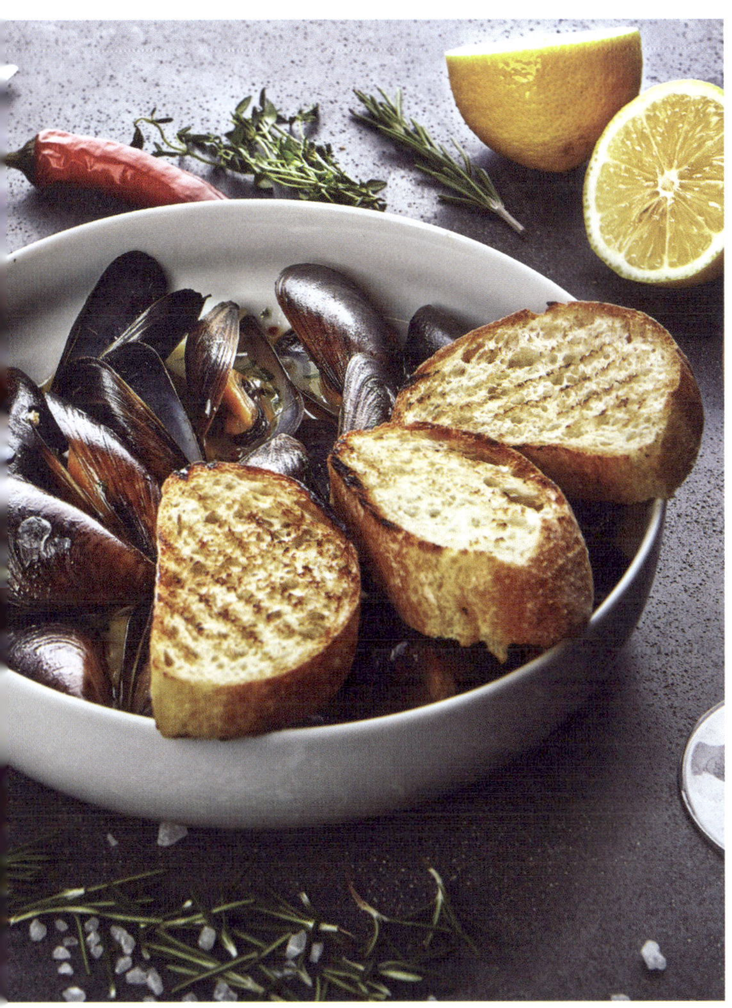

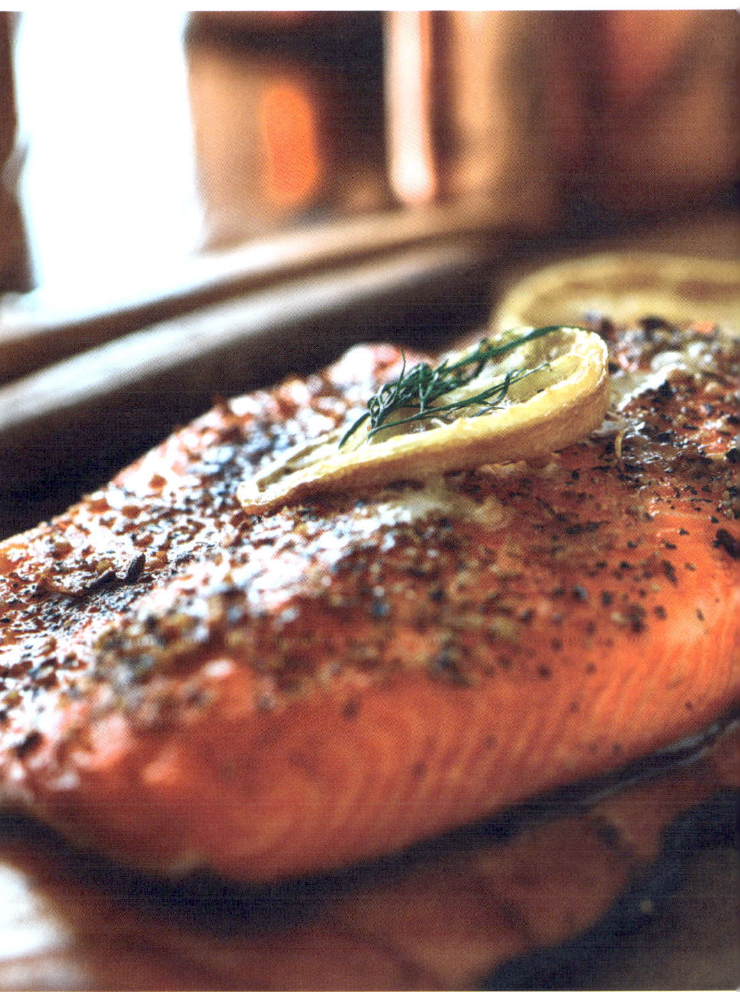

Mussels in White Wine

SERVES 4

COOK TIME: HIGH 25 MINS

GLUTEN FREE

Lemon Herb Salmon

SERVES 4

COOK TIME: LOW 2 HRS

GLUTEN FREE • DAIRY FREE

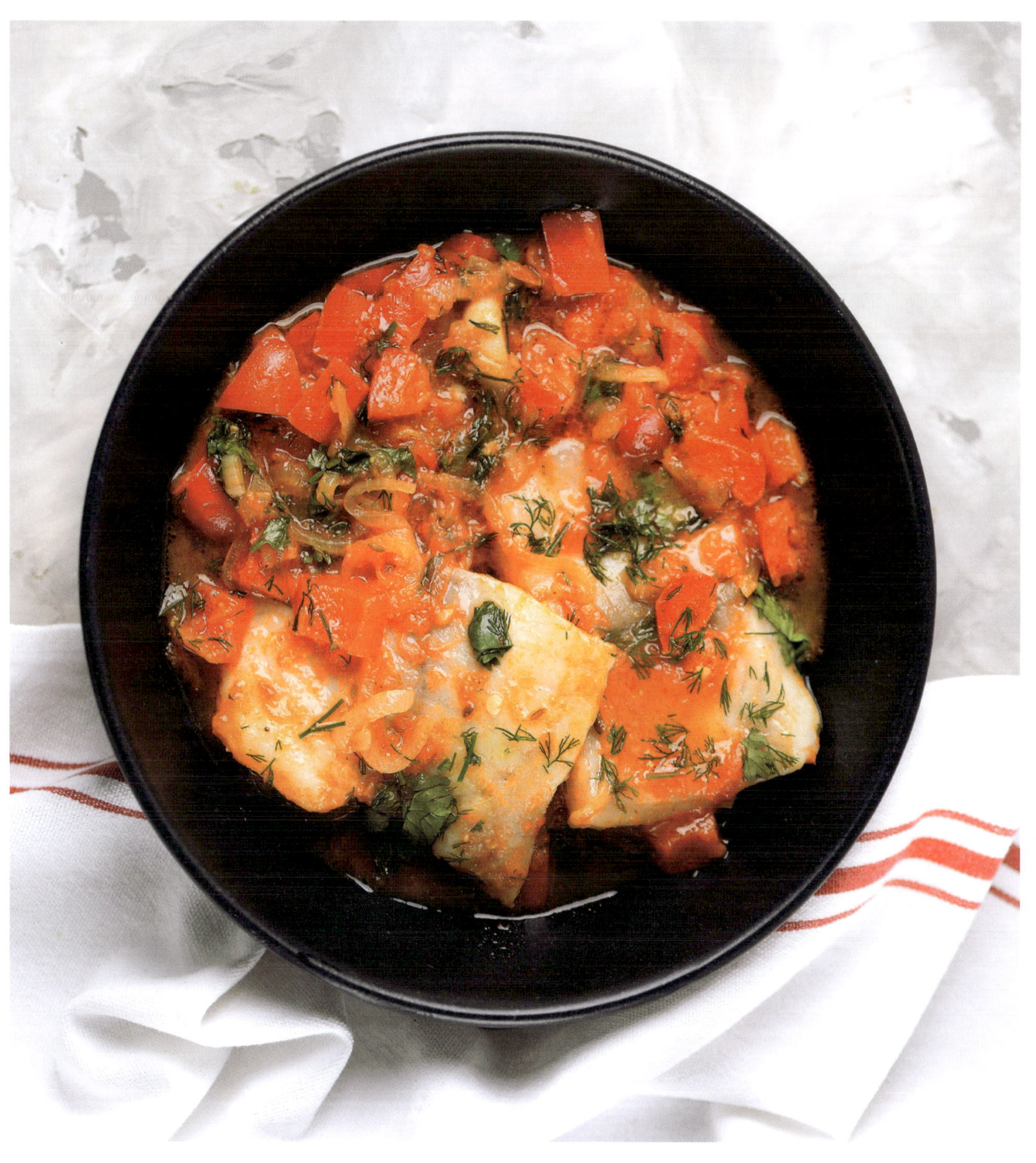

Fish with Tomato and Herb Sauce

SERVES 4

COOK TIME: HIGH 1½-2 HRS/LOW 3 HRS

GLUTEN FREE • DAIRY FREE

FISH WITH TOMATO AND HERB SAUCE

1 large onion, sliced
2 red capsicums, diced
2 cloves garlic, minced
1 x 400g can chopped tomatoes
500g firm white fish fillets
Salt and pepper to taste
½ cup (125ml) white wine
⅓ cup (80ml) chicken or vegetable stock
2 tbsps chopped dill
2 tbsps chopped coriander

Place onion, capsicum, garlic and tomatoes into slow cooker. Stir to combine.

Lay fish on top of vegetables. Season with salt and pepper then pour in wine and stock.

Cover and cook on low for 3 hours or on high for 1½-2 hours.

Gently stir through herbs and serve.

FISH SOUP WITH POTATO AND RICE

2 medium potatoes, peeled and chopped into small chunks

600g fish fillets (such as salmon) cut into bite-size chunks

1 tbsp tomato paste

1 tbsp turmeric

2 cups (500ml) chicken stock

1 cup (155g) basmati rice

2 tbsps cornflour

Fresh coriander, chopped, to garnish

Red chillies, chopped, to garnish

Place the potatoes at the bottom of the slow cooker. Add the fish, tomato paste, turmeric and stock.

Cover and cook on low for 4 hours. Add the rice and cook for 1 hour more. About 30 minutes before serving, stir in the cornflour until the soup has reached a thicker consistency.

Serve with a garnish of chopped coriander and red chillies if desired.

BRAZILIAN FISH STEW

2 x 400g cans chopped tomatoes

1 onion, roughly sliced

2 tsps tomato paste

3 tbsps fresh coriander, plus extra to garnish

Salt and pepper to taste

1kg white fish (such as snapper or barramundi)

1 x 400ml can coconut milk

Place in the slow cooker the tomatoes, onion, tomato paste, coriander and salt and pepper to taste. Stir well and cook on low for 2 hours.

Add the fish and cook for 1 hour or so until the fish is not quite completely cooked. Drain some of the liquid (the addition of the fish will make the mixture watery) then pour in the coconut milk and stir well. Cook for 1 hour more.

Serve with a garnish of fresh coriander.

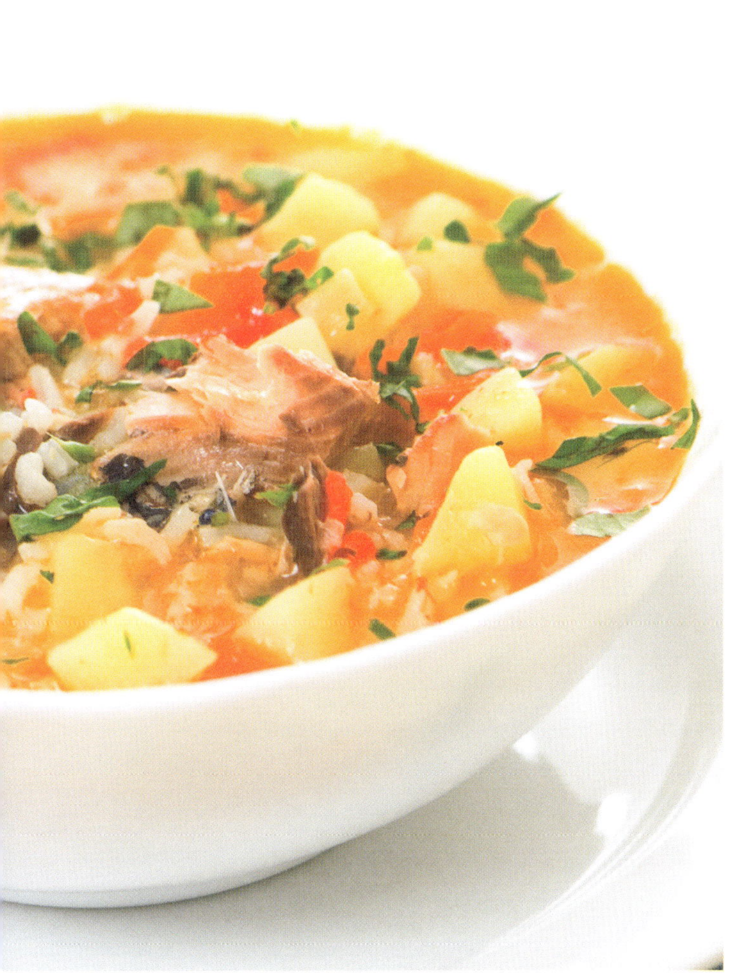

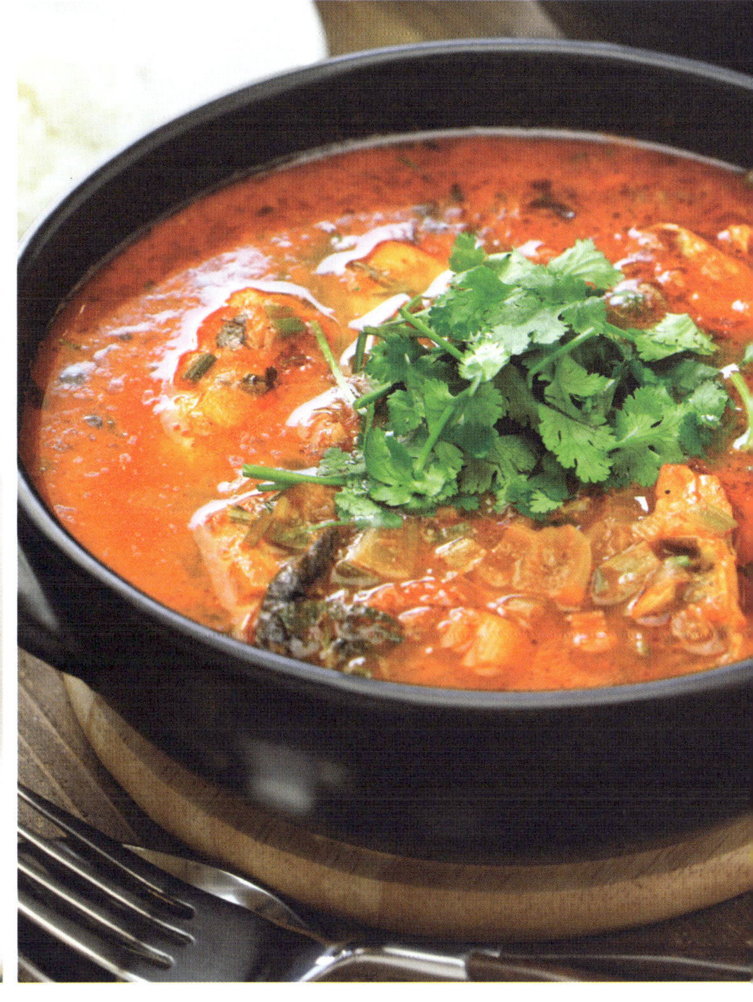

Fish Soup with Potato and Rice

SERVES 4

COOK TIME: LOW 5 HRS

GLUTEN FREE • DAIRY FREE

Brazilian Fish Stew

SERVES 4

COOK TIME: LOW 4 HRS

GLUTEN FREE • DAIRY FREE

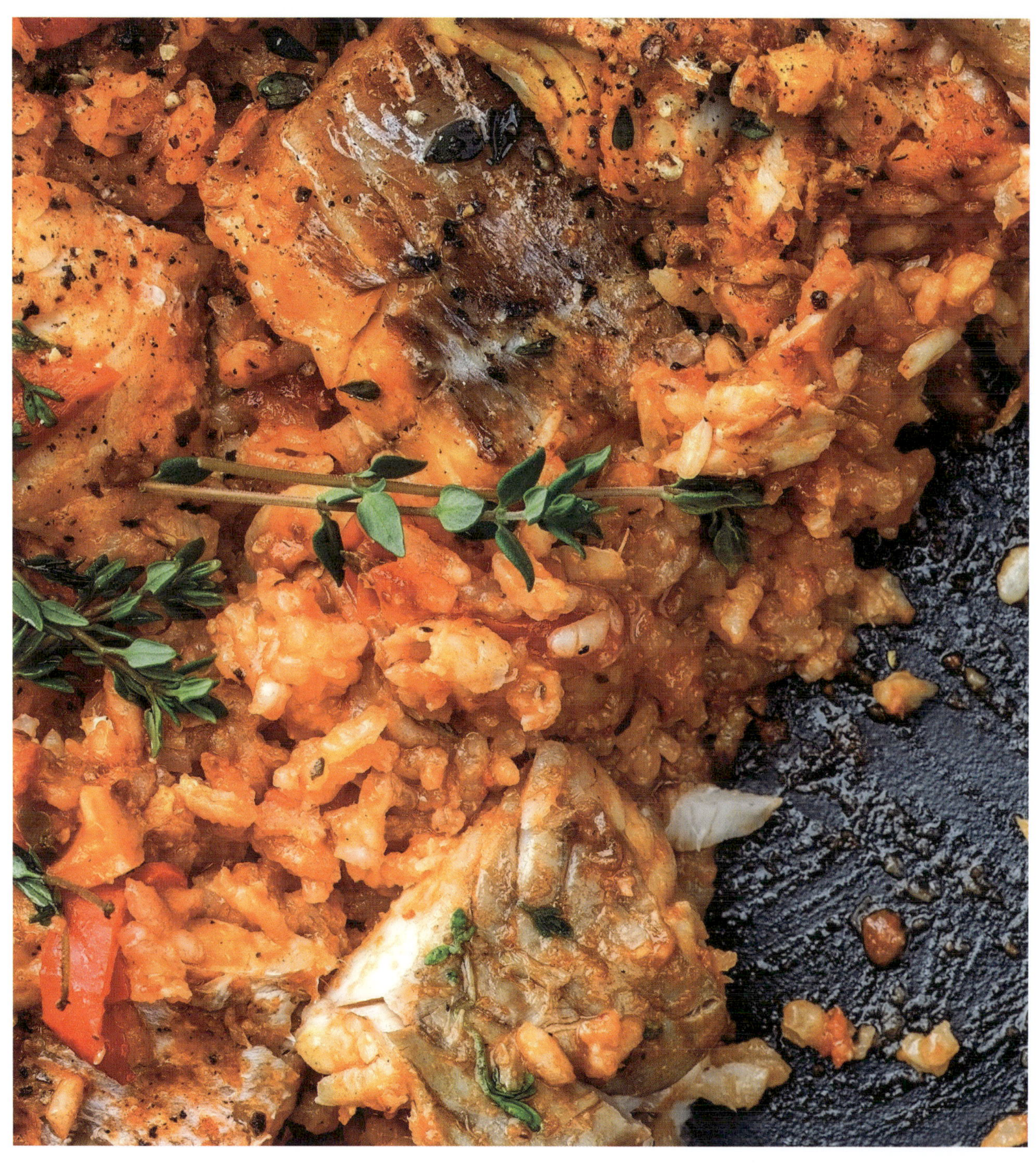

Fish Jambalaya

SERVES 4

COOK TIME: LOW 3 HRS 30 MINS

GLUTEN FREE • DAIRY FREE

FISH JAMBALAYA

400g white fish (such as Murray cod or Mahi Mahi), cut into bite-size chunks

2 x 400g cans chopped tomatoes

2 tsps Cajun seasoning

½ cup (125ml) water

Salt and pepper to taste

2 cups (330g) cooked white rice

300g prawns, deveined and tails removed

Fresh thyme, to garnish

Place the fish, tomatoes, Cajun seasoning and water in the slow cooker. Season to taste and stir well to combine.

Cover and cook on low for 4 hours and 30 minutes. About 20 minutes before serving, add the cooked rice and prawns.

Serve with a garnish of fresh thyme.

Chapter Four

Vegetables

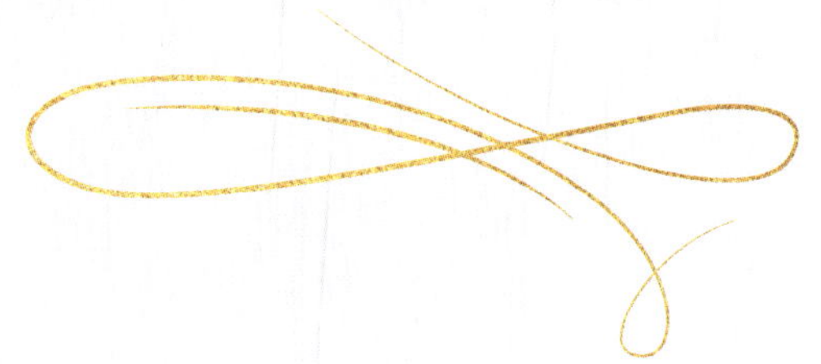

Pumpkin Soup with Roasted Hazelnuts

SERVES 4
COOK TIME: LOW 7 HRS
GLUTEN FREE

- 1kg pumpkin, chopped
- 1-2 onions, chopped
- 2 cups (500ml) chicken (or vegetable) stock
- 1 cup (125g) hazelnuts
- ½ cup (125ml) thickened cream (or sour cream)
- Pinch of nutmeg
- Salt and pepper to taste
- Fresh parsley, to garnish

Place the pumpkin, onion and stock in the slow cooker.

Cover and cook on low for 7 hours until pumpkin is soft.

Preheat the oven to 150°C.

Spread hazelnuts in an even layer on a baking tray and transfer to the oven. Bake for 10-15 minutes until deep brown and aromatic. Be careful not to burn. Remove from oven and set aside to cool slightly.

Using a clean tea towel, rub hazelnuts to loosen and shed skins. Roughly chop and set aside.

Blend cooked soup in the slow cooker with a stick blender or in batches with a stand blender.

Stir in cream and nutmeg. Season to taste.

Serve garnished with roasted hazelnuts and fresh parsley.

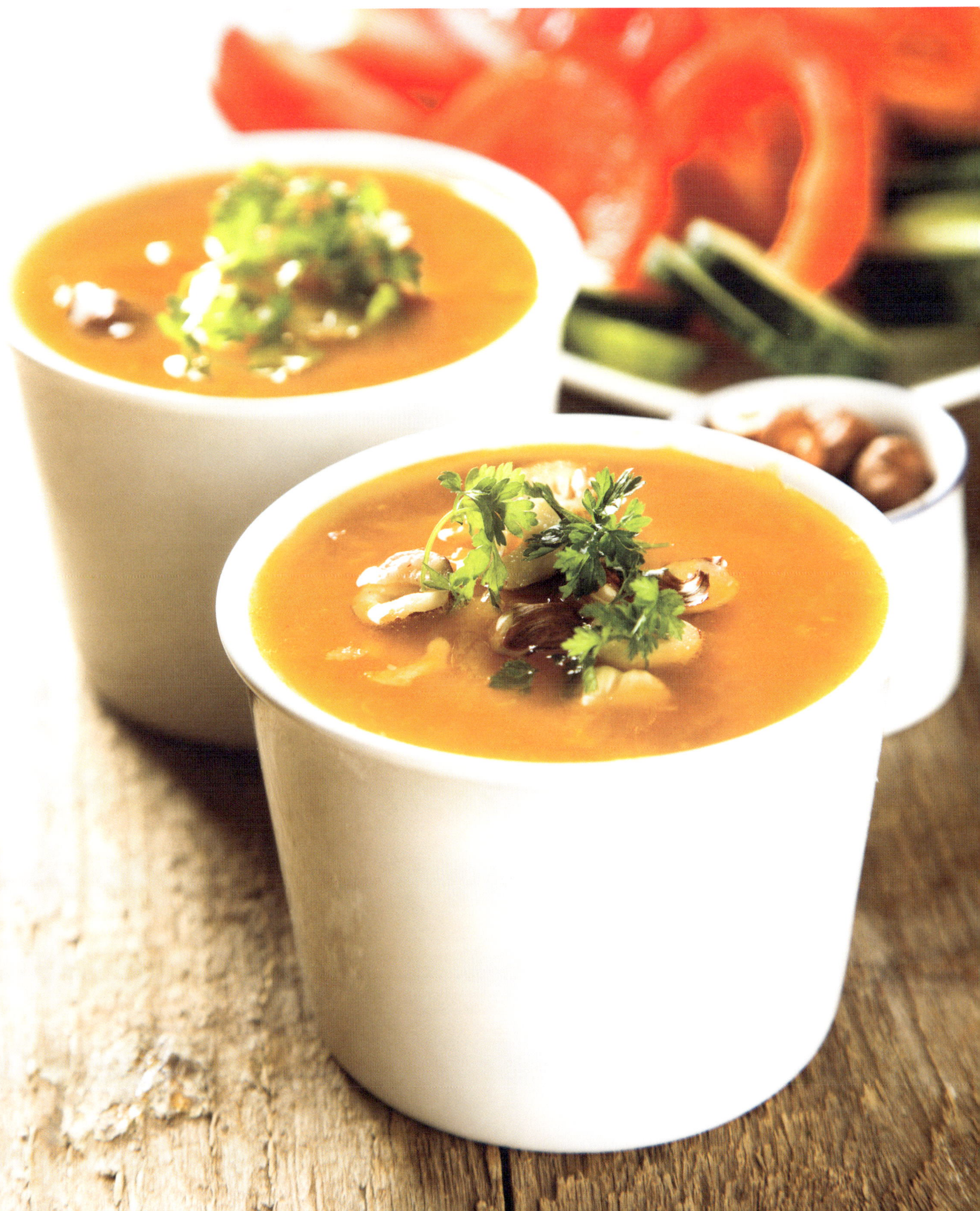

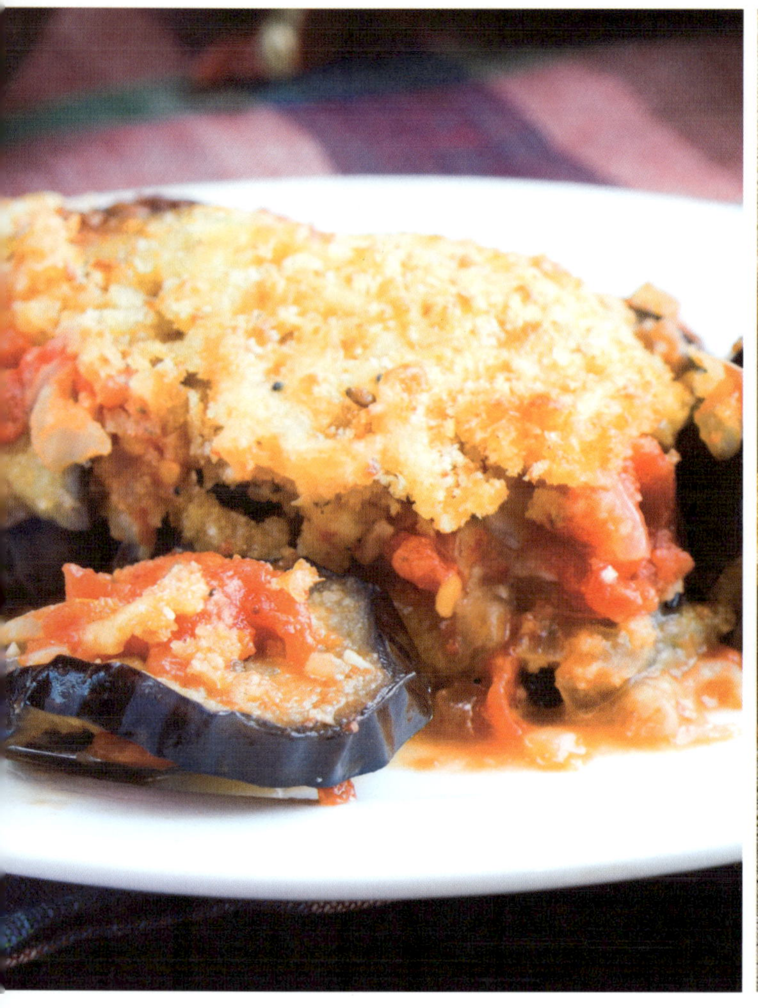

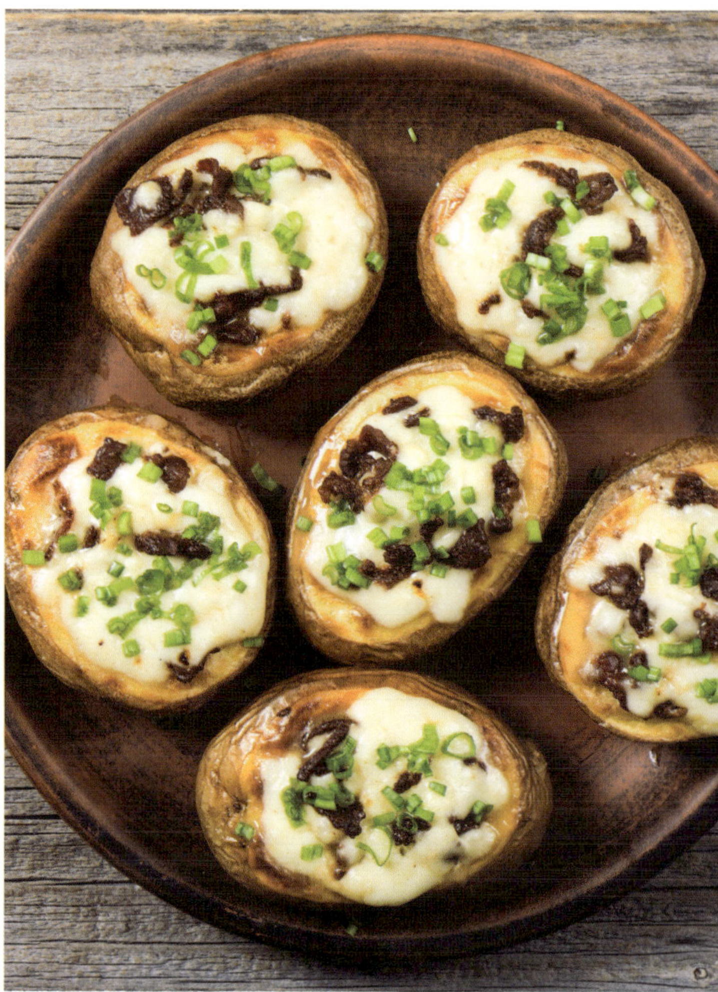

Vegetarian Moussaka

SERVES 4

COOK TIME: LOW 5 HRS + 15 MINS IN OVEN

Stuffed Baked Potatoes

SERVES 4

COOK TIME: HIGH 5-6 HRS/LOW 8 HRS

GLUTEN FREE

VEGETARIAN MOUSSAKA

1 large eggplant, chopped into cubes

1 large onion, finely chopped

1 zucchini, sliced

2 x 400g cans chopped tomatoes

3 cloves garlic, minced

Salt and pepper to taste

½ cup (60g) hard cheese (such as Cheddar, Parmesan or Swiss), grated

½ cup (60g) dried breadcrumbs

Place the eggplant, onion, zucchini, tomatoes and garlic in the slow cooker. Stir and season well. Cook on low for 5 hours or until the eggplant is tender.

Preheat the oven to 200°C.

When the moussaka is cooked, remove the insert from the slow cooker with the moussaka inside.

Sprinkle the cheese and the breadcrumbs on the top and cook in the oven for 15 minutes or until the cheese is melted and breadcrumbs are crispy.

STUFFED BAKED POTATOES

4 large potatoes

1 tsp salt

1 tbsp olive oil

1 red onion, chopped

1 tbsp olive oil

1 cup (125g) grated mozzarella or Cheddar cheese

2 tbsps chopped fresh chives

Rub each potato with salt and olive oil, then individually wrap each one tightly in foil.

Place into the base of slow cooker, cover and cook on low for 8 hours or on high for 5-6 hours. Unwrap potatoes and cut in half. Set aside.

Place onion in a frying pan with olive oil. Cook over medium-high heat for 8- 10 minutes, stirring regularly, until crispy. Set aside.

Sprinkle potatoes with grated cheese. Place under a hot grill and cook for 2 minutes until melted.

Remove from the grill. Top with crispy onion and chopped chives.

Vegetable Lasagne

SERVES 4

COOK TIME: LOW 4 HRS

3 large eggplants, sliced into 1cm-thick slices

4 tbsps olive oil

1 onion, chopped

4 cloves garlic, crushed

½ cup (125ml) Italian red wine

2 x 400g cans chopped tomatoes

Salt and pepper to taste

1 cup (15g) basil leaves

Olive oil cooking spray

250g instant lasagne sheets

350g mozzarella cheese, sliced

Brush eggplant slices with olive oil and cook on a hot grill pan over medium-high heat for 3 minutes each side.

Heat remaining oil in a saucepan over medium heat. Add onion and cook, stirring, for 3-5 minutes until soft. Add garlic and cook for 1 minute until fragrant. Add wine and tomatoes. Bring to the boil then reduce heat and simmer for 10 minutes. Season with salt and pepper. Tear basil leaves and stir through. Remove from heat and set aside.

Spray slow cooker with cooking spray. Cover base with tomato sauce. Top with lasagne sheets, more sauce, eggplant and mozzarella. Repeat for two more layers, then top with one final layer of lasagne sheets and sauce.

Cook, covered, on low for 4 hours.

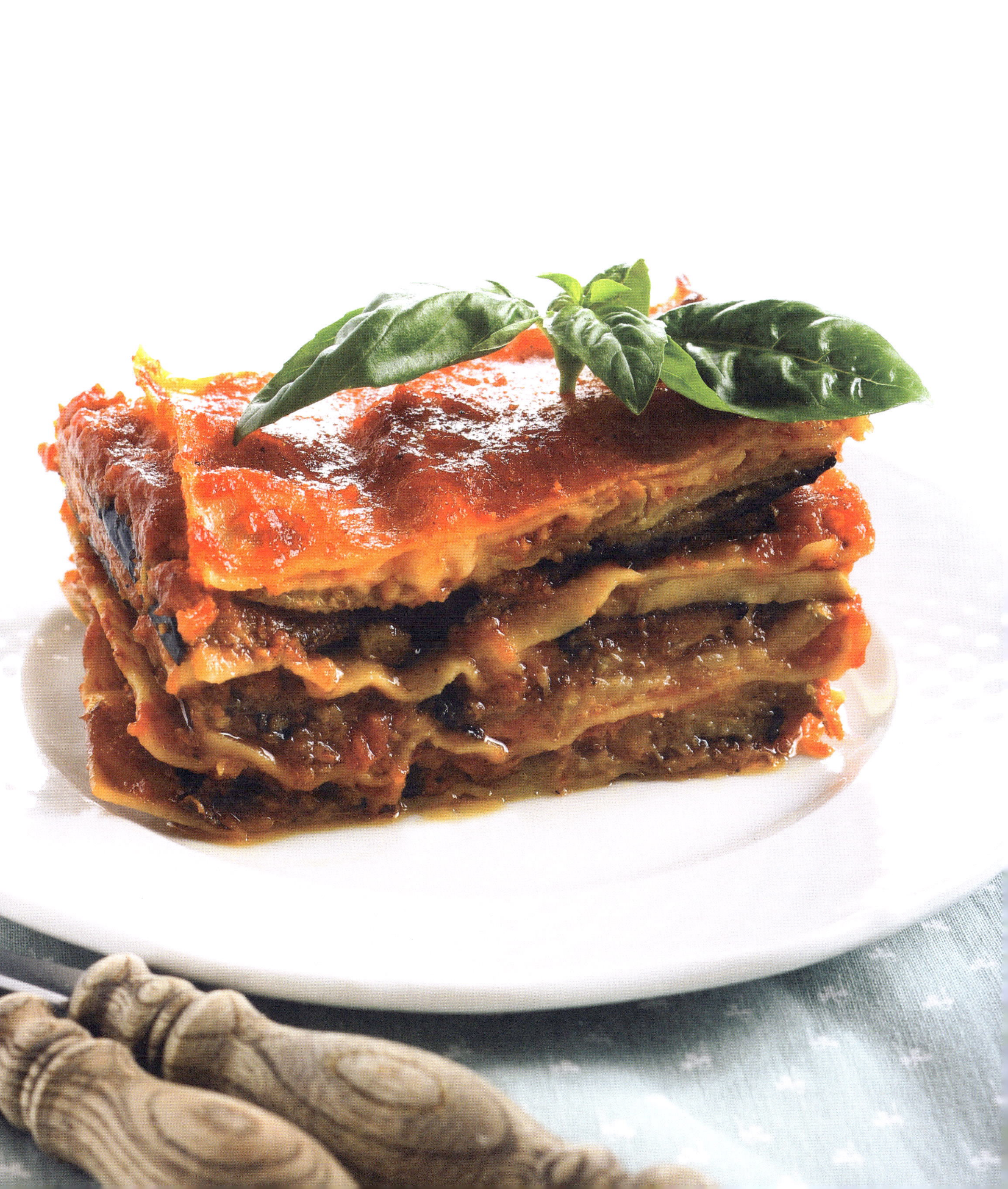

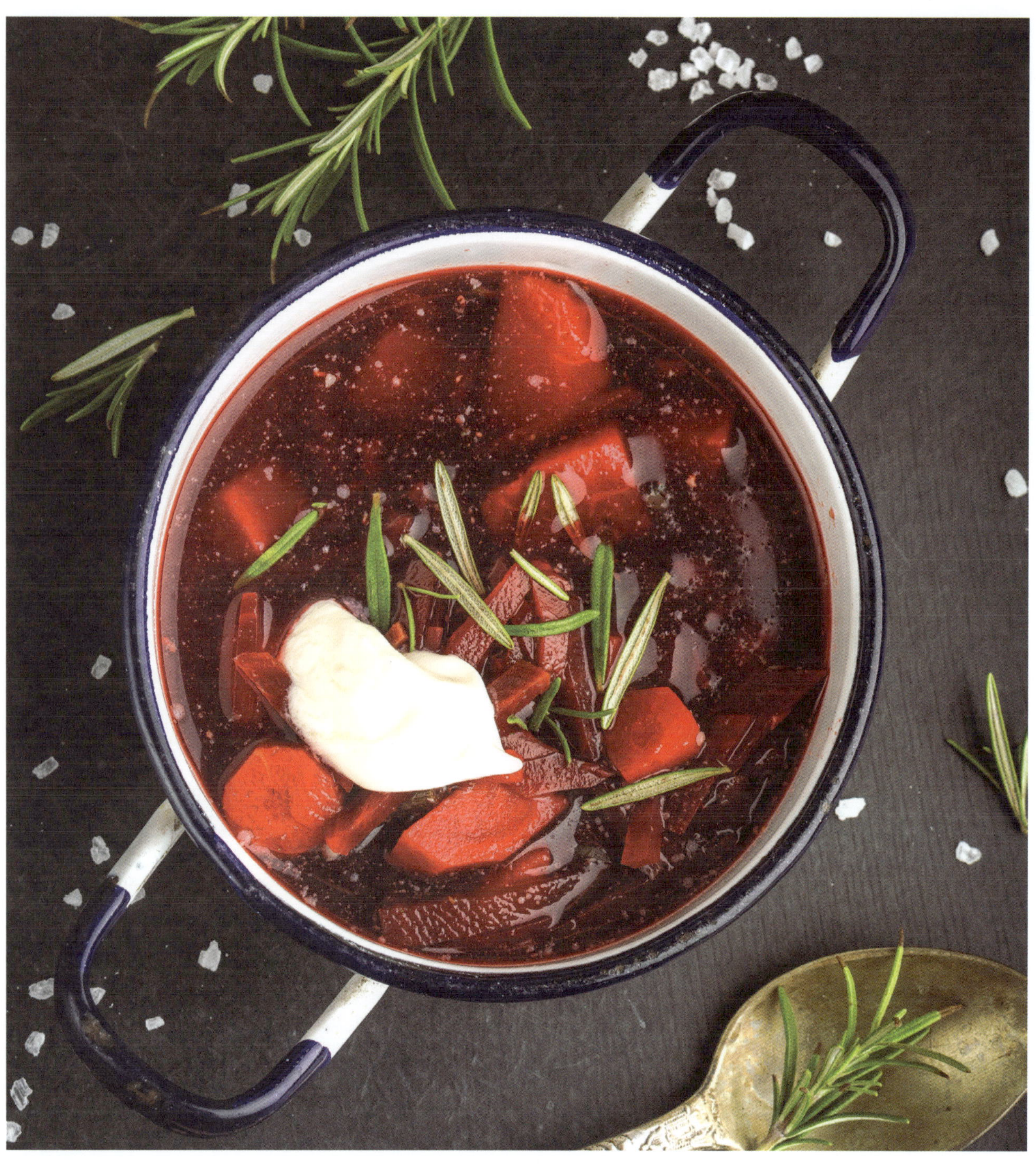

Russian Borscht

SERVES 4

COOK TIME: HIGH 4 HRS/LOW 8 HRS

GLUTEN FREE

RUSSIAN BORSCHT

2 tbsps olive oil
2 onions, finely chopped
4 stalks celery, diced
2 carrots, peeled and diced
4 cloves garlic, minced
1 tsp caraway seeds
½ tsp salt
½ tsp pepper
3 tbsps tomato paste
1 tbsp sugar
3 medium beetroots, peeled and diced
2 small potatoes, peeled and diced
¼ cup (10g) rosemary leaves (reserve some for garnish)
5 cups (1.25L) vegetable stock
2 tbsps fresh lemon juice
1 cup (250ml) sour cream
Rock salt, to garnish

Heat the oil in a frying pan over medium-high heat. Add onions, celery and carrots, and cook, stirring often, for 5 minutes, until softened.

Add the garlic, caraway seeds, salt and pepper and cook for a further 1 minute until aromatic.

Transfer the mixture to the slow cooker.

Add the tomato paste, sugar, beetroot, potato and rosemary. Add the stock and lemon juice. Stir.

Cover and cook on low for 8 hours, or on high for 4 hours, or until the vegetables are tender.

Ladle soup into bowls and top with the sour cream, rock salt and reserved rosemary leaves to serve.

VEGETABLE STEW

3 cloves garlic, chopped
1 medium onion, chopped
2 stalks celery, chopped
2 large zucchinis, cut into thick slices
½ head cauliflower, cut into florets
½ head broccoli, cut into florets
2 medium leeks, white part only, sliced
250g sliced mushrooms
1 x 400g can cannellini beans, drained and rinsed
500g potatoes, peeled and quartered
1½ cups (375ml) vegetable stock
4 Roma tomatoes, roughly chopped
1 bay leaf
Salt and pepper to taste

Add all ingredients to slow cooker. Season with salt and pepper. Stir to combine. Cover and cook on low for 5-6 hours.

LENTIL TAMARIND SOUP

2 tsps ghee or vegetable oil
1 large onion, finely chopped
2 cloves garlic, crushed
1½ tbsps ginger, grated
2 tsps ground cumin
1 tsp ground coriander
½ tsp turmeric
6 cups (1.5L) water
1½ tsps salt, or to taste
2 cups (370g) yellow lentils
3 tbsps tamarind concentrate
1 cup (200g) tomatoes, deseeded and finely chopped
1 x 400ml can coconut milk
3 tbsps lemon juice

Heat the ghee in a medium frying pan over medium-high heat.

Add the onion and fry for 5 minutes until soft and translucent. Add the garlic and fry for a further minute. Stir in the ginger, cumin, coriander and turmeric and stir for 1 more minute until fragrant. Pour in ¼ cup of the water and stir through, then transfer the contents of the pan to the slow cooker.

Add the rest of the ingredients, cover and cook on low for 8 hours.

Season to taste and serve hot.

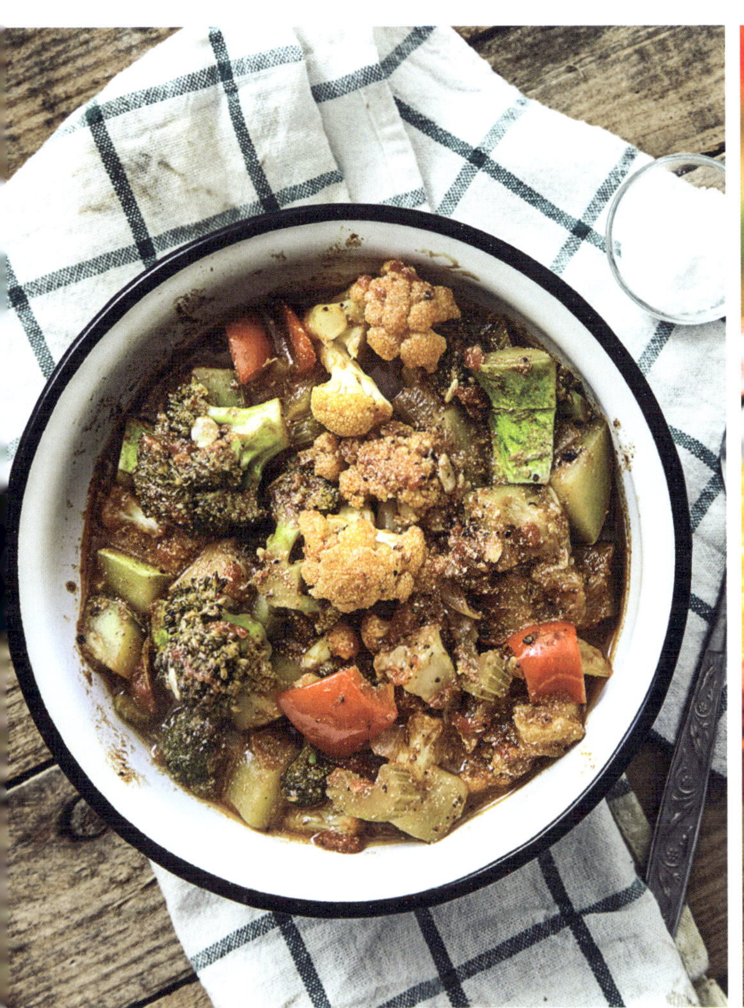

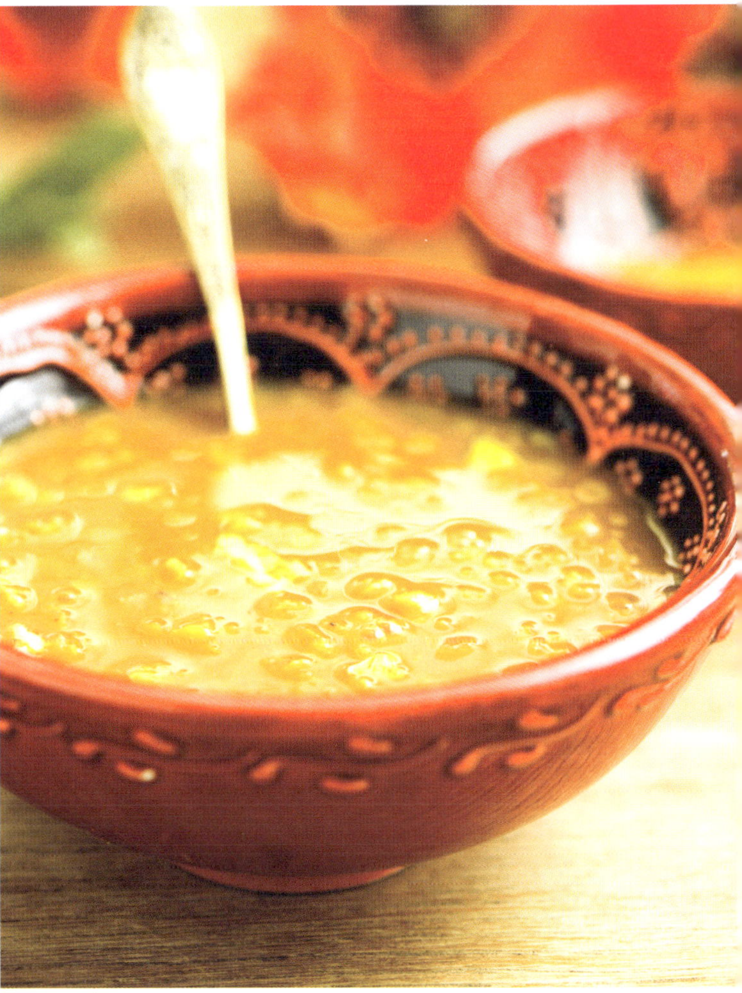

Vegetable Stew

SERVES 6

COOK TIME: LOW 5-6 HRS

GLUTEN FREE • DAIRY FREE

Lentil Tamarind Soup

SERVES 6

COOK TIME: LOW 8 HRS

GLUTEN FREE • DAIRY FREE

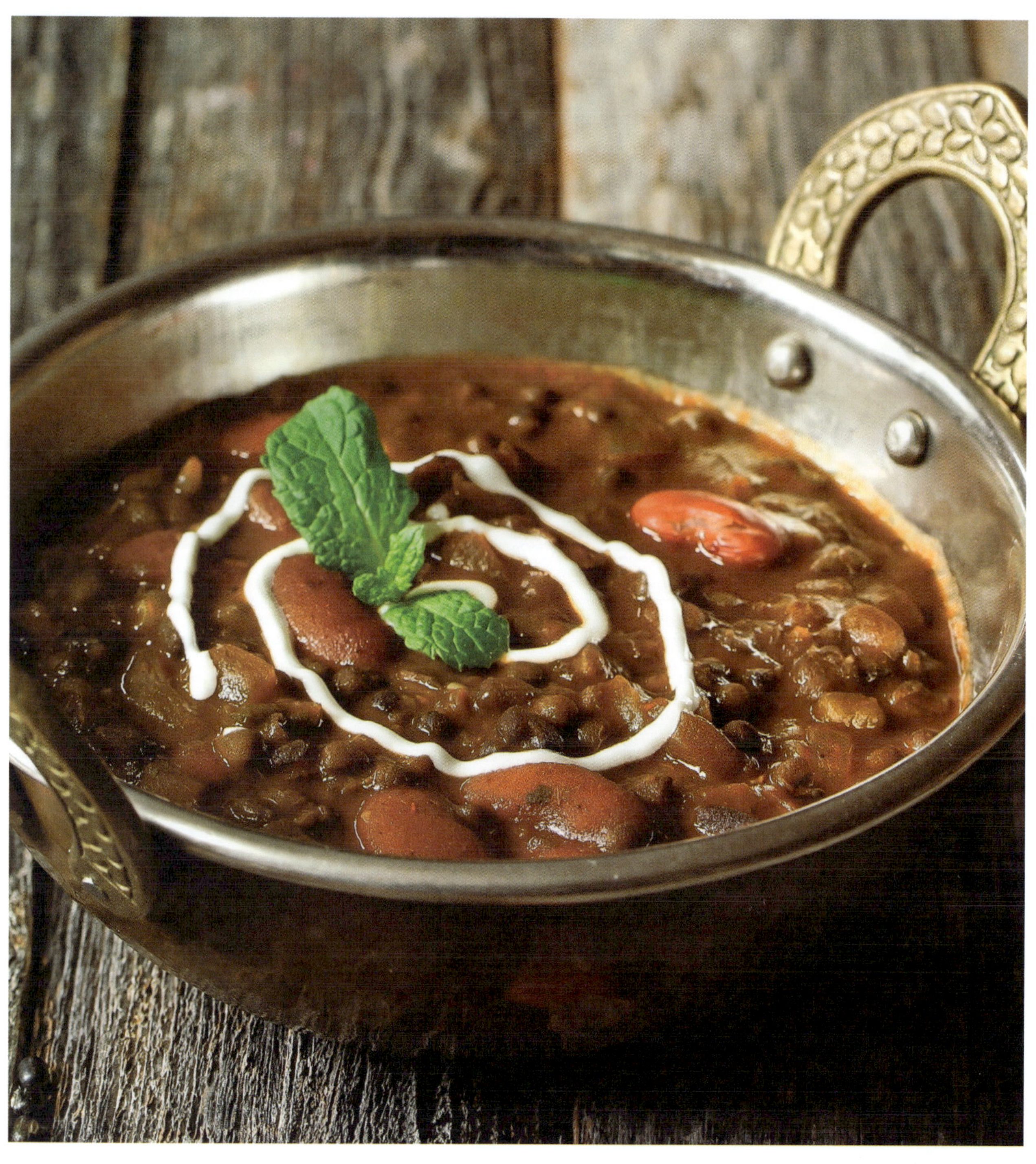

Lentil and Kidney Bean Curry

SERVES 4

COOK TIME: LOW 6 HRS

GLUTEN FREE • DAIRY FREE

LENTIL AND KIDNEY BEAN CURRY

1 onion, diced
3 cloves garlic, crushed
Medium piece ginger, peeled and grated
2 green bird's-eye chillies, finely chopped
1½ cups (375ml) crushed tomatoes and juice or passata
1 tbsp ground coriander
1 tbsp ground cumin
1½ tsps garam masala
1 x 400g can red kidney beans, drained and rinsed
1 cup (185g) brown lentils
1½ cups (375ml) vegetable stock
Salt and pepper to taste
Fresh mint and Greek yoghurt, to serve (optional)

Combine onion, garlic, ginger, chillies, tomatoes, spices, beans, lentils and stock in the slow cooker.

Season with salt and pepper and stir to combine.

Cover and cook on low for 6 hours.

Garnish with mint and drizzle with yoghurt to serve, if desired.

Broccoli Detox Soup

SERVES 4
COOK TIME: HIGH 4 HRS/LOW 8 HRS
GLUTEN FREE • DAIRY FREE

1 tbsp olive oil
1 medium onion, chopped
3 cloves garlic, chopped
1 carrot, chopped
1 stalk celery, chopped
1 large head broccoli, cut into florets
1 bay leaf
½ tsp dried basil
½ tsp dried thyme
½ tsp dried rosemary
1 tsp dried oregano
4 cups (1L) vegetable stock
Salt and pepper to taste
Pepitas and sesame seeds, to serve

Heat the olive oil in a frying pan on medium-high heat then add the onion, garlic, carrot and celery. Cook, stirring regularly, for 5 minutes until onions are golden.

Transfer to the slow cooker along with the broccoli, herbs and vegetable stock. Season with salt and pepper. Cover and cook on high for 4 hours or low for 8 hours.

Use a stick blender to blend until smooth and creamy.

Ladle into bowls and scatter with pepitas and sesame seeds to serve.

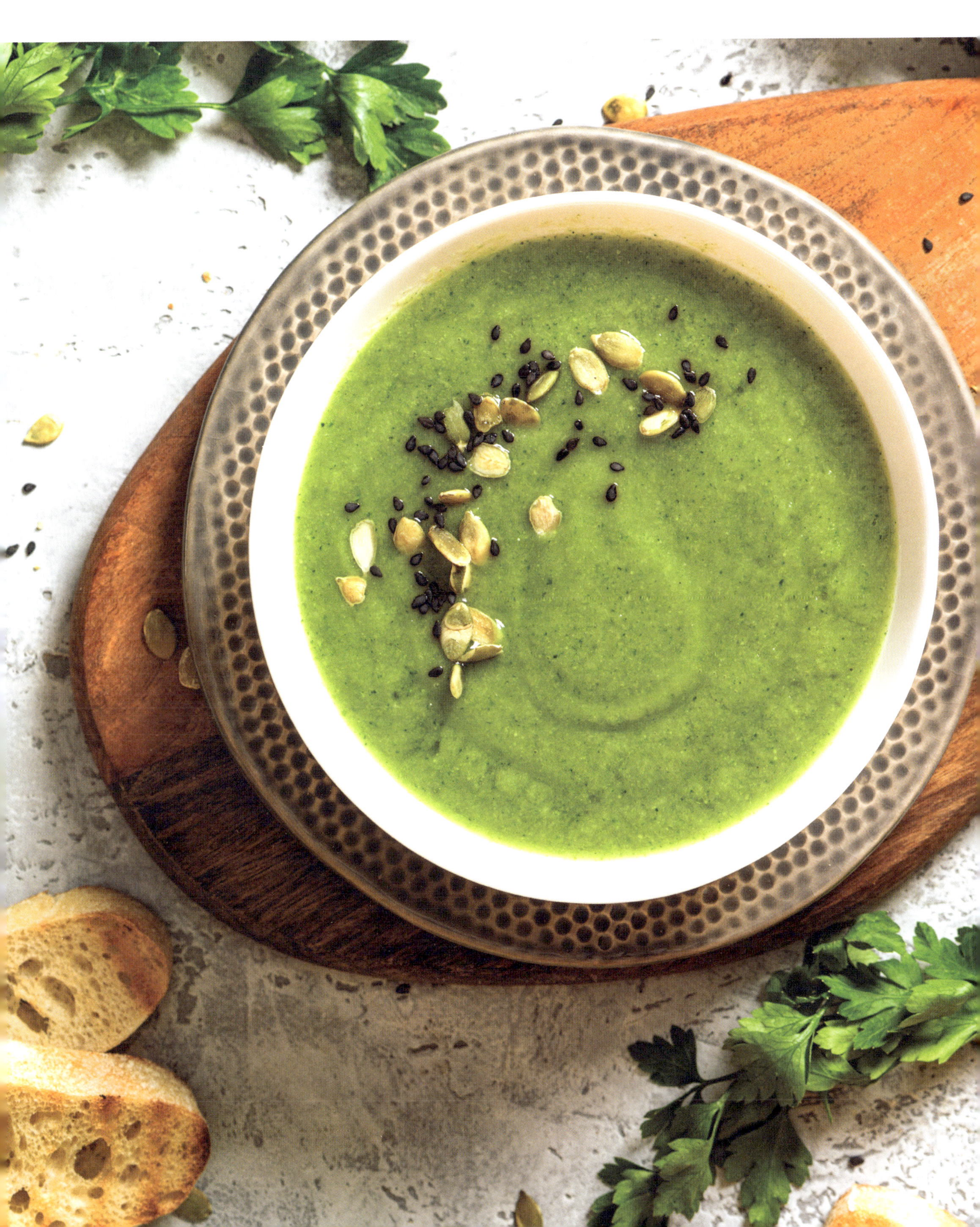

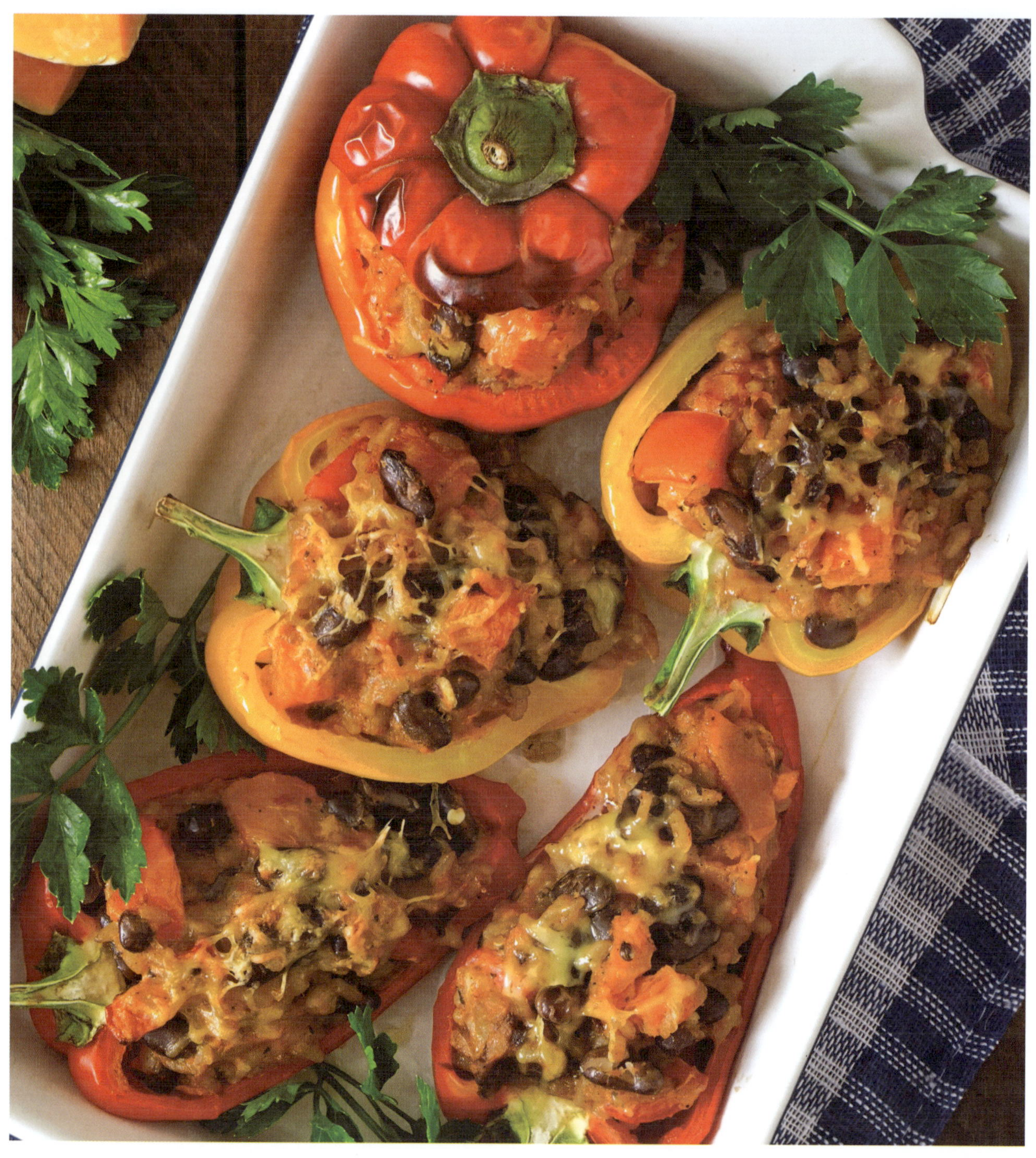

Quinoa Black Bean Stuffed Capsicums

SERVES 6

COOK TIME: HIGH 3 HRS/LOW 6 HRS

GLUTEN FREE

QUINOA BLACK BEAN STUFFED CAPSICUMS

6 capsicums

1 cup (170g) quinoa

1 x 400g can black beans, drained and rinsed

400g pumpkin, diced

1½ cups (340g) passata

1 tsp cumin

1 tsp chilli powder

1 tsp paprika

1 tsp dried oregano

2 tbsps chopped fresh parsley leaves

1 tsp onion powder

½ tsp garlic powder

1½ cups (185g) grated cheese

Salt and pepper to taste

½ cup (125ml) water

Either cut the tops off of the capsicums and scrape out the ribs and seeds, or cut the capsicums in half lengthways and scrape out in the same way.

In a large bowl, combine the quinoa, beans, pumpkin, passata, spices, herbs, seasonings and 1 cup of cheese. Season with salt and pepper. Fill each capsicum or capsicum half with the quinoa mixture. Place capsicum tops back in place if using whole capsicums.

Pour the water into the bottom of the slow cooker. Place the capsicums in the water. Cover and cook on low for 6 hours or on high for 3 hours.

Remove lid, scatter remaining cheese over the tops of the capsicums. Cover and cook for 10 minutes to melt the cheese.

TOMATO SOUP

2 x 400g cans whole peeled plum tomatoes
1 x 400ml jar passata
1½ cups (375ml) vegetable stock
3 cloves garlic, minced
1 onion, diced
1 red capsicum, diced
2 tbsps tomato paste
1½ tsps dried oregano
1 tsp sugar
½ tsp salt + more to season
½ tsp pepper + more to season
⅓ cup (80ml) cream
⅓ cup (15g) chopped fresh basil
1½ cups (45g) croutons

Place tomatoes into the slow cooker. Stir in passata, vegetable stock, garlic, onion, capsicum, tomato paste, oregano, sugar, salt and pepper.

Crush tomatoes into chunks using the back of a spoon. Cover and cook on low for 8 hours or on high for 4 hours.

Blend with a stick blender until smooth. Stir in cream and basil. Season with salt and pepper to taste.

Serve immediately with croutons.

JACKFRUIT TACOS

1 onion, diced
4 cloves garlic, minced
2 x 400g cans jackfruit, drained and rinsed
1 tbsp coconut sugar
1 tsp oregano
1 tsp cumin
1 tsp chilli powder
½ tsp smoked paprika
½ cup (125ml) fresh orange juice
1 tsp each salt and pepper or to taste
24 corn taco shells
¼ iceberg lettuce, shredded
Guacamole, salsa, chipotle mayonnaise and fresh coriander leaves or your choice of toppings, to serve

In the slow cooker, stir together onion, garlic and jackfruit.

Combine coconut sugar, oregano, cumin, chilli powder, smoked paprika, orange juice, salt and pepper in a small bowl. Pour over jackfruit mixture.

Cover and cook on low for 7-9 hours or on high 3-4 hours.

Shred jackfruit with two forks.

Fill tacos with lettuce and with jackfruit filling. Top with your choice of toppings.

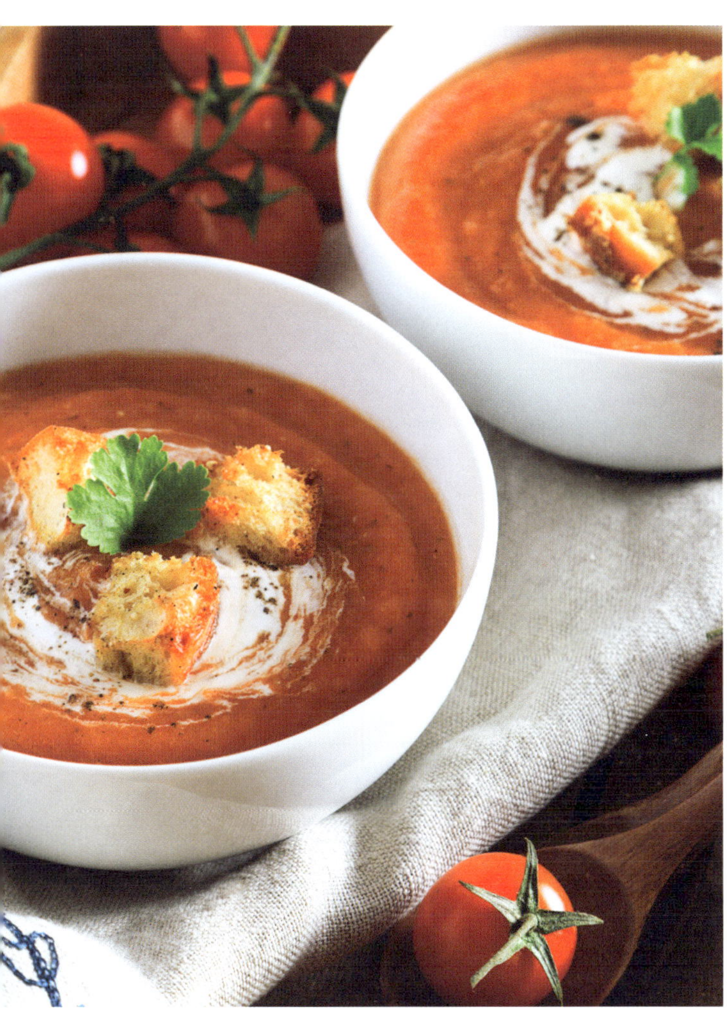

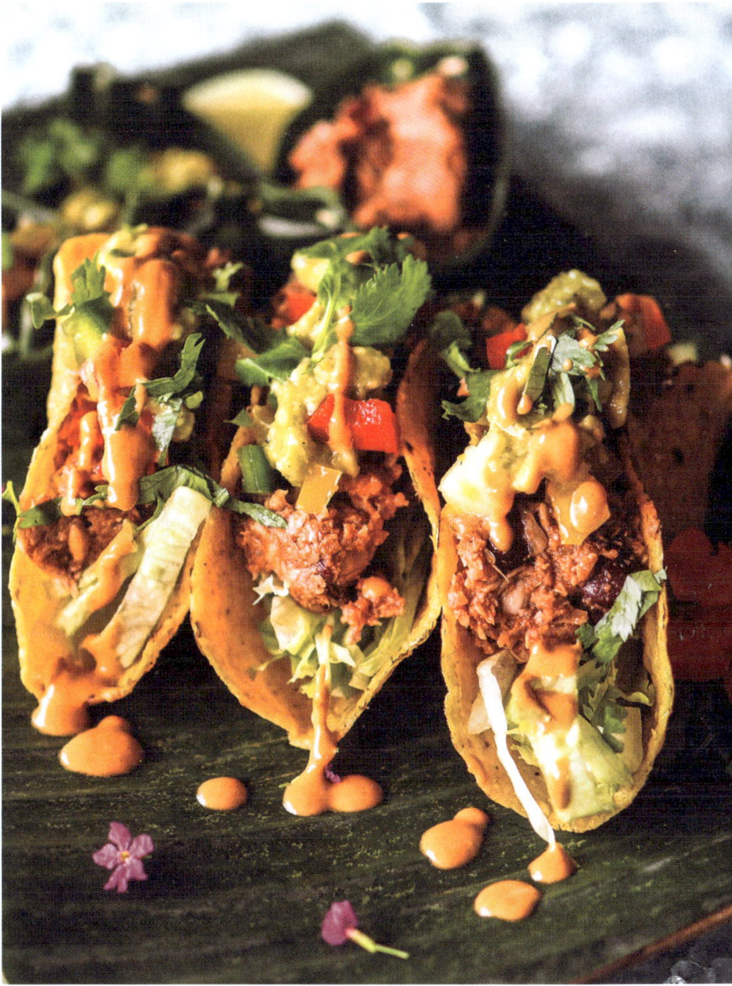

Tomato Soup

SERVES 8

COOK TIME: HIGH 4 HRS/LOW 8 HRS

Jackfruit Tacos

SERVES 8

COOK TIME: HIGH 3-4 HRS/LOW 7-9 HRS

GLUTEN FREE • DAIRY FREE

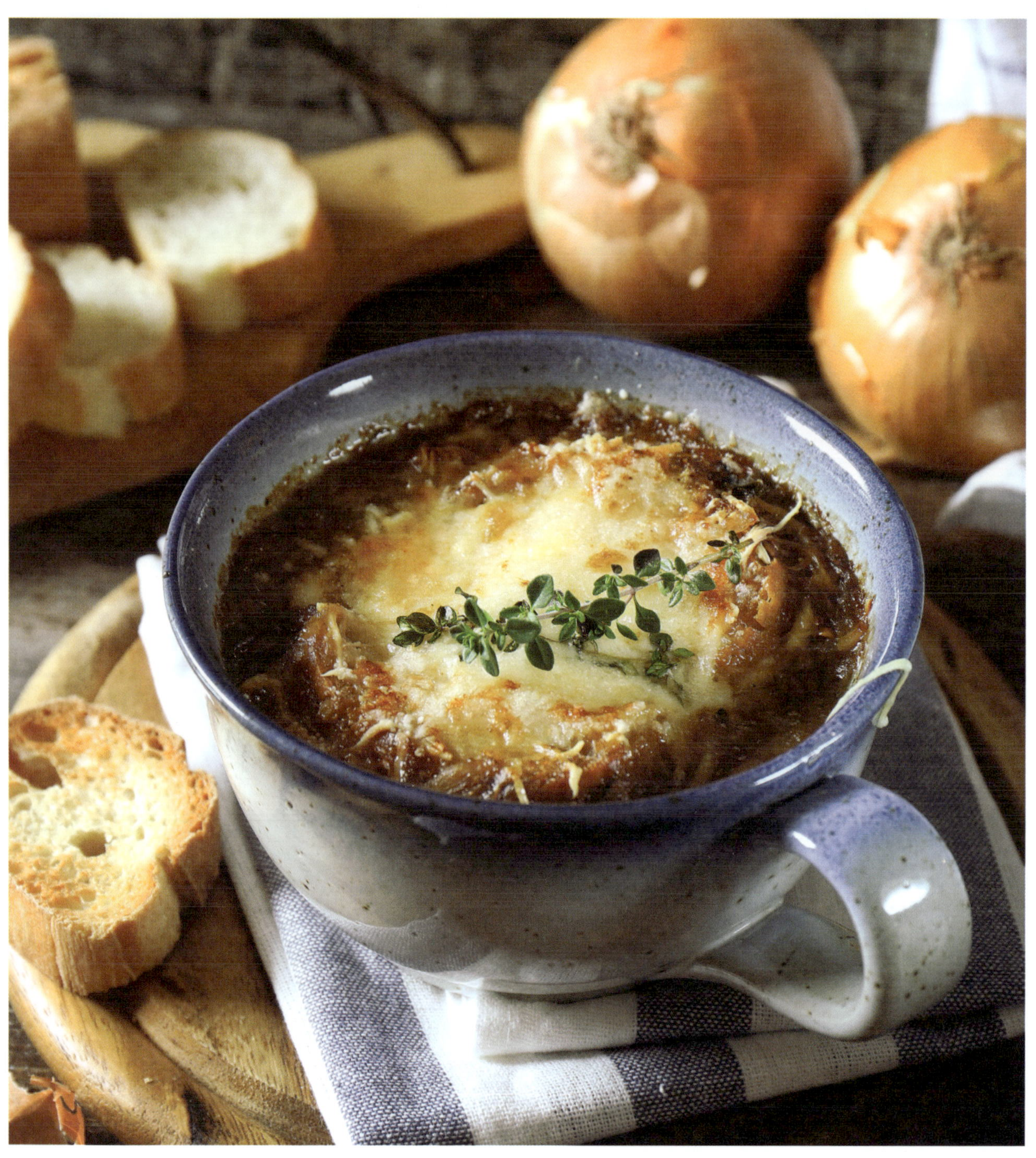

French Onion Soup

SERVES 8

COOK TIME: HIGH 4-6 HRS/LOW 8-10 HRS

FRENCH ONION SOUP

6 tbsps butter
4 large brown onions, sliced
1 tbsp sugar
2 cloves garlic, minced
½ cup (125ml) cooking sherry
7 cups (1.75L) beef stock
¼ tsp dried thyme
1 bay leaf
1 tsp salt, or to taste
8 slices French bread
1 cup (125g) grated Gruyere or mozzarella cheese

Heat butter in a large, heavy pan over medium-high heat. Add onions and cook, stirring regularly, for 3-5 minutes until soft and translucent. Sprinkle onions with sugar and reduce heat to medium. Cook, stirring constantly, until onions are soft and browned, at least 30 minutes. Stir in garlic and cook until fragrant, about 1 minute.

Stir sherry into onion mixture and scrape up any brown bits from the bottom of the pan with a spatula. Transfer onions into the slow cooker and add beef stock, thyme and bay leaf. Season to taste with salt.

Cover and cook on high for 4-6 hours or low for 8-10 hours.

Place bread slices under a hot grill for 1-2 minutes each side until golden.

Top bread slices with cheese and return to grill for a couple of minutes until cheese is melted.

Divide soup between bowls and top each with a piece of cheesy toast.

Red Lentil Dahl

SERVES 6

COOK TIME: HIGH 4-5 HRS/LOW 8-10 HRS

GLUTEN FREE • DAIRY FREE

1 tsp cumin seeds
1 tsp brown mustard seeds
½ tsp fennel seeds
1 tsp coriander seeds
1 tsp fenugreek seeds
1 tbsp ghee, peanut oil or coconut oil
1 onion, diced
2 cloves garlic, minced
Medium piece fresh ginger, grated
1½ tsps ground turmeric
¾ cup (135g) red lentils
¾ cup (135g) yellow split peas or use all red lentils
1 x 400g can diced tomatoes
3 cups (750ml) vegetable stock
3 green cardamom pods, crushed
1 bay leaf
1 tsp salt
¼ tsp pepper
Boiled basmati rice or naan bread to serve

Heat a small frying pan over medium heat. Add cumin, mustard, fennel, coriander and fenugreek seeds to the pan. Shake or stir the seeds for 1-2 minutes until fragrant. Remove from heat and set aside to cool.

Heat ghee or oil in a frying pan over medium-high heat. Add onion and cook for 3-5 minutes, stirring regularly, until soft and translucent. Add garlic, ginger, turmeric and toasted seeds. Cook for 30 seconds until fragrant.

Scrape out the pan into the slow cooker. Add red lentils, split peas, tomatoes, vegetable stock, cardamom pods and bay leaf. Season with salt and pepper. Stir well to combine.

Cover and cook on low for 8-10 hours or high for 4-5 hours.

Serve with boiled basmati rice or naan bread.

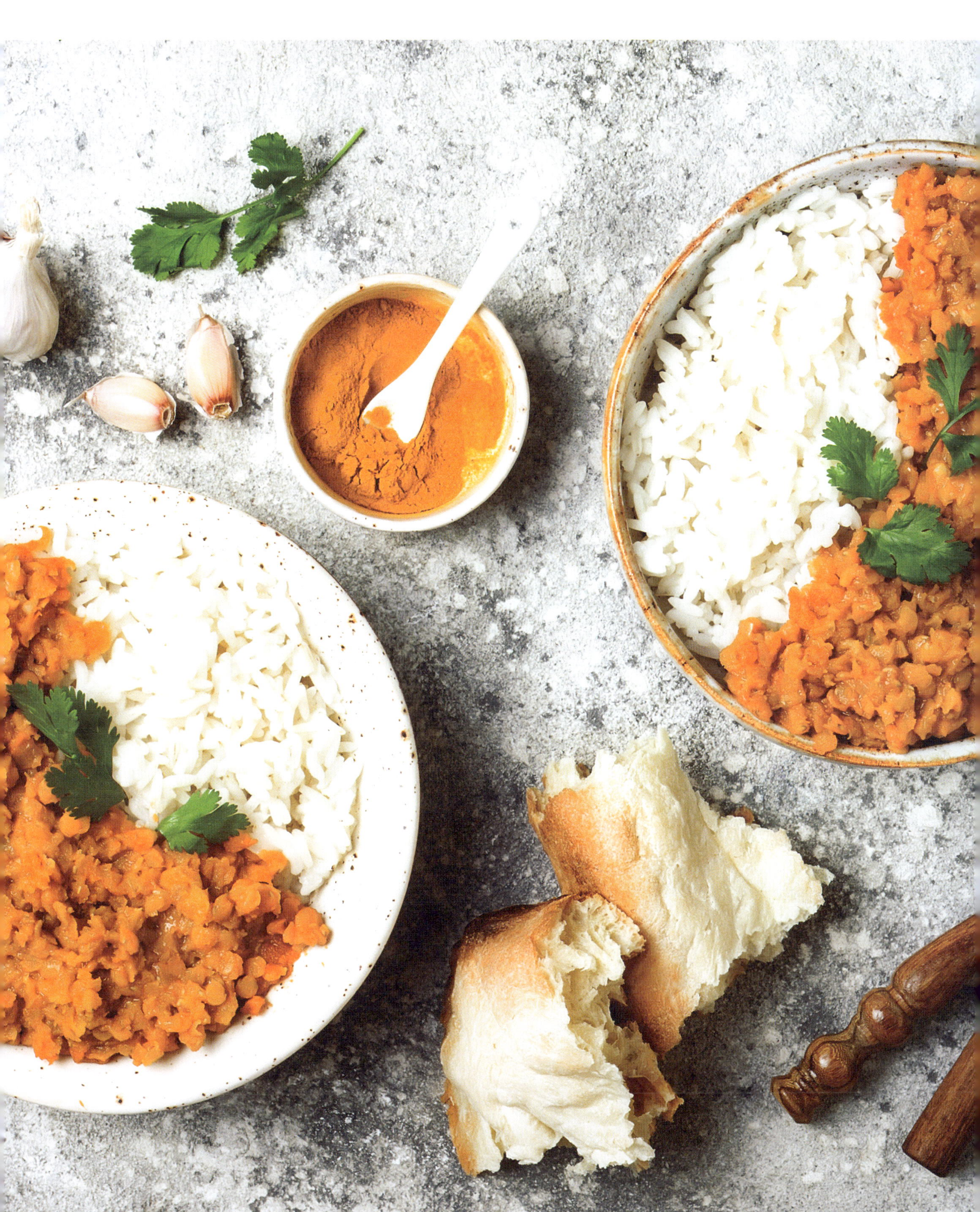

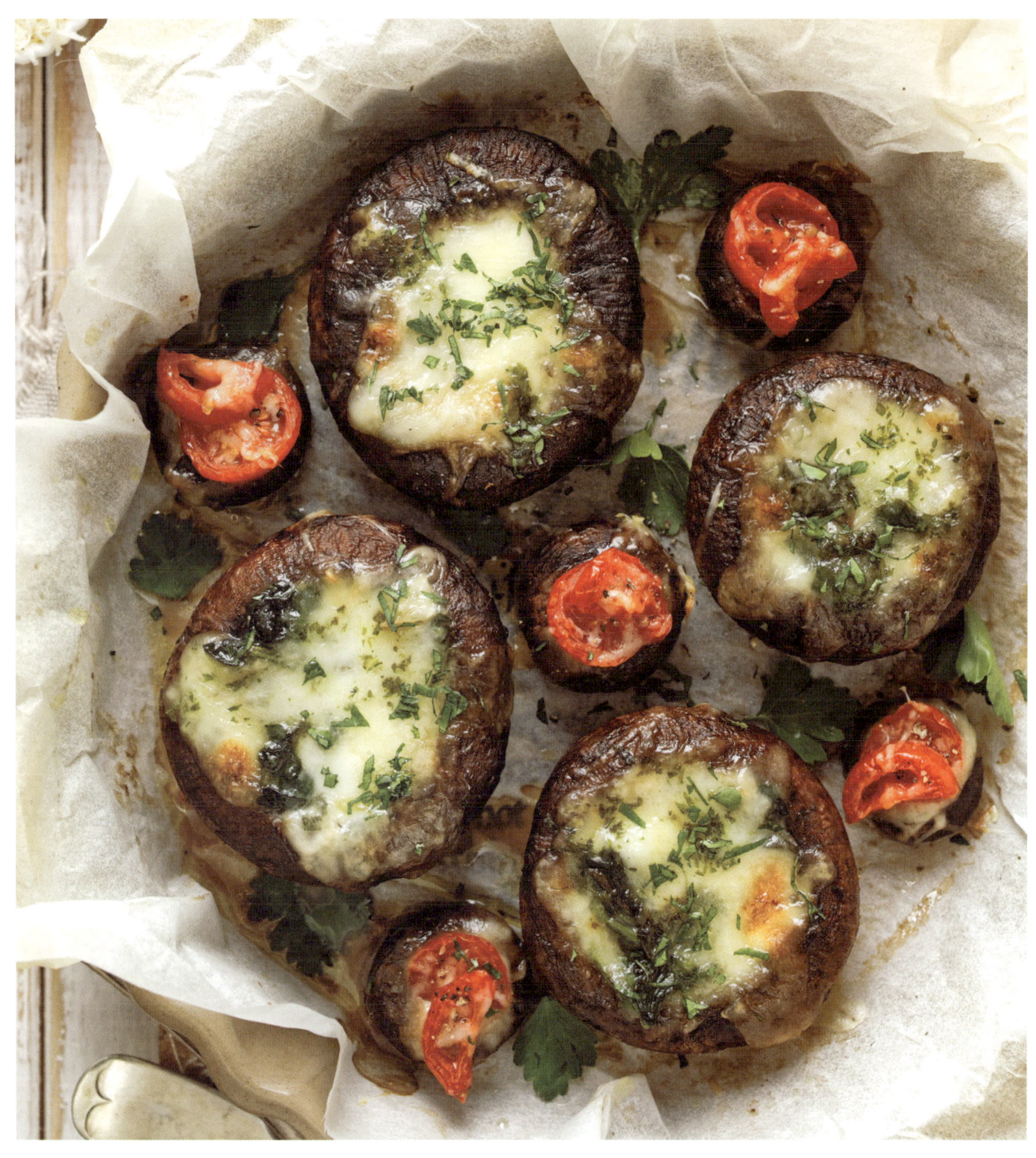

Stuffed Mushrooms

SERVES 4

COOK TIME: HIGH 3 HRS

GLUTEN FREE

STUFFED MUSHROOMS

4 large portobello mushrooms, stalks removed
4-8 chestnut mushrooms, stalks removed
1 clove garlic, minced
3 tbsps olive oil
4 tbsps finely chopped parsley
1½ tsps lemon zest
⅛ tsp chilli powder
1 cup (100g) grated pecorino
2-4 cherry tomatoes, halved

Place a large sheet of foil on a work surface and cover with a sheet of greaseproof paper.

Place the mushrooms stalk-side up on the greaseproof paper.

In a bowl mix together garlic, olive oil, 2 tablespoons parsley, lemon zest and chilli. Brush the mushrooms with the mixture.

Sprinkle mushrooms with cheese and scatter over remaining parsley. Top smaller mushrooms with cherry tomato halves.

Lift the corners of the foil and pinch together at the top to form a tent over the mushrooms. Pinch the sides closed to form a sealed package.

Transfer to slow cooker and cook on high for 3 hours until mushrooms are cooked through and the cheese is melted.

Barley Risotto with Mushrooms and Pumpkin

SERVES 4

COOK TIME: HIGH 2-3 HRS

- 3 tbsps butter
- 1 tbsp olive oil
- ½ cup (50g) finely chopped spring onion
- 350g button mushrooms
- 350g butternut pumpkin, diced
- 1½ cups (300g) pearl barley
- 1 tsp salt + more to taste
- ½ tsp pepper + more to taste
- ¼ cup (60ml) dry white wine (or water)
- ½ cup (50g) grated carrot
- 4 cups (1L) chicken stock
- 1 cup (100g) finely grated Parmesan cheese
- ¼ cup (10g) finely chopped fresh dill

Heat 1 tablespoon butter and oil in a large deep-sided frying pan over medium-high heat. Add the spring onions and cook, stirring, for 2-3 minutes until tender. Add mushrooms and pumpkin and fry for 2 minutes until the mushrooms start to soften.

Add barley to the pan. Add salt and pepper and cook for a further minute until starting to turn golden. Pour in the white wine (or water) and cook, stirring, for 1-2 minutes, until the liquid evaporates. Transfer the barley mixture to the slow cooker.

Add the carrot and stock to the slow cooker. Stir gently to combine.

Cover and cook on high for 2-3 hours until the liquid is absorbed and the barley and pumpkin are tender. Remove the lid and stir in half of the cheese and the remaining 2 tablespoons butter. Season to taste.

Serve hot, garnished with the remaining cheese and dill.

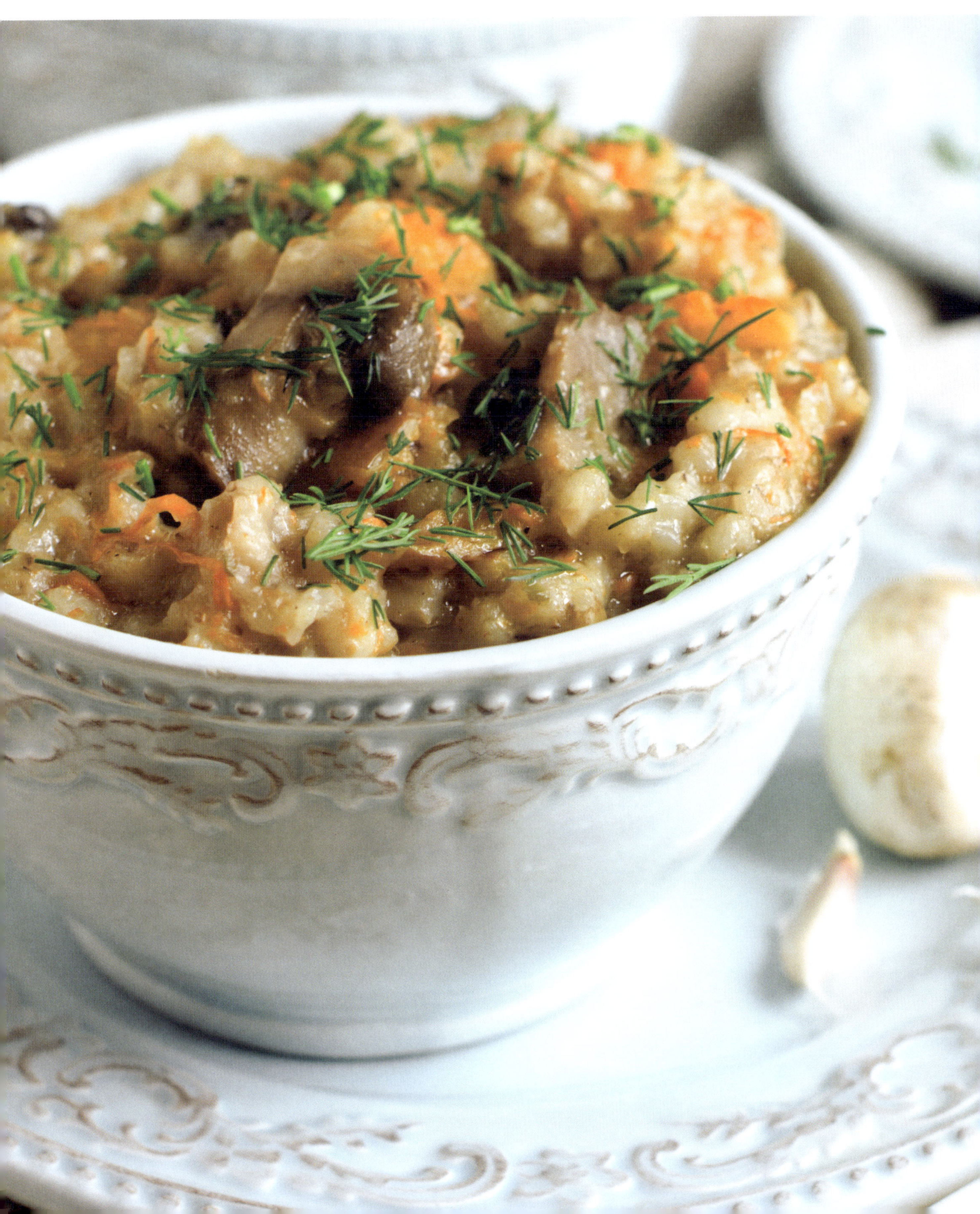

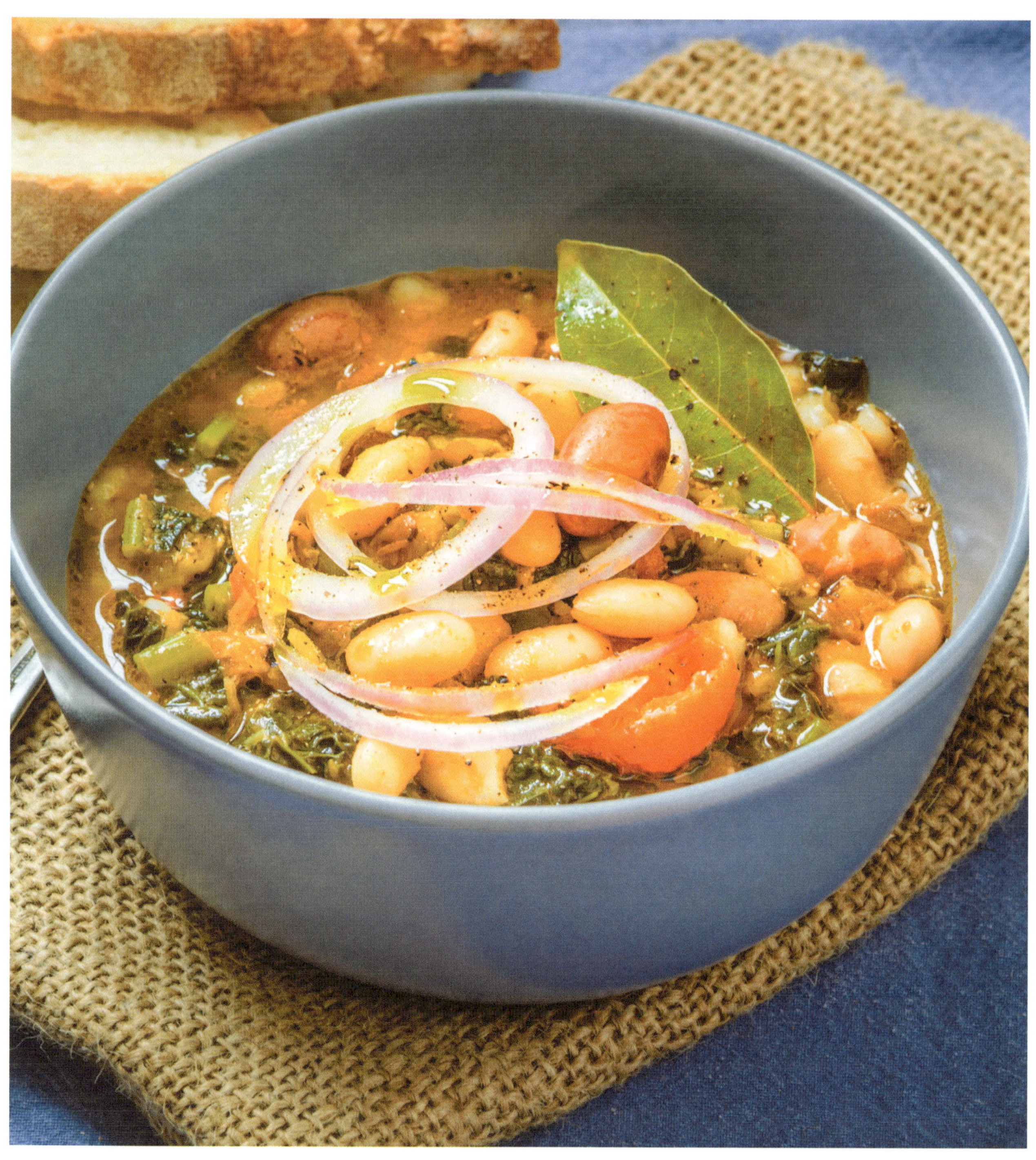

Ribollita

SERVES 6

COOK TIME: LOW 8 HRS

DAIRY FREE

RIBOLLITA

75g pancetta, diced
1 large onion, finely chopped
2 stalks celery, finely chopped
1 carrot, finely chopped
1 bulb fennel, finely chopped
3 cloves garlic, crushed
500g cherry tomatoes
2 sprigs fresh rosemary
4 bay leaves
½ tsp dried chilli flakes
8 cups (2L) water
400g cavolo nero, shredded coarsely
1 x 400g can cannellini beans, drained and rinsed
1 x 400g can mixed beans, drained and rinsed
½ cup (20g) coarsely chopped fresh basil
250g sourdough bread, torn into chunks
Salt and pepper to taste
Olive oil, to serve
Sliced red onion, to serve

Combine pancetta, onion, celery, carrot, fennel, garlic, tomatoes, rosemary, bay leaves, chilli and water in the slow cooker. Cook, covered, on low for 8 hours.

Add the cavolo nero, beans, basil and bread to the soup and stir to combine. Cook, covered, on high for about 20 minutes or until cavolo nero is wilted.

Season to taste, drizzle with olive oil and scatter with red onion to serve.

NOTE: *for a vegetarian version of this dish, simply omit the pancetta.*

HOT AND SOUR SOUP

8 cups (2L) vegetable stock
¼ cup (60ml) soy sauce (or tamari)
¼ cup (60ml) rice wine vinegar
½ cup (75g) canned bamboo shoots, thinly sliced
3 carrots, julienned or cut into long thin strips
350g mushrooms, sliced
Medium piece fresh ginger, grated
1 red chilli, deseeded and chopped
1 tbsp Sriracha
1 tsp white pepper
1 tsp sugar
350g firm tofu, cut into 1cm-thick slices
2 spring onions, sliced

Pour stock into the slow cooker. Stir in soy sauce, rice wine vinegar, bamboo shoots, carrots, mushrooms, ginger, chilli, Sriracha, white pepper, sugar and tofu.

Cover and cook on low for 6-8 hours or high for 3-4 hours.

Spoon into bowls and garnish with spring onions to serve.

BUFFALO CAULIFLOWER

1 cup (250ml) water
1 cup (225g) passata
¾ cup (185ml) barbecue sauce
4 tbsps butter, melted
1 vegetable stock cube, crumbled
2 tbsps hot sauce (such as Sriracha)
2 cloves garlic, minced
1 head cauliflower, cut into florets
2 tbsps chopped parsley, to serve
2 tbsps toasted sesame seeds, to serve

Stir together water, passata, barbecue sauce, butter, stock cube, hot sauce and garlic in slow cooker. Add cauliflower and stir to coat.

Cover and cook on high for about 2 hours.

Remove from slow cooker and arrange on a baking tray.

Place under a hot grill for 1-2 minutes.

Sprinkle with parsley and sesame seeds to serve.

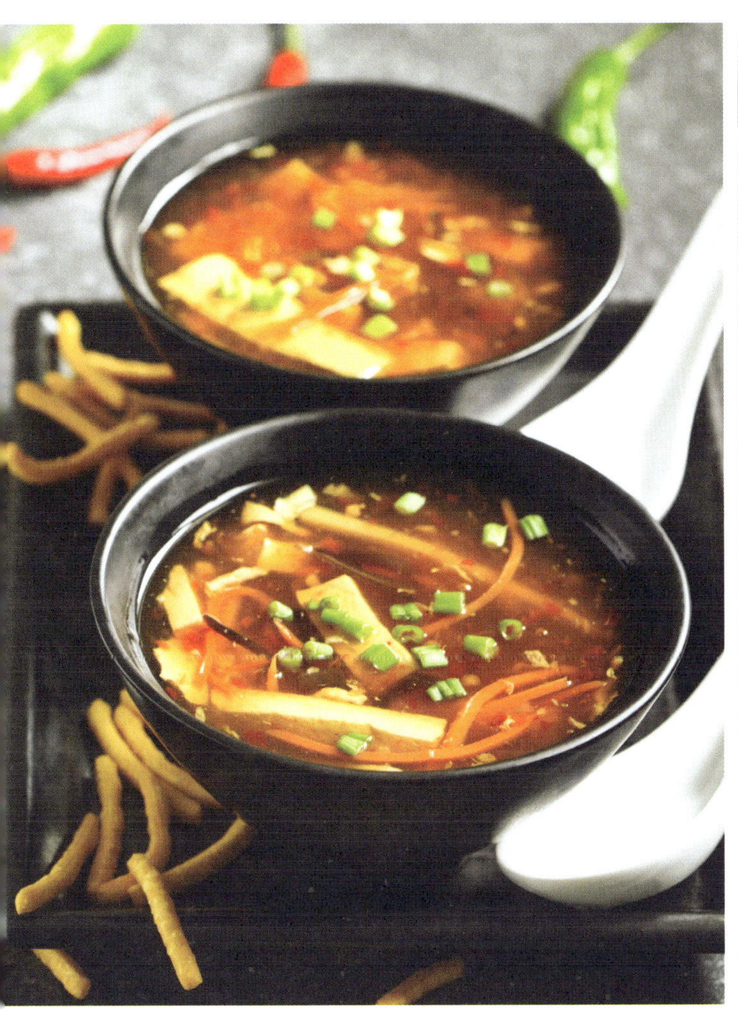

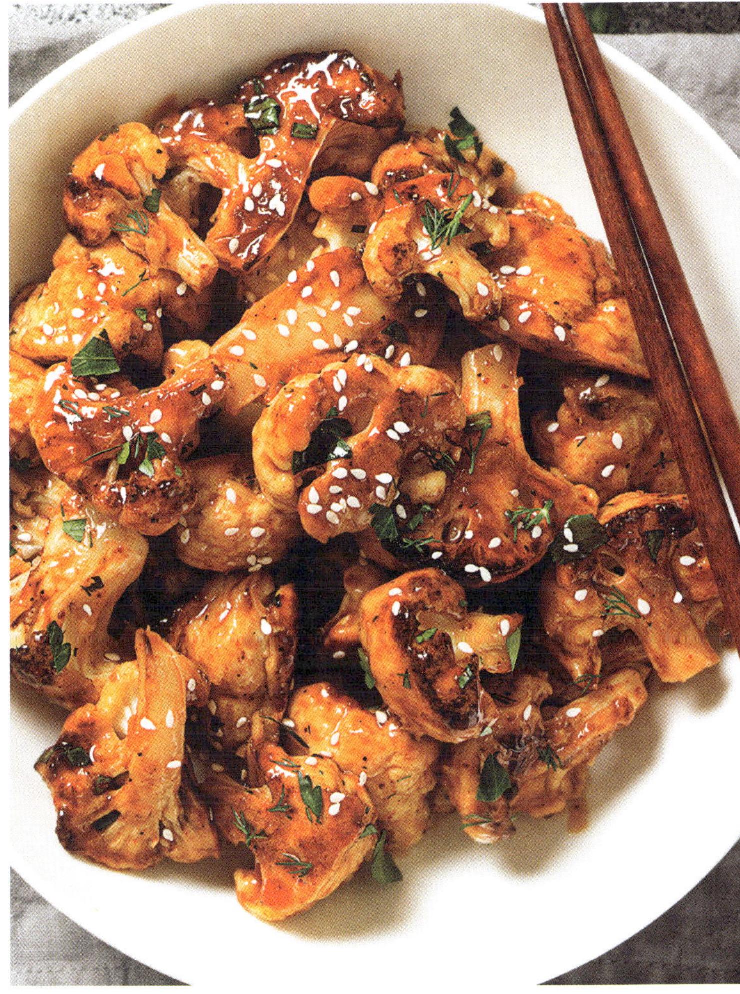

Hot and Sour Soup

SERVES 4-6

COOK TIME: HIGH 3-4 HRS/LOW 6-8 HRS

GLUTEN FREE • DAIRY FREE

Buffalo Cauliflower

SERVES 6

COOK TIME: HIGH 2 HRS

GLUTEN FREE • DAIRY FREE

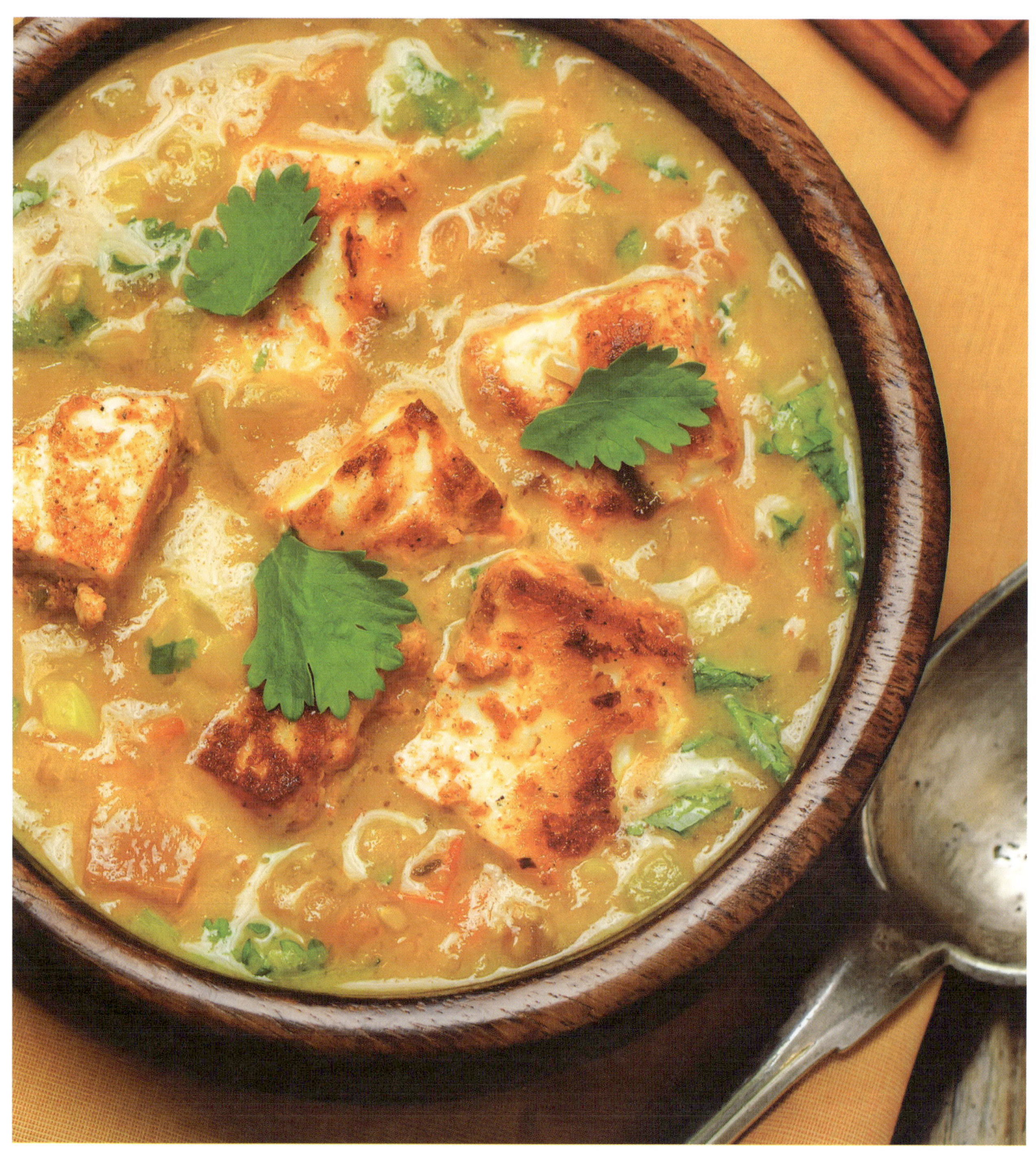

Paneer Tikka Masala

SERVES 4

COOK TIME: HIGH 4½-5 HRS

GLUTEN FREE

PANEER TIKKA MASALA

450g paneer cheese, cut into bite-size cubes
1 onion, chopped
2 yellow or red capsicums, cut into chunks
2 cloves garlic, minced
Small piece ginger, minced
2 x 400g tins chopped tomatoes
2 tsps smoked paprika
1½ tsps ground cumin
1 tsp ground turmeric
1 tsp ground coriander
Salt and pepper to taste
4 tbsps double cream
Fresh coriander leaves, to serve

Place paneer, onion, capsicum, garlic, ginger, tomatoes, paprika, cumin, turmeric and coriander into the slow cooker. Season with salt and pepper. Stir to combine.

Cover and cook on high for 4½–5 hours.

Add the cream and mix well. Top with fresh coriander to serve.

Stuffed Tomatoes

SERVES 4-5
COOK TIME: LOW 2-4 HRS
GLUTEN FREE

10 vine-ripened tomatoes
1 cup (250g) ricotta
¼ cup (25g) grated Parmesan
1 clove garlic, minced
2 tbsps fresh chopped basil
1⅔ cups (50g) baby spinach, chopped
Salt and pepper to taste
¼ cup (60ml) water
2 tbsps olive oil
Chopped chives, to serve

Cut the tops off the tomatoes and set aside. Use a small sharp spoon to scoop out the core and seeds of each tomato. Discard.

In a large bowl place ricotta, Parmesan, garlic, basil and spinach. Season with salt and pepper and mix well.

Spoon mixture into each tomato and place the tops back on the tomatoes.

Pour water into slow cooker then carefully place tomatoes in the water. Drizzle olive oil over tomatoes.

Cover and cook on low for 2-4 hours.

Scatter with chives to serve.

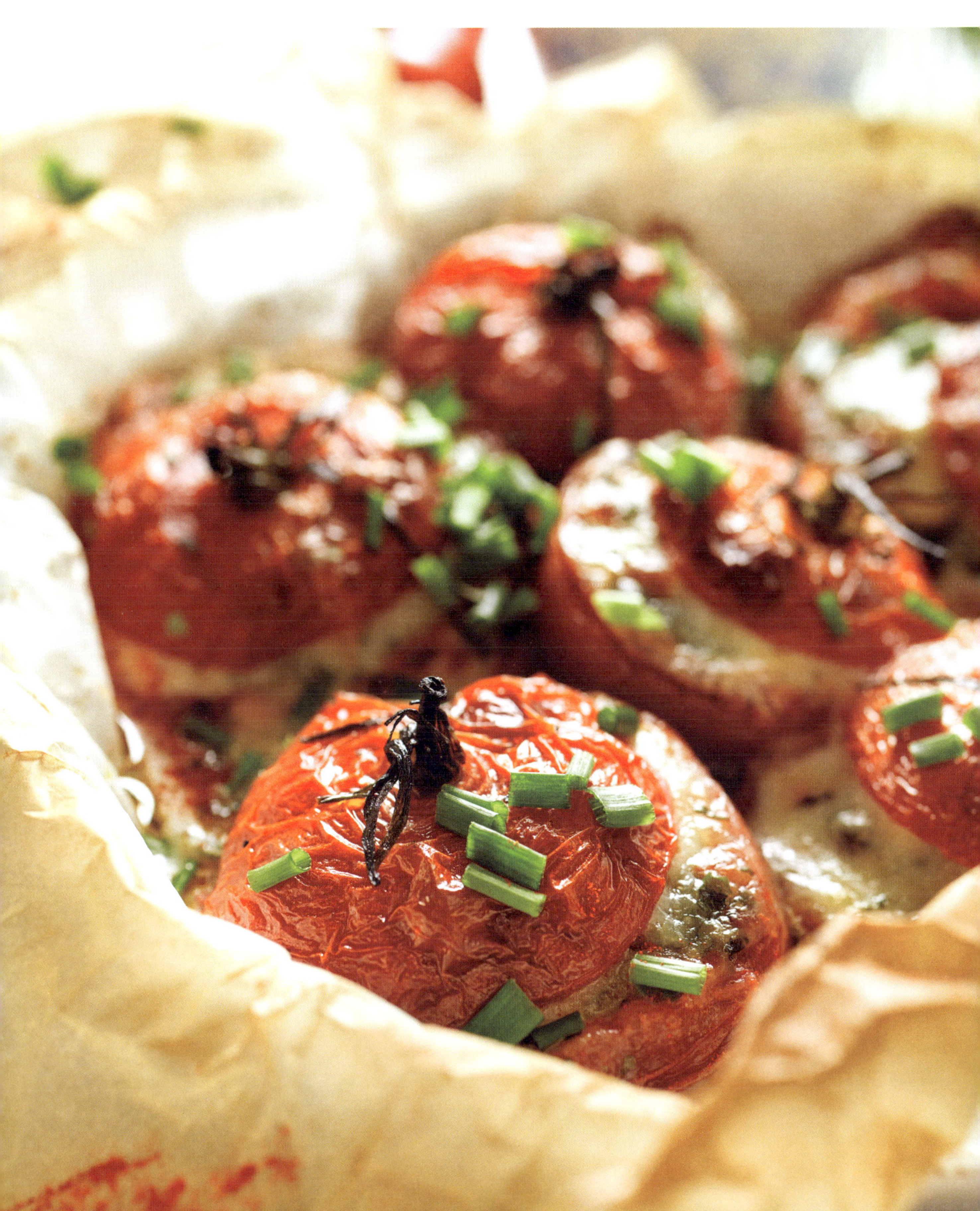

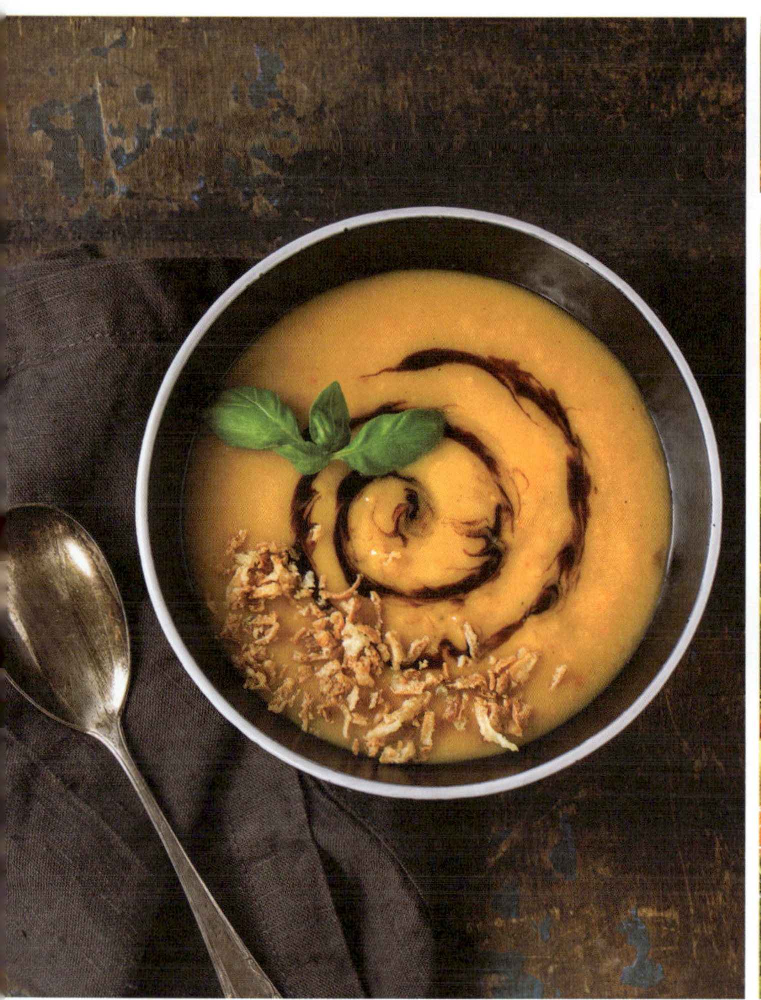

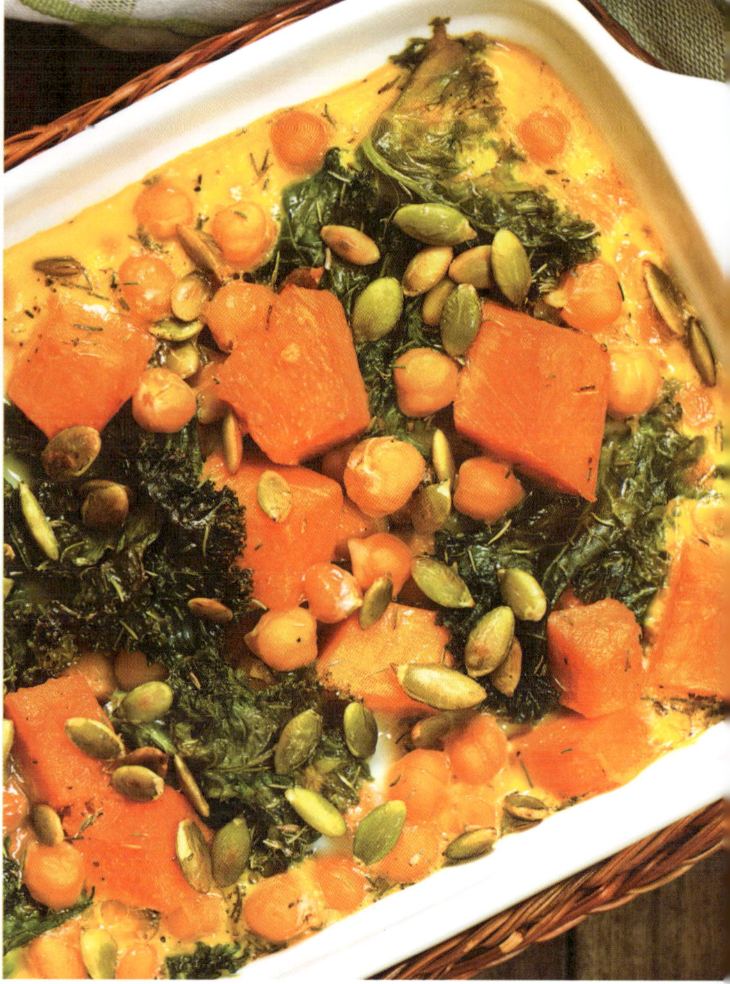

Sweet Potato Soup

SERVES 4

COOK TIME: HIGH 4 HRS/LOW 6 HRS

GLUTEN FREE • DAIRY FREE

Pumpkin, Kale and Chickpea Casserole

SERVES 4

COOK TIME: HIGH 4 HRS/LOW 8 HRS

GLUTEN FREE • DAIRY FREE

SWEET POTATO SOUP

2 tbsps olive oil

1 onion, chopped

2 stalks celery, sliced

2 medium carrots, chopped

3 cloves garlic, minced

1.5kg sweet potatoes, roughly chopped

5 cups (1.25L) vegetable stock

Salt and pepper to taste

¼ cup (60ml) balsamic glaze

¼ cup (15g) crispy shallots

Heat oil in a frying pan over medium heat. Add onion, celery, carrot and garlic. Cook for 10 minutes, stirring regularly, until vegetables are tender.

Transfer to slow cooker along with sweet potato and stock. Season with salt and pepper.

Cover and cook on low for 6 hours or on high for 4 hours.

Blend until smooth using a stick blender.

Spoon into bowls. Drizzle with balsamic glaze and scatter with crispy shallots to serve.

PUMPKIN, KALE AND CHICKPEA CASSEROLE

600g pumpkin, peeled, seeded and cut into 3cm cubes

1 x 400g can chickpeas, drained

2 tbsps tomato paste

1 tsp turmeric

3 cups (750ml) vegetable stock

1 bunch kale, hard stems removed, coarsely chopped

Toasted pepitas, to garnish

Combine the pumpkin, chickpeas, tomato paste, turmeric and stock in the slow cooker.

Cover and cook on high for 4 hours or low for 8 hours. Add the kale with 30 minutes or 1 hour left of cooking respectively.

Serve with a garnish of toasted pepitas.

Cabbage Rolls

SERVES 4

COOK TIME: LOW 7-9 HRS

12 large savoy cabbage leaves

1 large egg, beaten

1 cup (225g) + ¼ cup (60g) tomato passata

½ small onion, finely chopped

1 tsp salt

¼ tsp pepper

1kg beef mince

1 cup (165g) cooked rice

¼ cup (60ml) vegetable stock

1 tbsp brown sugar

1 tbsp lemon juice

1 tsp Worcestershire sauce

2 tbsps finely chopped fresh parsley

1 tbsp finely chopped fresh dill

1 cup (250ml) sour cream (or Greek yoghurt)

Prepare a large bowl of boiling water. Immerse cabbage leaves in water for about 3 minutes or until limp. Drain and set aside.

In a large bowl combine egg, ¼ cup of passata, onion, salt, pepper, beef and cooked rice.

Place about ¼ cup of the meat mixture in the centre of each cabbage leaf. Tuck in each short end and roll lengthwise. Place seam-side down in the slow cooker.

Combine the 1 cup passata, stock, brown sugar, lemon juice and Worcestershire sauce in a small mixing bowl and whisk to combine. Pour the mixture over the cabbage rolls.

Cover and cook on low for 7-9 hours.

Serve warm, garnished with parsley, dill and sour cream.

NOTE: ***cabbage is the hero in this dish, but note that it contains beef mince so is not suitable for vegetarians.***

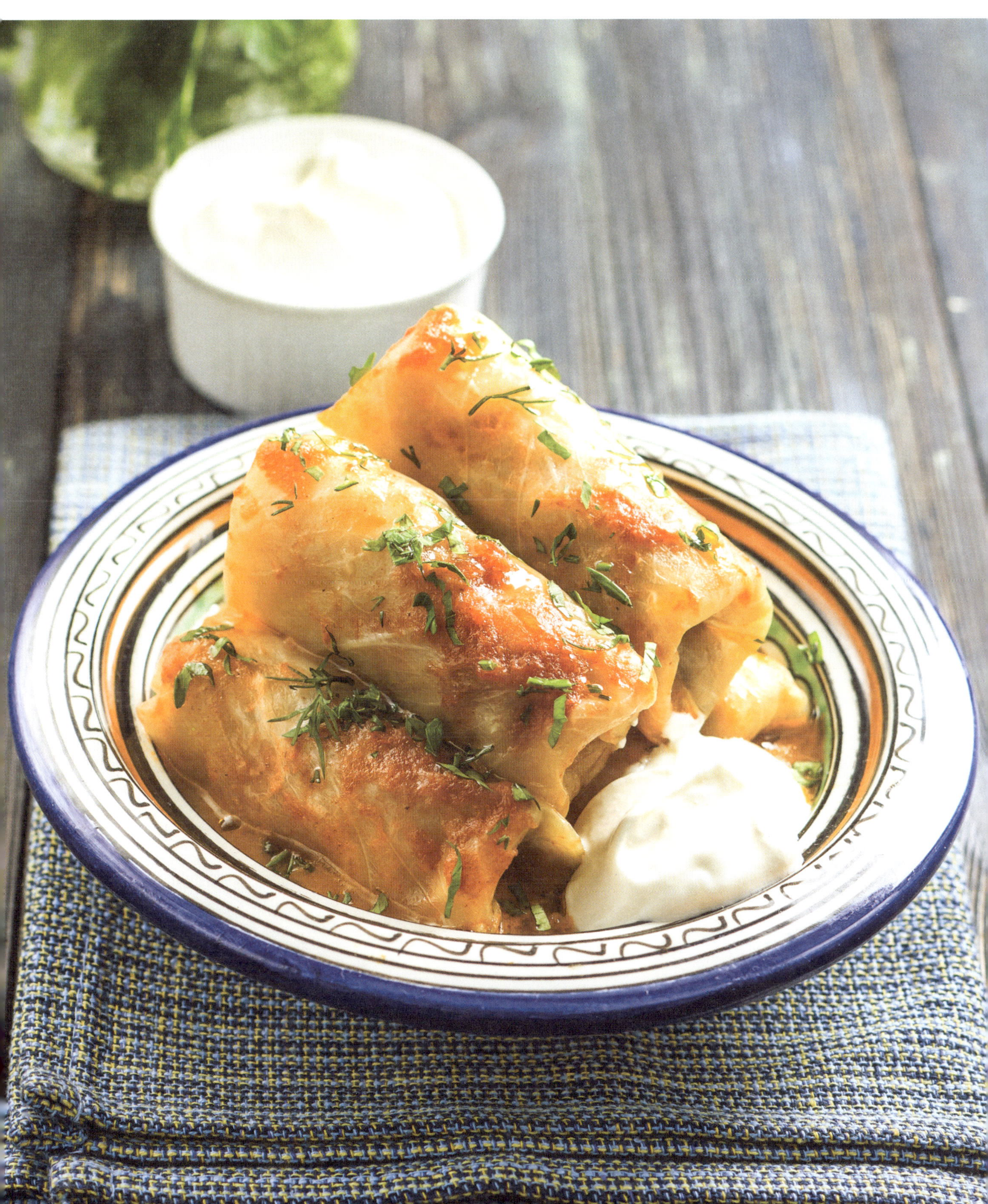

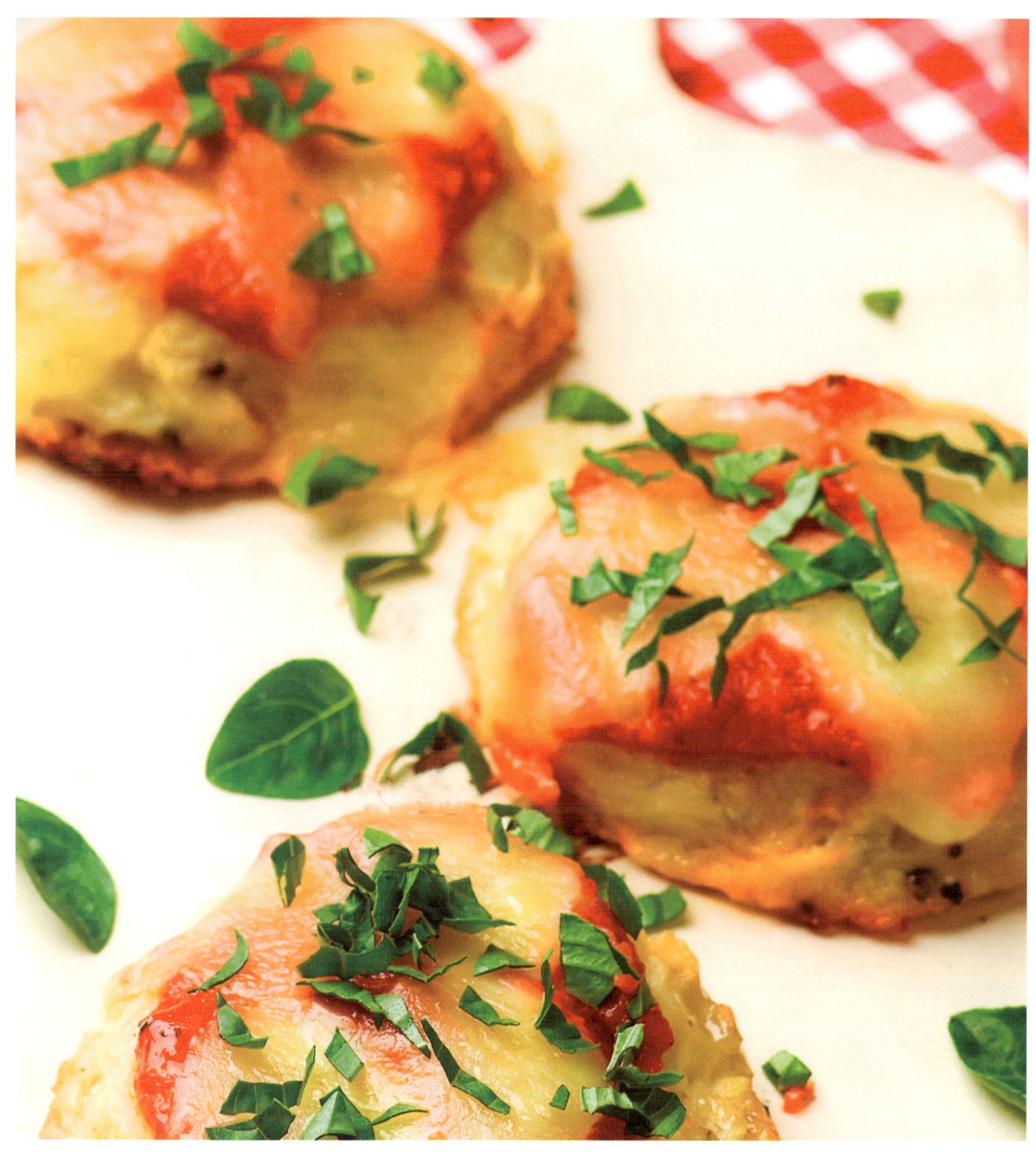

Cheese and Tomato Pizzettes on Cauliflower Base

SERVES 4

COOK TIME: HIGH 2 HRS

GLUTEN FREE

CHEESE AND TOMATO PIZZETTES ON CAULIFLOWER BASE

1 cauliflower head, roughly chopped
2 tbsps olive oil
1 egg white
⅔ cup (80g) mozzarella cheese, grated
¼ cup (25g) Parmesan cheese, grated
3 large tomatoes, thickly sliced
1 cup (125g) Cheddar cheese, grated
Salt and pepper to taste

Place the cauliflower in a blender or food processor and pulse until it is finely chopped.

In a mixing bowl combine the cauliflower with the oil, egg white, mozzarella and Parmesan. Using hands, form the mixture into mini pizza bases.

Place tomato slices on each base and sprinkle generously with Cheddar. Arrange the pizzas in the base of the slow cooker and cook on high for 2 hours or until the cheese is melted and the crust browned.

Season with salt and pepper to serve.

LEEK AND POTATO SOUP

500g Sebago potatoes, peeled and diced
4 leeks, sliced, white and light green parts only
4 cups (1L) vegetable stock
2 tbsps butter
1 tsp chopped thyme leaves
1 tsp salt
¼ tsp pepper
¼ cup (60ml) sour cream

Place the potatoes, leeks, stock, butter, thyme, salt and pepper in the slow cooker and stir to combine. Cover and cook on high for 4 hours or on low for 8 hours.

Use a stick blender, or transfer the soup in batches to a stand blender, and blend until smooth.

Add the sour cream and whisk to combine.

Ladle into bowls to serve.

QUINOA WITH EGGPLANT AND TOMATO

1½ cups (250g) quinoa
1 tbsp olive oil
3 cups (750ml) vegetable stock
1 eggplant, diced
2 cloves garlic, minced
Salt and pepper to taste
300g cherry tomatoes, halved
Fresh coriander, chopped, to garnish

Rinse the quinoa then place it in the slow cooker. Add the olive oil and stir through to coat the quinoa. Stir in the stock, eggplant and garlic and season well with salt and pepper.

Cook on high for 3 hours or low for 6 hours. Add the tomatoes with 30 minutes left of cooking.

Stir through chopped coriander before serving if desired.

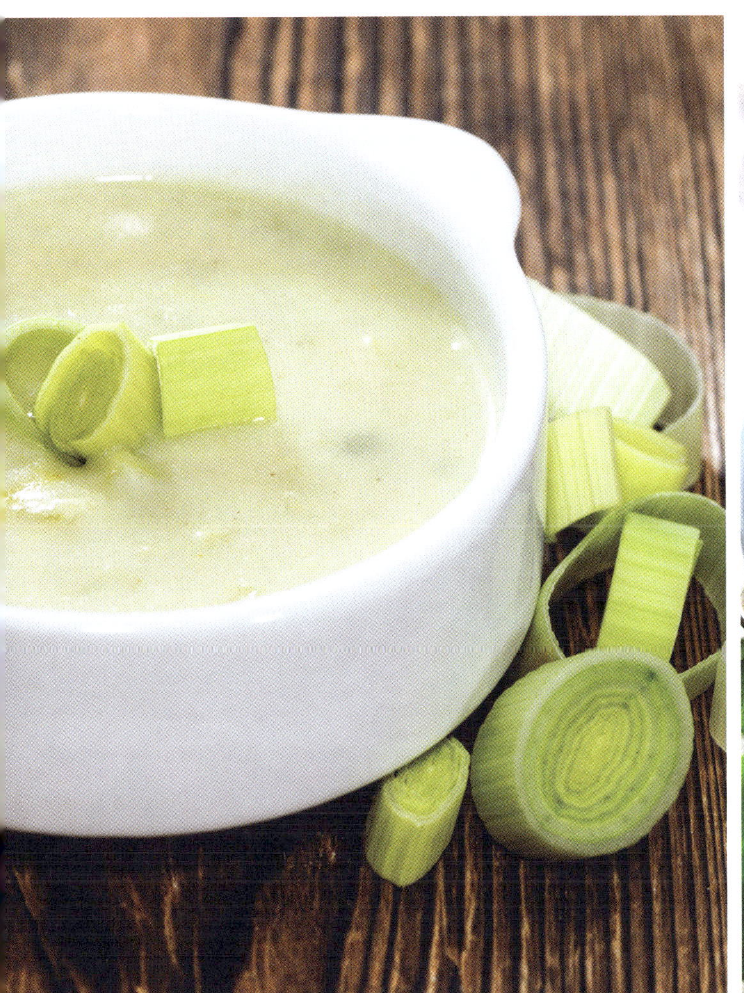

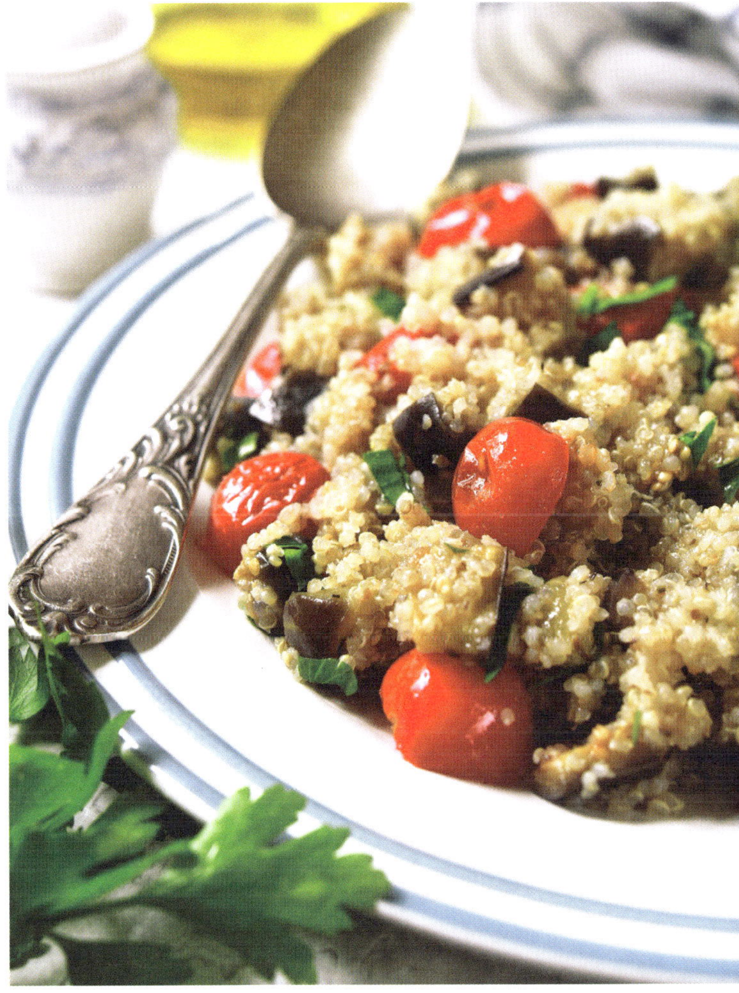

Leek and Potato Soup

SERVES 4-6

COOK TIME: HIGH 4 HRS/LOW 8 HRS

GLUTEN FREE

Quinoa with Eggplant and Tomato

SERVES 4

COOK TIME: HIGH 3 HRS/LOW 6 HRS

GLUTEN FREE • DAIRY FREE

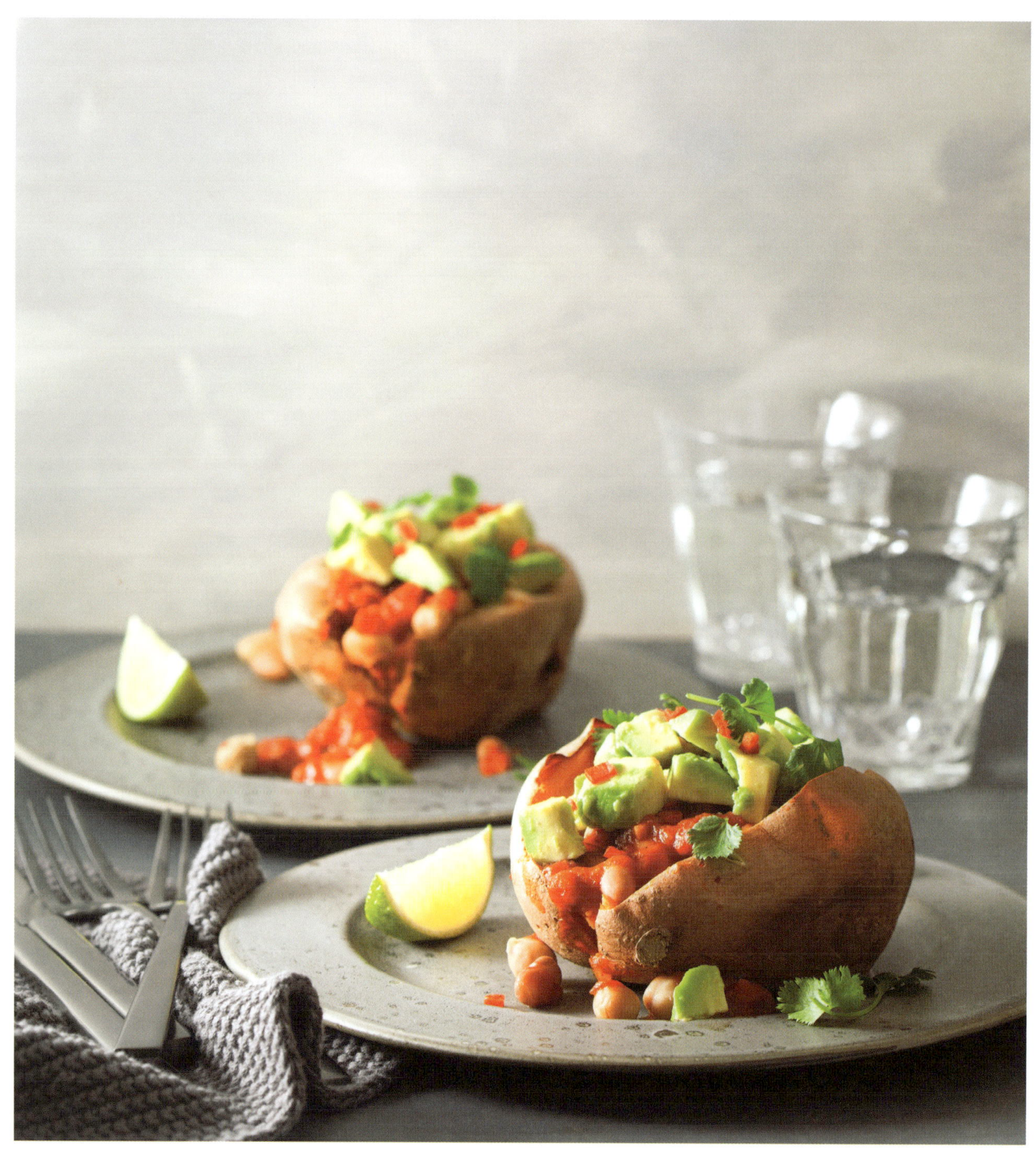

Baked Sweet Potatoes with Warm Chickpea Salsa

SERVES 4

COOK TIME: HIGH 3-3½ HRS/LOW 6-7 HRS

GLUTEN FREE • DAIRY FREE

BAKED SWEET POTATOES WITH WARM CHICKPEA SALSA

4 medium sweet potatoes
1 tbsp olive oil
1 red onion, finely chopped
2 cloves garlic, minced
½ tsp dried chilli flakes
2 tsps ground cumin
1 tsp ground paprika
1 x 400g can chopped tomatoes
1 x 400g can chickpeas including the chickpea water
Salt and pepper to taste
1 avocado, diced
¼ cup (5g) fresh coriander leaves
1 lime, cut into wedges

Scrub sweet potatoes and place in one layer in slow cooker; cover and cook on low for 6-7 hours or on high for 3-3½ hours.

Meanwhile heat olive oil in a large frying pan over medium-high heat. Add red onion and cook, stirring, for 3-5 minutes, until soft and translucent. Add garlic, chilli, cumin and paprika. Cook for 1 minute until fragrant.

Add tomatoes, chickpeas and ½ cup chickpea water. Bring to the boil, then simmer for 15-20 minutes. Season with salt and pepper.

When sweet potatoes are cooked, cut in half and spoon in chickpea salsa. Top with diced avocado and coriander leaves. Squeeze over lime juice to serve.

Spinach and Feta Cannelloni

SERVES 4

COOK TIME: LOW 3 HRS

2 tbsps butter

2 tbsps plain flour

1⅔ cups (410ml) milk

Salt and pepper to taste

2 pinches nutmeg

1 pkt frozen spinach, thawed and squeezed dry

1¼ cups (315g) ricotta cheese

1 egg, whisked

1 clove garlic, minced

10 cannelloni tubes

350g mozzarella cheese, torn

¼ cup (25g) grated Parmesan cheese

Melt butter in a large pan over medium heat. Add flour and whisk to a thick paste.

After a few seconds, add milk a little at a time, whisking continually until milk starts to boil. When all milk is added reduce heat to low and keep whisking until sauce starts to thicken.

When sauce is thick enough to coat a spoon, season with salt, pepper and a pinch of nutmeg to taste. Remove from heat and set aside.

In a bowl, stir together spinach, ricotta cheese, egg and garlic. Season with salt and pepper and a pinch of nutmeg. Using a piping bag, pipe mixture into cannelloni tubes to fill.

Spread a thin layer of white sauce over base of slow cooker. Place stuffed cannelloni in one layer on top of sauce. Sprinkle with pieces of mozzarella and top with a thicker layer of white sauce, ensuring pasta is completely covered. Sprinkle with Parmesan cheese.

Cover and cook on low for 3 hours.

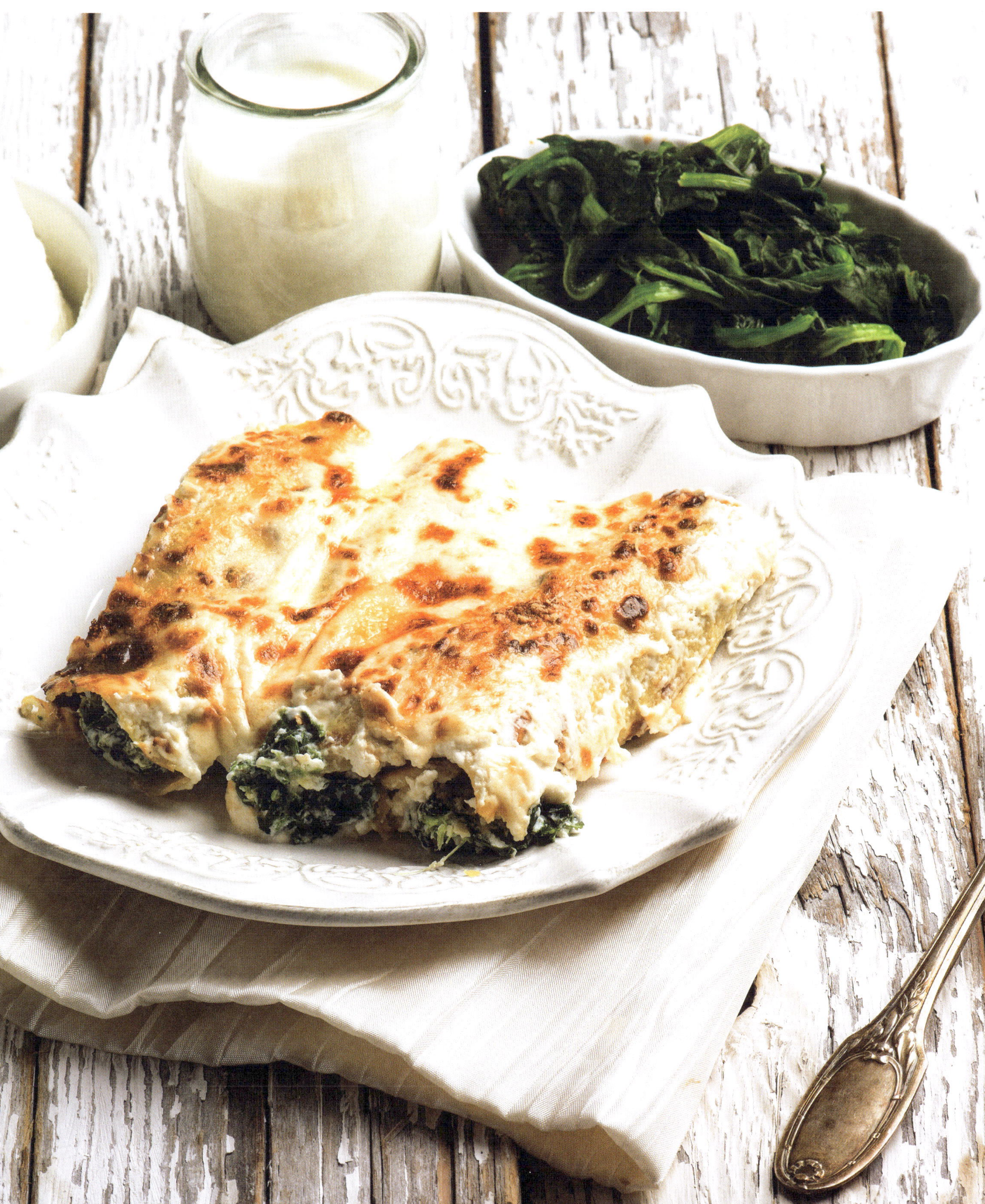

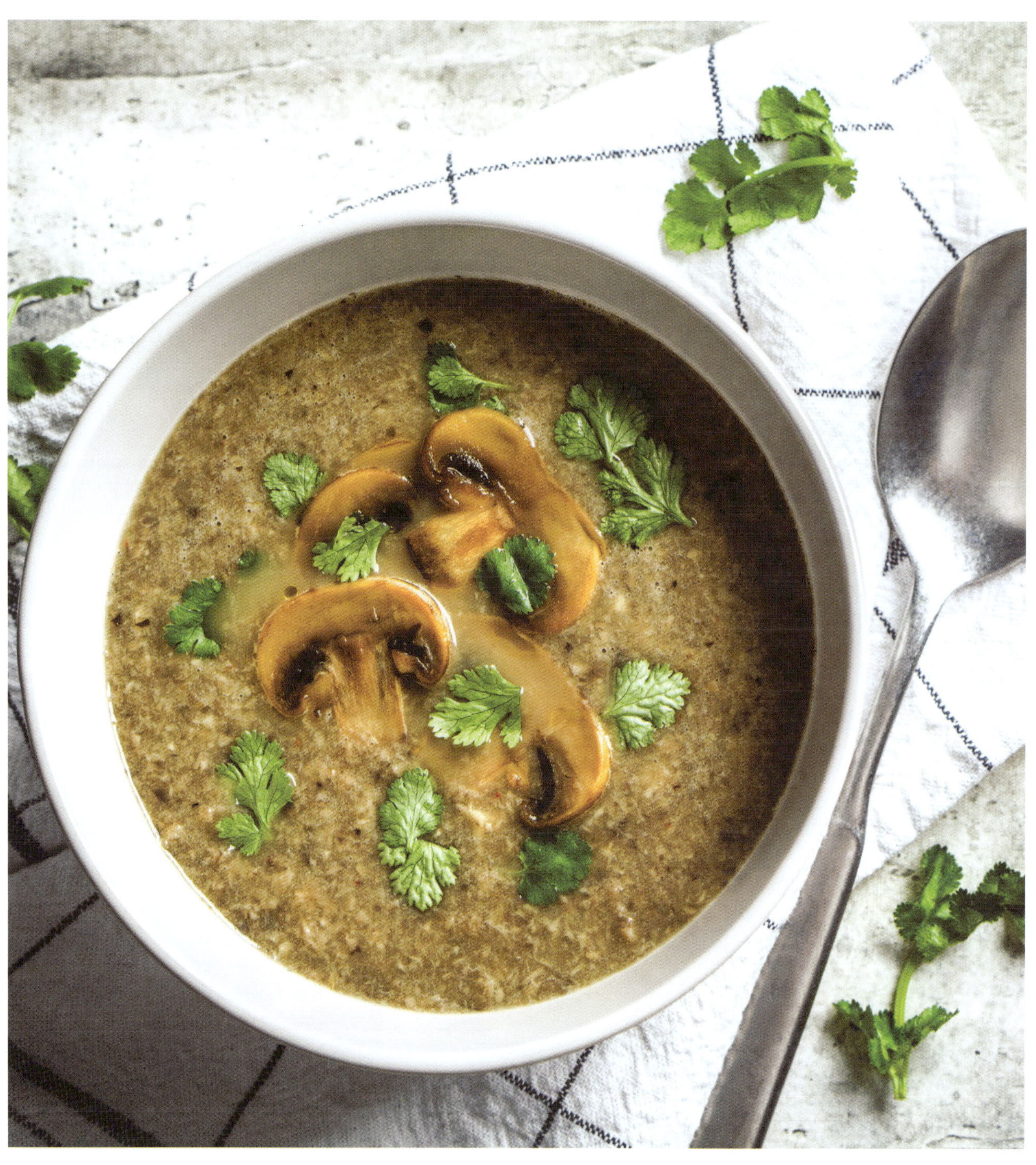

Mushroom Soup

SERVES 4

COOK TIME: LOW 4-5 HRS

GLUTEN FREE

MUSHROOM SOUP

750g chestnut mushrooms, sliced
4 tbsps unsalted butter, melted
½ tsp salt
1 medium onion, diced
2 cloves garlic, minced
2 cups (500ml) vegetable stock
2 tbsps dry sherry
10g dried porcini mushrooms
½ tsp pepper
½ tsp dried thyme
¼ tsp dried tarragon
½ cup (125ml) cream
2 tsps fresh lemon juice
Coriander leaves, to garnish

Preheat oven to 190°C. Line a baking tray with greaseproof paper.

Place mushrooms on prepared baking try. Drizzle with melted butter, sprinkle with salt and toss to combine. Spread into a single layer. Roast for 15-17 minutes until mushrooms are tender and most of the liquid has evaporated.

Set aside a few mushroom slices for garnish if you wish.

Transfer remaining mushrooms and their liquid to the slow cooker. Add onion, garlic, stock, sherry, porcini mushrooms, pepper, thyme and tarragon, and stir to combine. Cover and cook on low for 3-4 hours.

Use a stick blender, or transfer the soup in batches to a stand blender, and blend until smooth.

Return soup to the slow cooker and cook on low for 1-2 hours. Stir in cream and lemon juice, then ladle into bowls and serve topped with reserved mushrooms and fresh coriander leaves.

Potato Gratin

SERVES 8
COOK TIME: HIGH 4-5 HRS
GLUTEN FREE

1.2kg potatoes, peeled
1½ cups (375ml) thickened cream
3 cloves garlic, minced
1 sprig thyme, leaves picked
1 tbsp chopped fresh rosemary leaves
Pinch of nutmeg
Salt and pepper to taste
1 cup (125g) grated Cheddar cheese
¼ cup (25g) freshly grated Parmesan

Use a mandoline or sharp knife to cut potatoes into 3mm-thick slices.

In a medium saucepan, whisk together cream, garlic, thyme, rosemary and nutmeg over medium heat, for 2 minutes, until hot.

Add a layer of potatoes to slow cooker in an overlapping pattern; season with salt and pepper. Pour ⅓ cup cream mixture over potatoes; sprinkle with Cheddar. Repeat with remaining potato slices, cream mixture and Cheddar to create more layers.

Cover and cook on high for 4-5 hours, or until potatoes are tender. Sprinkle with Parmesan. Cover and cook on high for about 5 minutes.

Remove lid and let potatoes rest for 15 minutes, allowing the sauce to thicken as it sits.

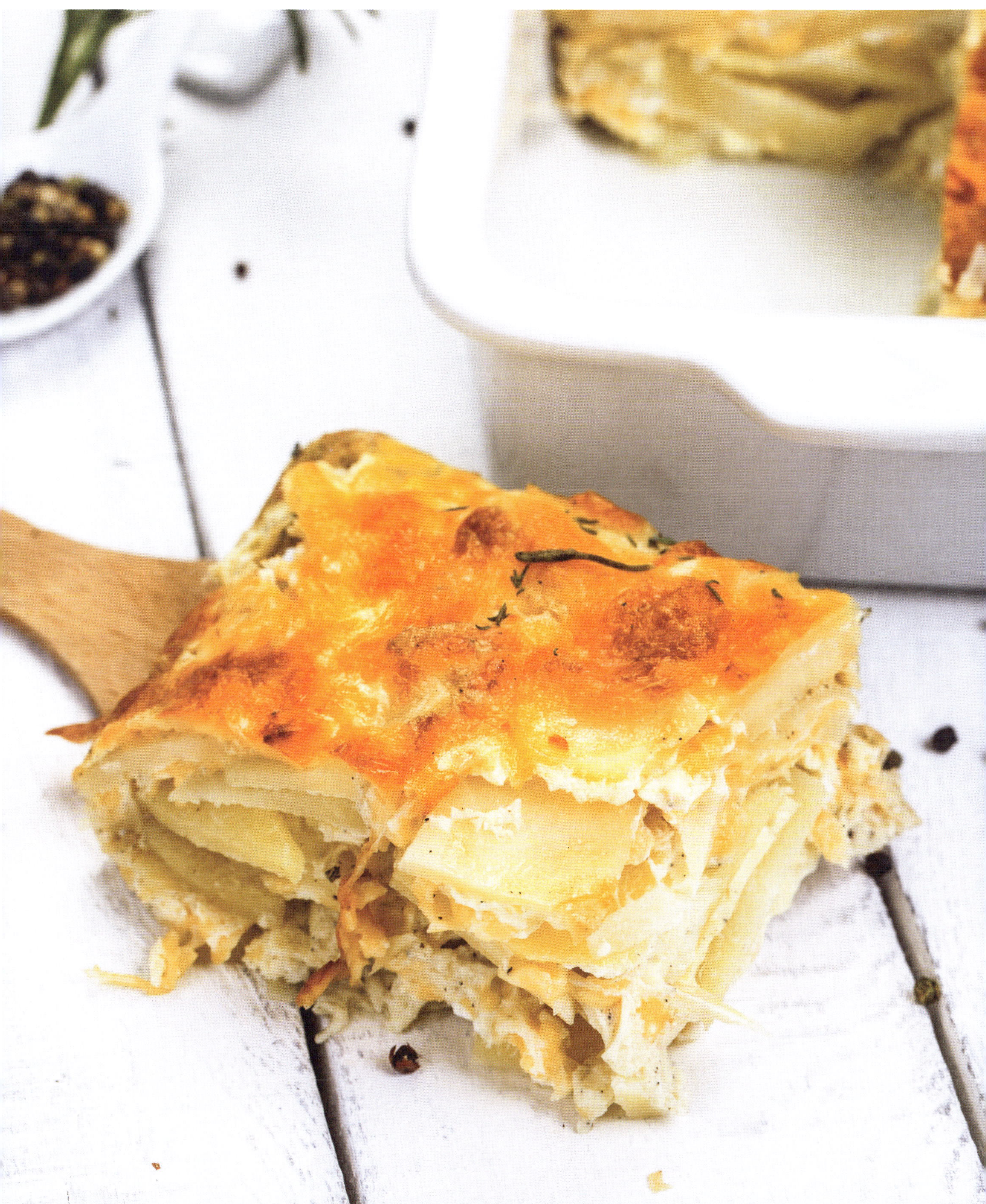

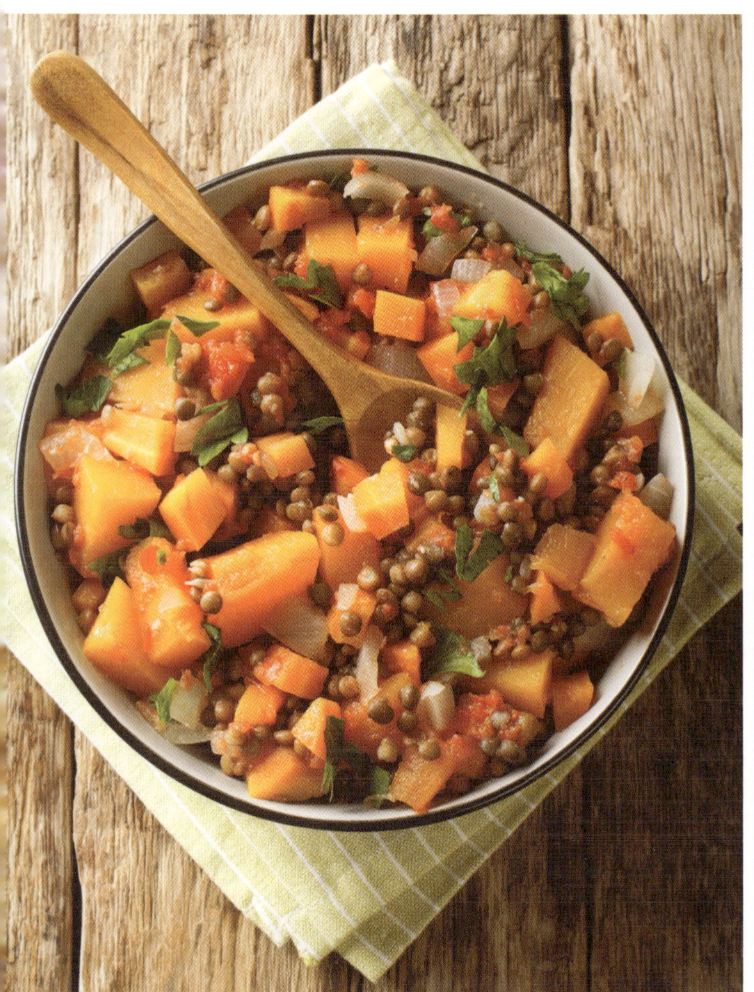

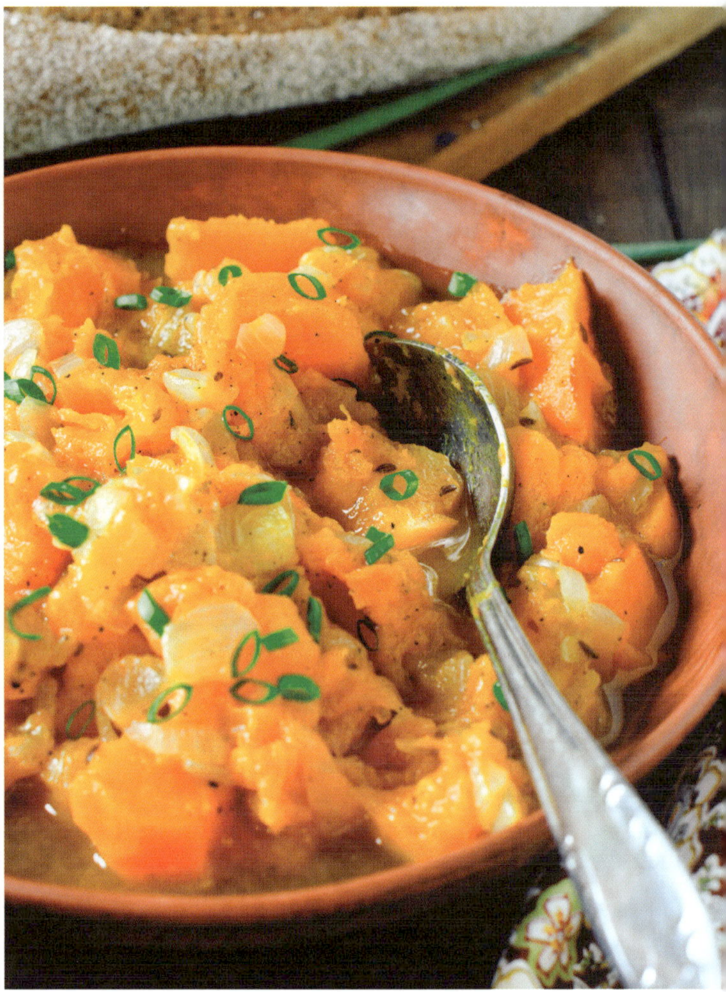

Pumpkin and Lentil Stew

SERVES 6

COOK TIME: LOW 5-6 HRS

GLUTEN FREE • DAIRY FREE

Spiced Pumpkin Stew

SERVES 4

COOK TIME: LOW 6 HRS

GLUTEN FREE • DAIRY FREE

PUMPKIN AND LENTIL STEW

500g pumpkin, cut into bite-size pieces

1 cup (185g) green lentils

1 large onion, chopped

4 cups (1L) vegetable stock

2 Roma tomatoes, chopped

2 tbsps tomato paste

Juice of 1 lime

1 tbsp cumin

1 tbsp ground ginger

1 tsp turmeric

1 tsp nutmeg

Salt and pepper to taste

Chopped fresh coriander, to serve

Place pumpkin, lentils, onion, stock, tomatoes, tomato paste, lime juice, cumin, ginger, turmeric and nutmeg in slow cooker. Season with salt and pepper. Stir to combine.

Cover and cook on low for 5-6 hours.

Scatter with chopped coriander to serve.

SPICED PUMPKIN STEW

1kg pumpkin, peeled, seeded and cut into bite-size chunks

1 large onion, finely chopped

3 cups (750ml) vegetable stock

1 tsp nutmeg

1 tbsp cumin seeds

1 tsp turmeric

Salt and pepper to taste

Fresh chives, chopped, to garnish

Place the pumpkin, onion, stock, nutmeg, cumin seeds and turmeric in the slow cooker.

Cook on low for 6 hours or until the pumpkin is tender. Season with salt and pepper and serve with a garnish of fresh chives.

Eggplant Parmigiana

SERVES 4
COOK TIME: LOW 5 HRS
GLUTEN FREE

4 tbsps olive oil
1 large onion, finely chopped
3 cloves garlic, minced
1 tbsp tomato paste
1 tsp caster sugar
½ cup (10g) basil leaves, torn
1 tsp dried oregano
1 cup (250ml) white wine
1kg cherry tomatoes, halved
½ cup (125ml) vegetable stock
Salt and pepper to taste
1 large eggplant, cut into 1cm-thick rounds
¼ cup (35g) capers, drained and rinsed
1⅔ cups (200g) grated mozzarella cheese
½ cup (50g) grated Parmesan cheese
Thyme sprigs, to serve

Heat 2 tablespoons oil in a large saucepan over medium-low heat. Add onion and cook, stirring occasionally, for 3-5 minutes until onions are soft and translucent. Stir in garlic, tomato paste and sugar and cook, stirring continuously, for 1-2 minutes. Add herbs, wine, tomatoes and stock. Season with salt and pepper. Bring to the boil then reduce heat and simmer for 10 minutes. Remove from heat and set aside.

Heat a grill pan over medium heat. Brush eggplant with remaining olive oil and place on grill pan. Grill for 2-3 minutes on each side, or until grill marks are visible. Remove from the pan and set aside.

Spoon half of the sauce into base of slow cooker. Top with eggplant slices. Spoon remaining sauce on top of eggplant slices. Scatter with capers and sprinkle with the cheeses.

Cook on low for 5 hours. Scatter with thyme sprigs to serve.

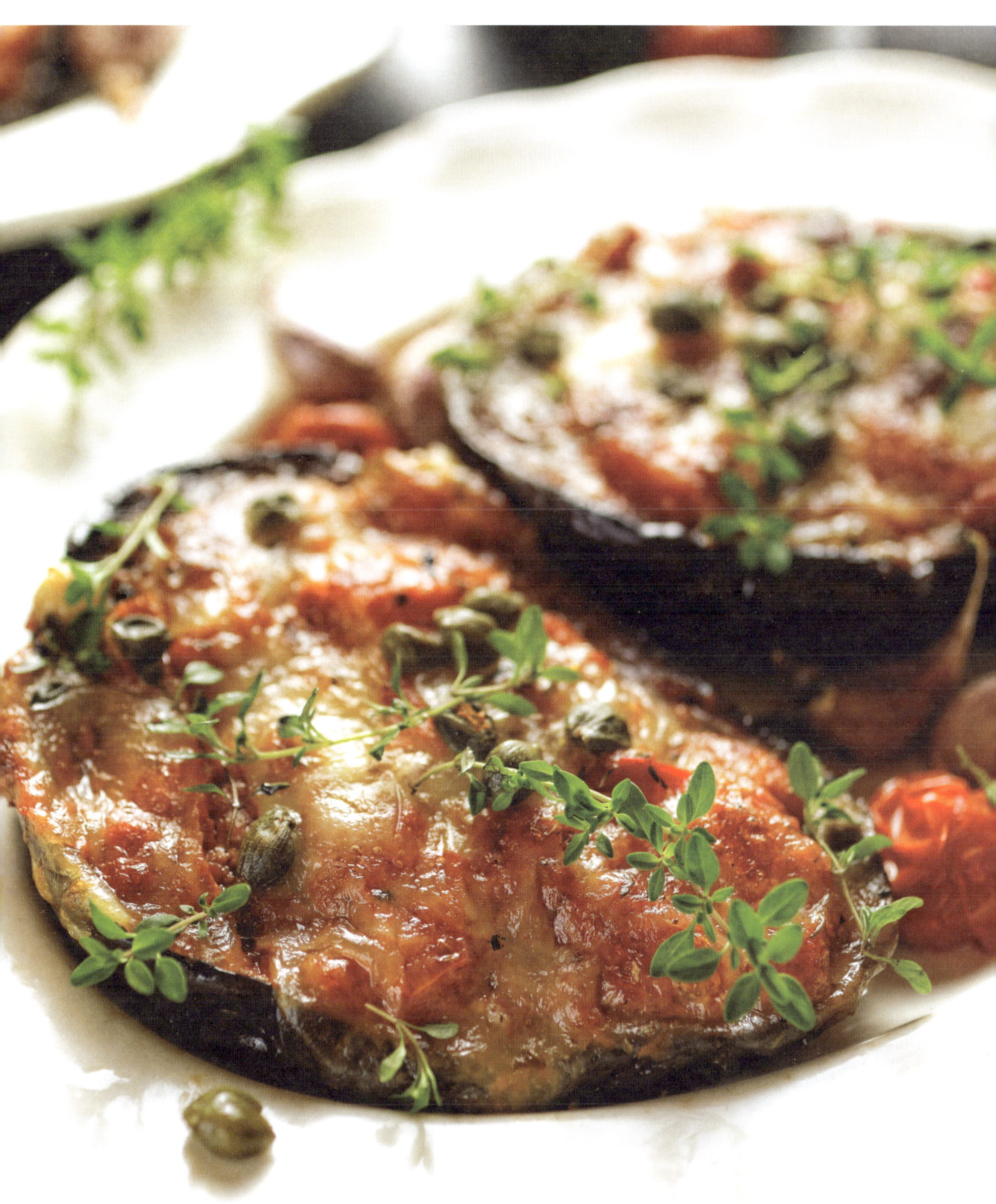

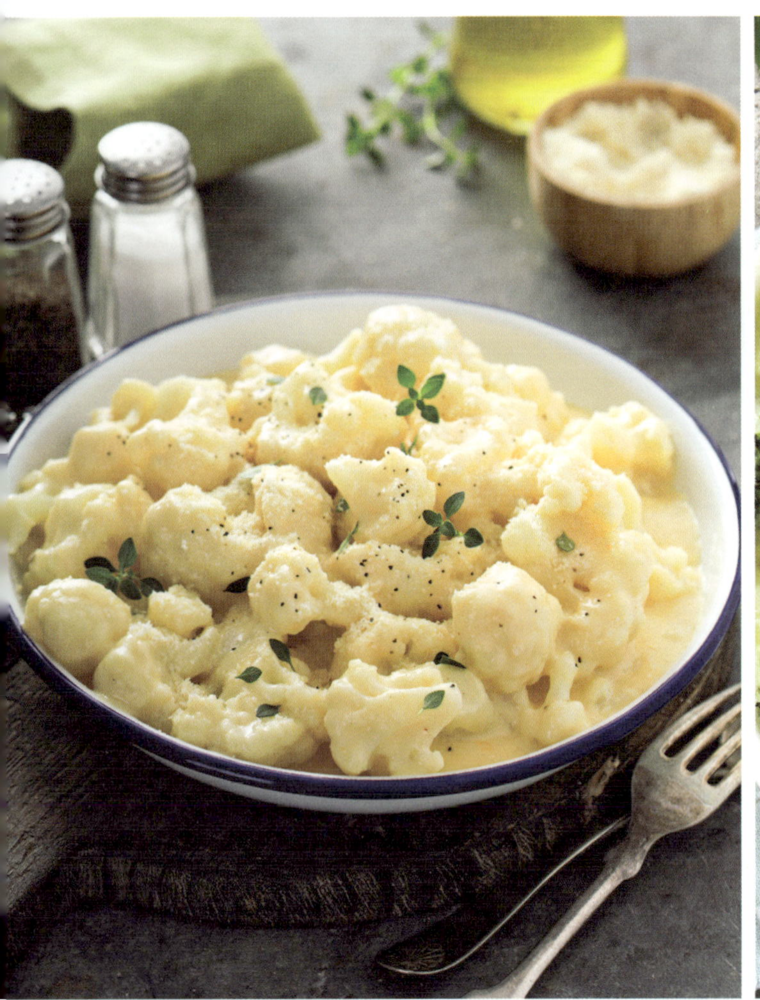

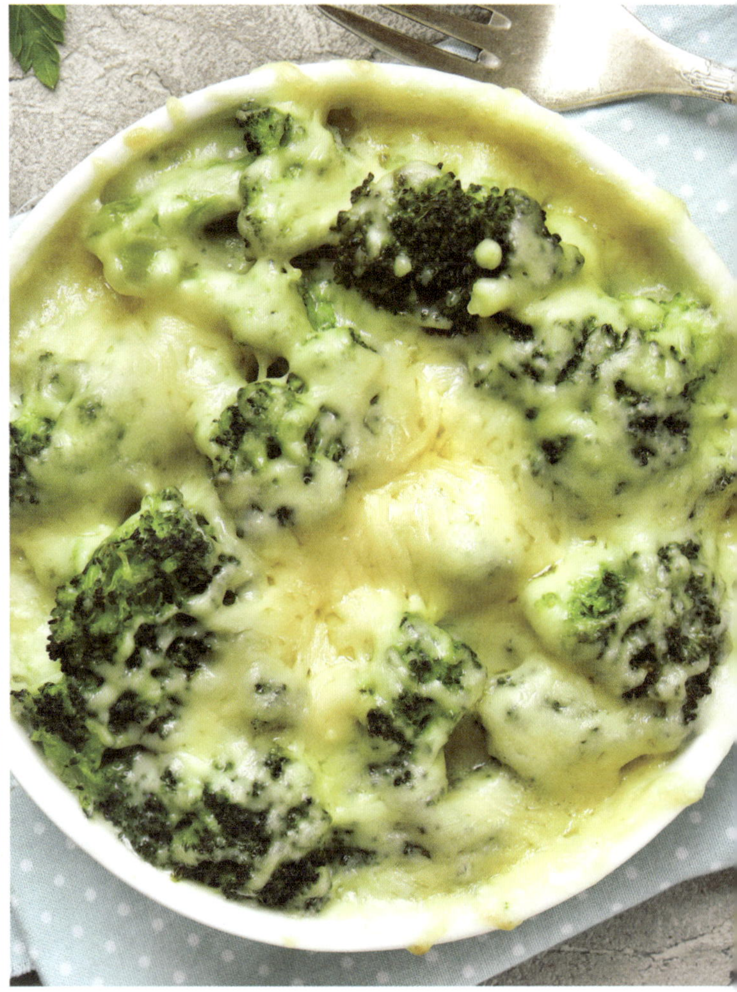

Cauliflower Cheese

SERVES 6

COOK TIME: LOW 3 HRS

Broccoli Bake

SERVES 4

COOK TIME: HIGH 3 HRS

GLUTEN FREE

CAULIFLOWER CHEESE

50g butter
3 tbsps plain flour
2 cups (500ml) milk
Salt and pepper to taste
1½ cups (185g) grated Cheddar cheese
1 head cauliflower, cut into florets
1 onion, finely chopped
½ cup (50g) grated Parmesan cheese
Fresh thyme leaves, to serve

Melt butter in a large pan over medium heat. Add flour and whisk to a thick paste. After a few seconds, add milk a little at a time, whisking continually until milk starts to boil. When all milk is added, reduce heat to low and keep whisking until sauce starts to thicken. When sauce is thick enough to coat a spoon, season with salt and pepper. Remove from heat and stir in cheese until melted.

Place cauliflower and onion into slow cooker. Pour over sauce and stir gently to coat.

Sprinkle with Parmesan cheese.

Cover and cook on low for 3 hours.

Sprinkle with thyme leaves and season with salt and pepper to serve.

BROCCOLI BAKE

500g frozen broccoli florets
1 x 410g can cream of celery soup
2 spring onions, finely chopped
Salt and pepper to taste
2 cups (250g) grated Cheddar cheese

Add broccoli, soup and spring onions to slow cooker. Season with salt and pepper. Gently stir to combine.

Cover and cook on high for 2½ hours.

Add cheese. Cover and cook for 30 minutes on high until cheese is melted.

Cheese and Vegetable Loaf

SERVES 10

COOK TIME: HIGH 2 HRS 30 MINS

1 cup (250ml) milk
1 tbsp lemon juice
2½ cups (310g) self-raising flour
2 tsps baking powder
1½ cups (185g) grated Cheddar cheese
½ cup (50g) grated Parmesan cheese
¼ cup (5g) basil leaves, chopped
4 cloves garlic, minced
1 zucchini, finely diced
1 carrot, finely diced
1 small eggplant, finely diced
Pinch of salt and pepper
1 egg, beaten

Preheat the slow cooker for 20 minutes on high.

Grease and line the slow cooker with baking paper or grease and line a loaf tin that fits inside your slow cooker. If using a loaf tin place in slow cooker on top of two egg rings or an upturned saucer.

In a small bowl add milk and lemon juice and set aside for 5-10 minutes.

In a large bowl add flour, baking powder, cheeses, basil, garlic, zucchini, carrot, eggplant, salt and pepper. Stir well to combine.

Pour prepared milk mixture into flour and vegetable mixture and stir with a wooden spoon until a dough forms.

Mould into an oval shape and carefully place in your slow cooker, or shape into a loaf shape and place in loaf tin.

Score the top of the loaf twice. Brush with beaten egg.

Cover the slow cooker with a cotton tea towel, place lid on slow cooker and fold the tea towel back over the lid.

Cook on high for 2½ hours until an inserted skewer comes out clean.

Remove and allow to cool slightly before slicing with a large sharp bread knife and serving warm with butter.

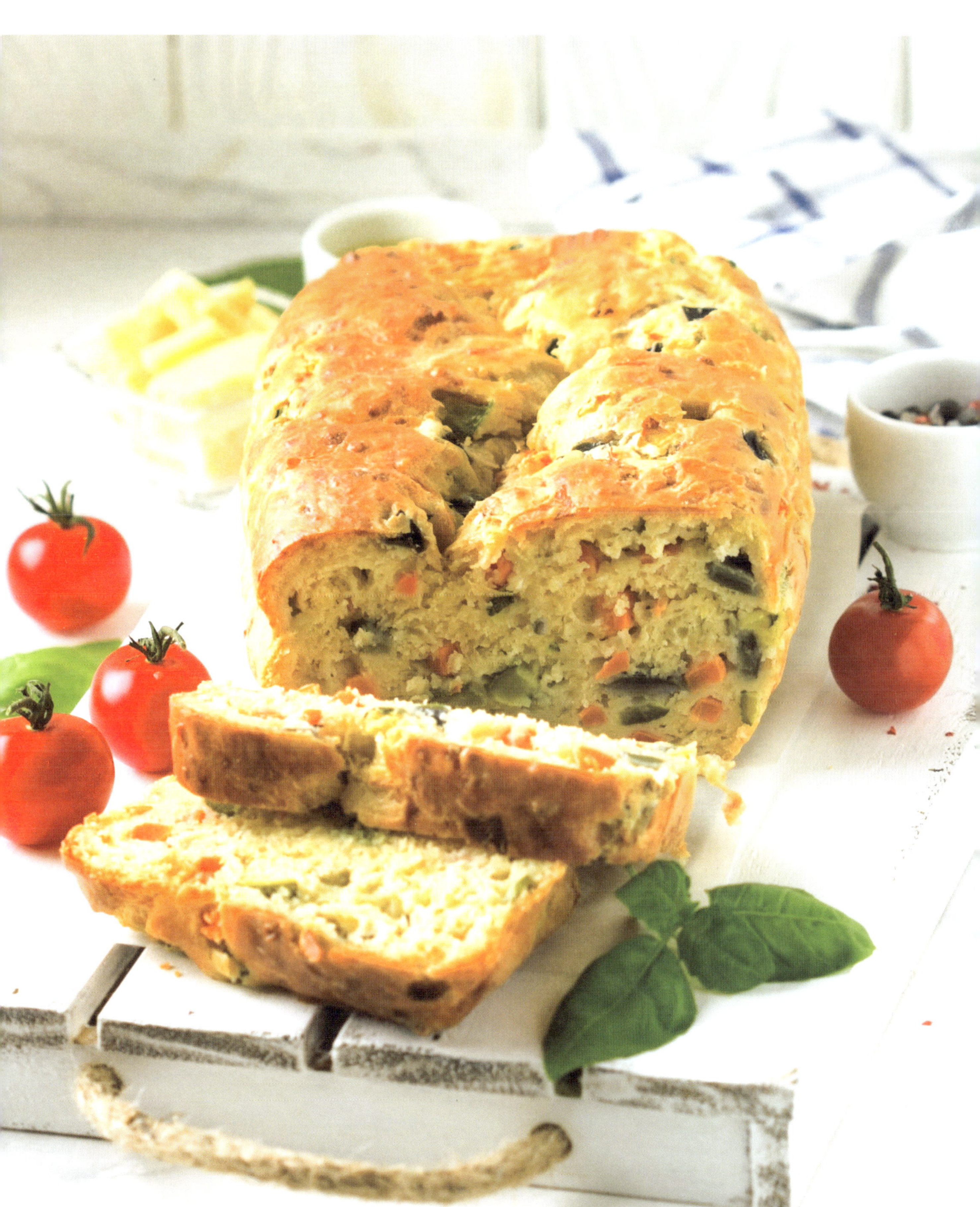

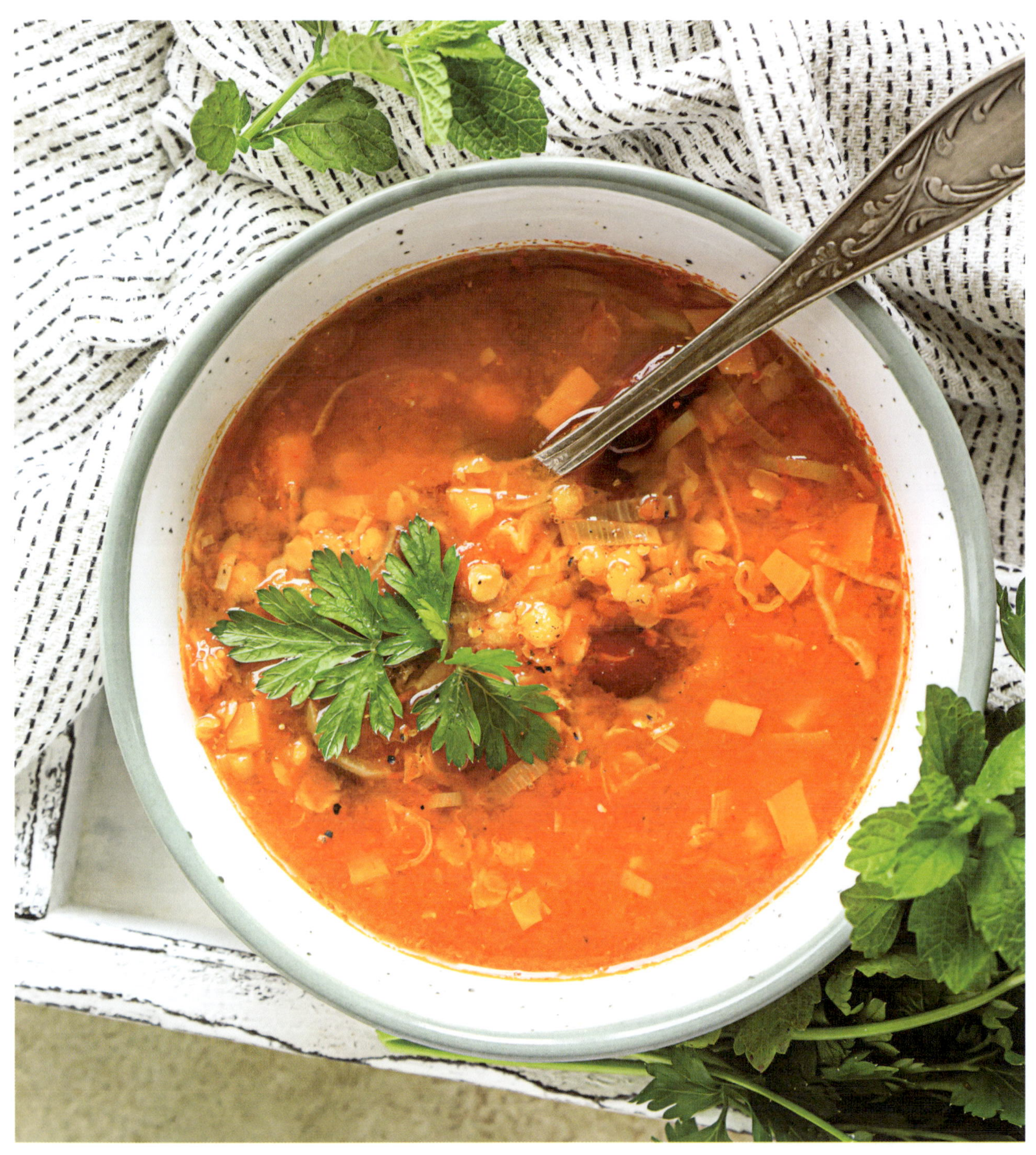

Red Lentil Soup

SERVES 4

COOK TIME: 4 HRS 30 MINS

GLUTEN FREE • DAIRY FREE

RED LENTIL SOUP

2 tsps olive oil
1 onion, diced
1 leek, sliced
2 carrots, diced
2 stalks celery, diced
2 cloves garlic, thinly sliced
Small piece fresh ginger, finely chopped
3 tsps ground cumin
3 tsps ground coriander
1½ cups (275g) red lentils
4 cups (1L) vegetable stock
2 cups (500ml) water
Salt and pepper to taste
1 x 400g can kidney beans, drained and rinsed

Heat oil in a large non-stick frying pan over medium heat. Add onion, leek, carrot and celery. Cook, stirring often, for 5-8 minutes or until soft. Add garlic, ginger, cumin and coriander. Cook, stirring regularly, for 1 minute until fragrant. Transfer to the slow cooker.

Add lentils, stock and water. Season with salt and pepper. Cover and cook on low for 4 hours or until thickened. Add kidney beans and cook for 30 minutes more.

Spoon into bowls to serve.

Marsala Mushrooms

SERVES 2-4
COOK TIME: LOW 8 HRS
GLUTEN FREE

1 tbsp butter + more for greasing
4 rashers bacon, finely chopped
1 tsp maple syrup
700g Swiss or button mushrooms, trimmed and halved
⅓ cup (50g) diced shallots
2 cloves garlic, finely chopped
2 tbsps chopped fresh parsley
¼ cup (60ml) sweet Marsala
¼ cup (60ml) chicken stock
Salt and pepper to taste
½ cup (125ml) thickened cream
1 tsp cornflour
Parmesan cheese, grated, to serve
2 tbsps chives, chopped

Heat butter in a small frying pan over medium-high heat. Add bacon and maple syrup and fry for 8 minutes until crispy. Remove from the pan and drain on paper towels.

Grease the base of the slow cooker. Arrange mushrooms across the bottom. Sprinkle with shallots, garlic and parsley.

In small bowl, mix Marsala and chicken stock; pour over mushrooms. Season with salt and pepper.

Cover and cook on low for 8 hours.

About 30-60 minutes before end of cook time, in a small bowl, stir cream with cornflour to dissolve. Pour mixture into slow cooker and gently stir to combine.

Serve with a sprinkle of Parmesan, bacon and chives.

NOTE: *mushrooms are the hero in this dish, but note that it contains bacon and chicken stock so is not suitable for vegetarians.*

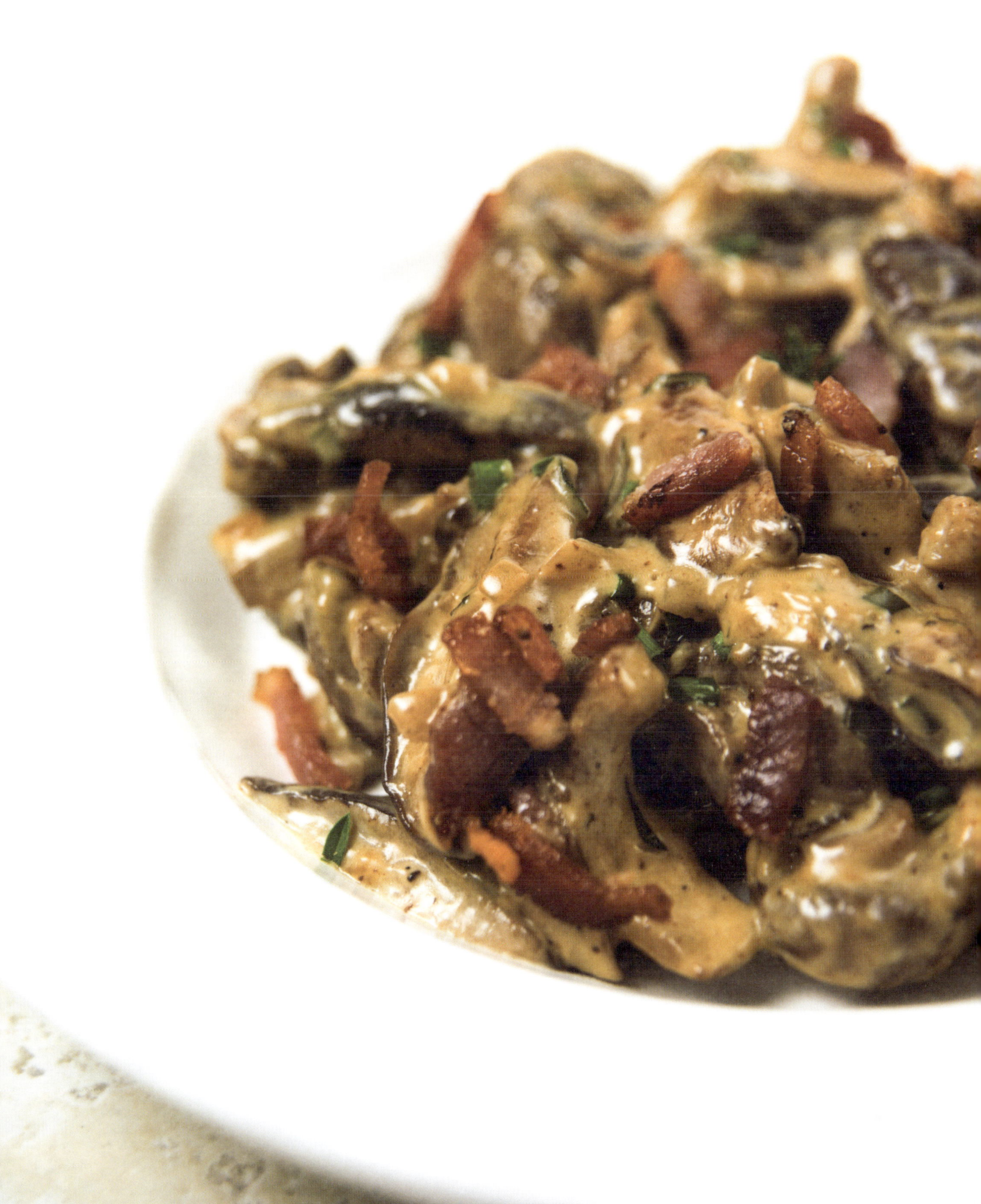

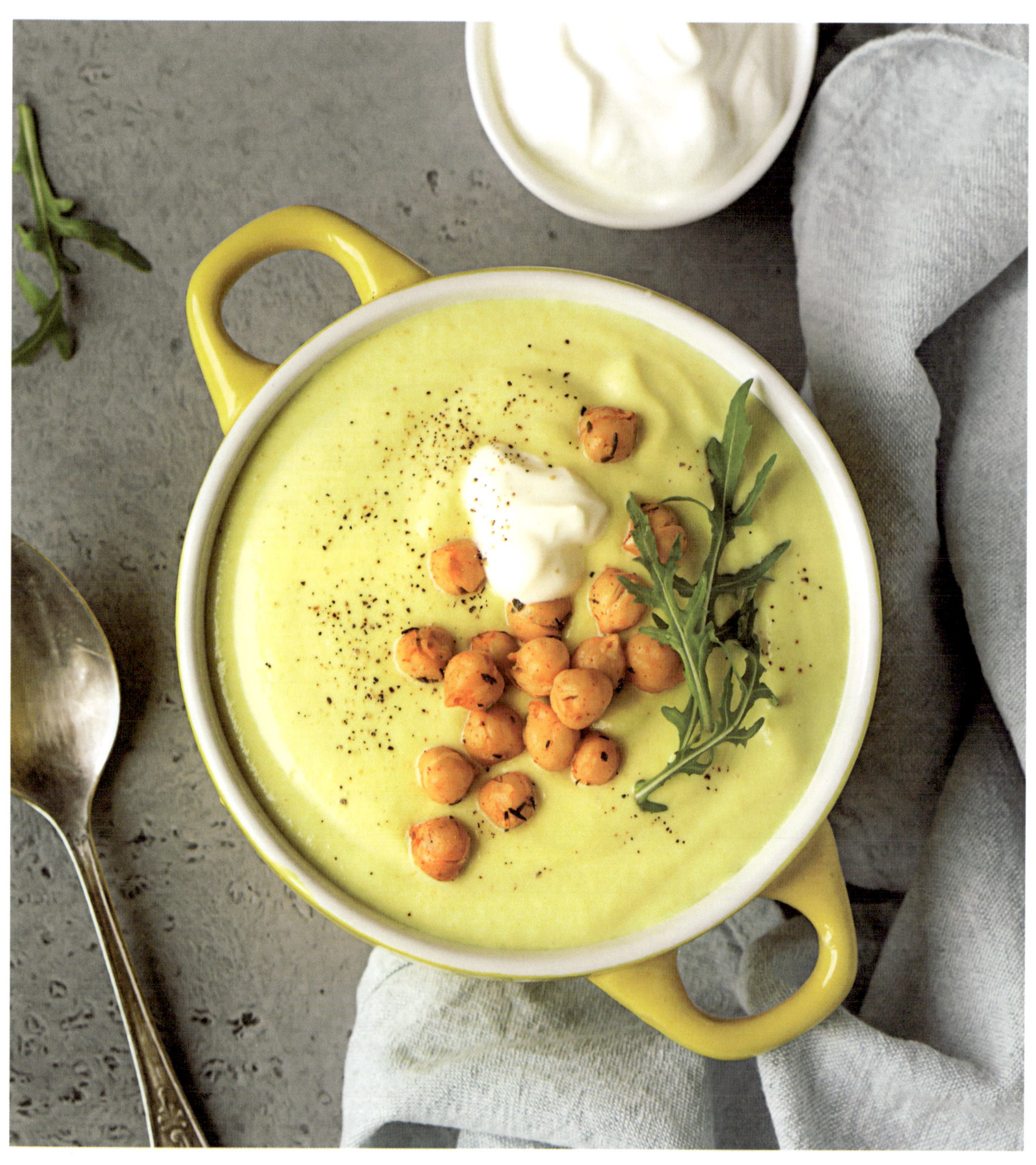

Curried Cauliflower Soup

SERVES 4

COOK TIME: HIGH 4 HRS/LOW 6-8 HRS

GLUTEN FREE • DAIRY FREE

CURRIED CAULIFLOWER SOUP

1 onion, diced
3 cloves garlic, minced
2 carrots, diced
2 stalks celery, diced
1 medium potato, peeled and diced
1 head cauliflower, cut into florets
3 tbsps curry powder
⅛ tsp cayenne pepper
Salt and pepper to taste
4 cups (1L) vegetable stock
⅓ cup (80ml) Greek yoghurt (optional)
Roasted chickpeas, to serve (optional)

Place the onion, garlic, carrots, celery, potato and cauliflower into the slow cooker. Sprinkle with curry powder and cayenne and season with salt and pepper.

Pour in stock.

Cover and cook on high for 4 hours or on low for 6-8 hours.

Using a stick blender, blend the soup until smooth and creamy.

Spoon into bowls. Season with salt and pepper and top with a dollop of yoghurt, if using. Garnish with roasted chickpeas if desired.

Coconut Stew with Quinoa and Vegetables

SERVES 6

COOK TIME: LOW 4 HRS

GLUTEN FREE • DAIRY FREE

1 x 400ml can coconut cream

4 cups (1L) vegetable stock

1 tbsp minced fresh ginger

2 tbsps green curry paste

1 tbsp fish sauce

1 tbsp grated palm sugar

1 onion, thinly sliced

1 large sweet potato, peeled and cubed

1 red capsicum, cut into long strips

1 eggplant, cubed

1 bunch Chinese broccoli, stems and leaves separated and roughly chopped

1 cup (180g) fresh edamame (optional)

½ cup (80g) quinoa

Salt and pepper to taste

1 tbsp fresh lime juice

2 tbsps chopped chives, to garnish

2 tbsps coriander leaves, to garnish

4 lime wedges, to serve

Place all ingredients except lime juice and garnishes in the slow cooker.

Cover and cook on low for 4 hours, or until the sweet potato is tender.

Stir through the lime juice and season to taste.

Ladle into bowls and garnish with chives and coriander and a lime wedge on the side.

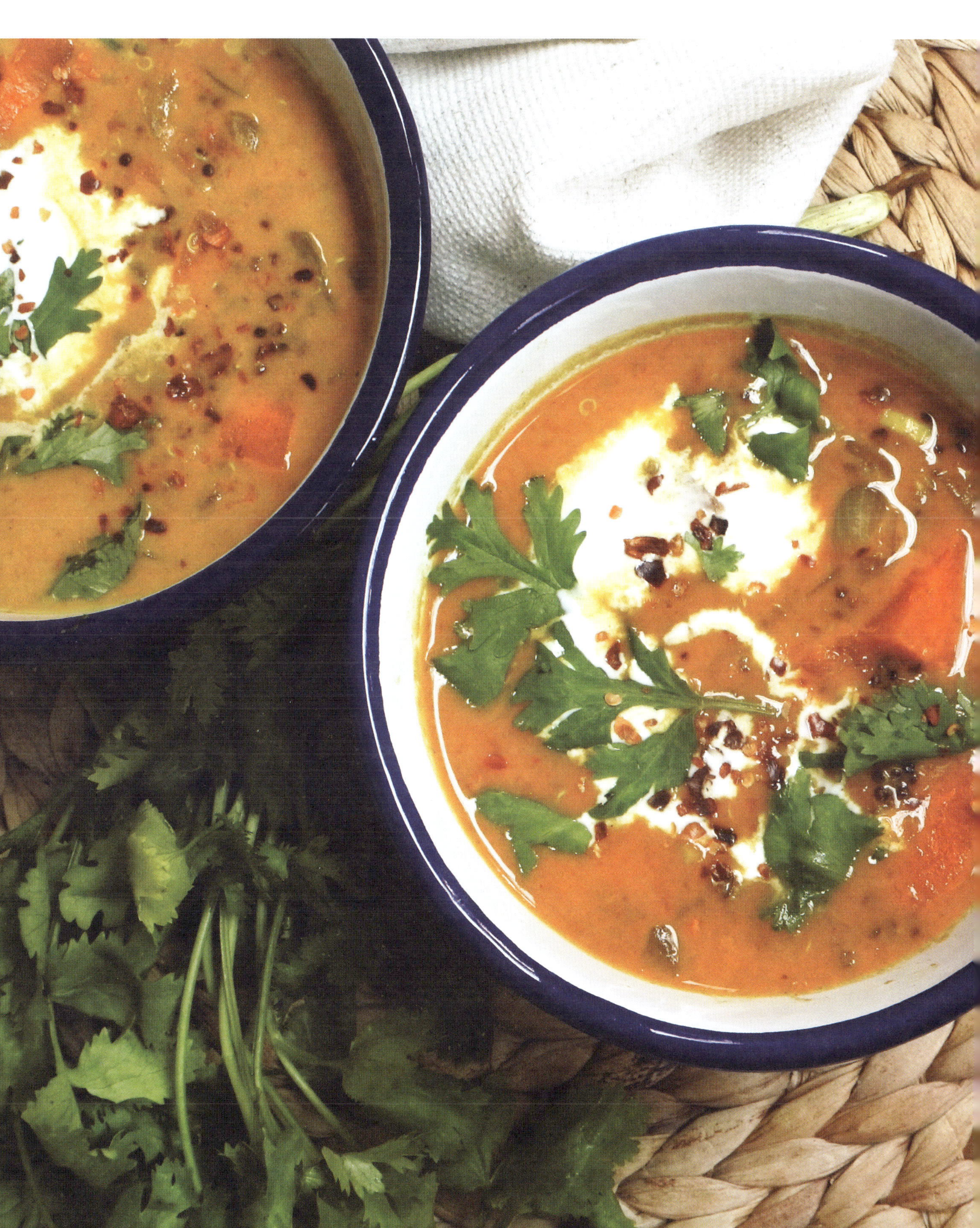

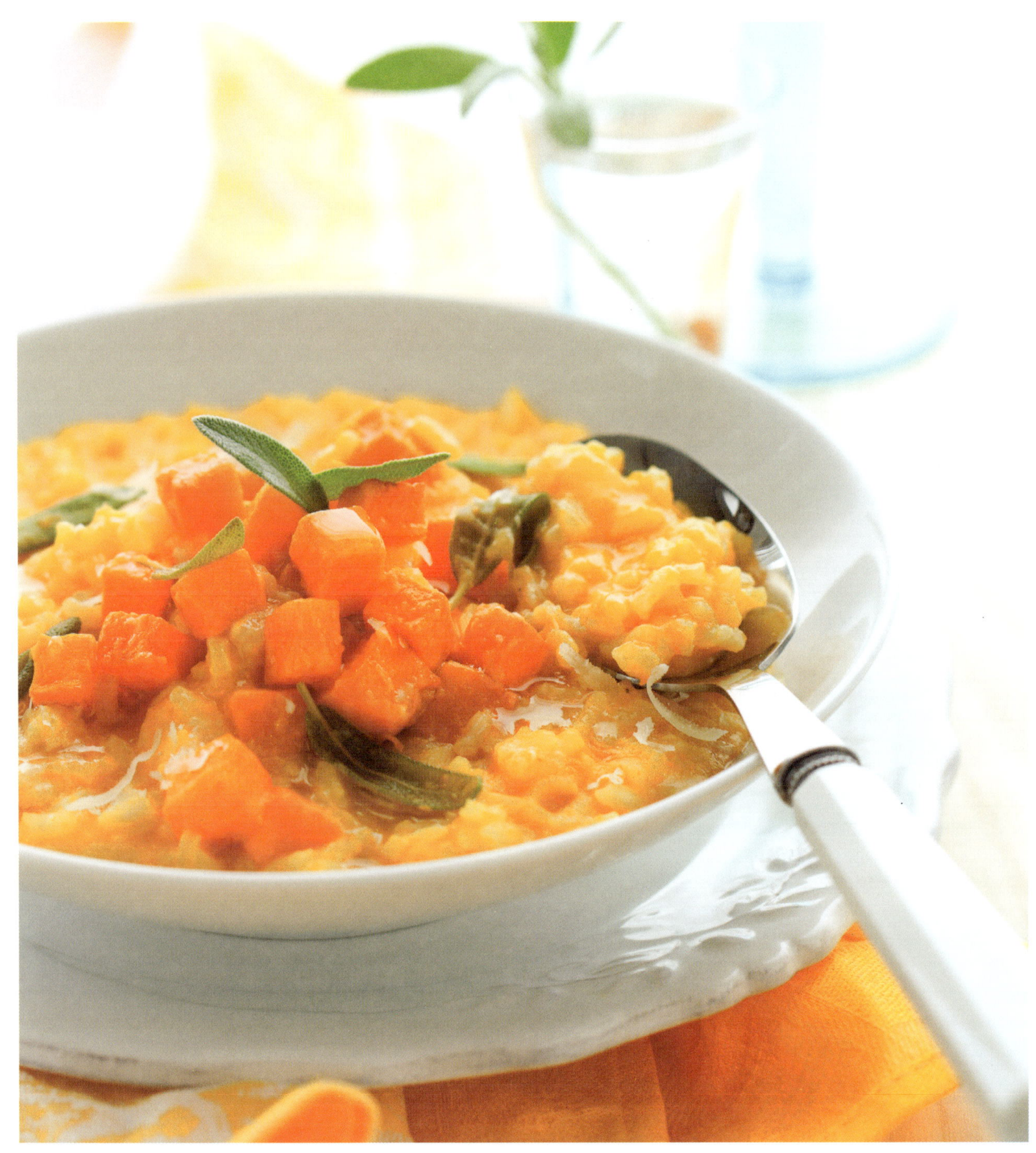

Pumpkin Risotto

SERVES 4

COOK TIME: 45 MINS OVEN + HIGH 1 HR 30 MINS

GLUTEN FREE • DAIRY FREE

PUMPKIN RISOTTO

- 1 small butternut pumpkin, diced
- 3 tbsps olive oil
- Salt and pepper to taste
- 2 tsps dried sage
- ½ cup (75g) chopped onion
- 1 tbsp crushed garlic
- 1½ cups (235g) Arborio rice
- 4 cups (1L) vegetable stock or water
- ½ cup (10g) fresh sage leaves, to garnish

Preheat the oven to 180°C.

Drizzle the pumpkin with 2 tablespoons olive oil and sprinkle with salt, pepper and sage. Transfer to the oven to roast for 45 minutes until soft. Remove from the oven and set aside to cool slightly.

Transfer half of the pumpkin to a blender and pulse until a puree forms. Set aside.

Heat 1 tablespoon olive oil in a medium frying pan over a medium-high heat. Add the onion and cook, stirring occasionally, for 3-5 minutes until soft and translucent. Add the garlic and cook for a further minute, until fragrant. Stir in the Arborio rice and cook for an additional 2-3 minutes.

Transfer the rice and onion mixture to a lightly greased slow cooker. Stir in the vegetable stock, 2 teaspoons salt, 1 teaspoon pepper and pumpkin puree.

Cover the slow cooker and cook on high for 1½ hours, until the rice is tender. Stir in the retained roast pumpkin pieces. Add salt and pepper to taste, before serving garnished with fresh sage.

Chapter Five

Baked and Sweets

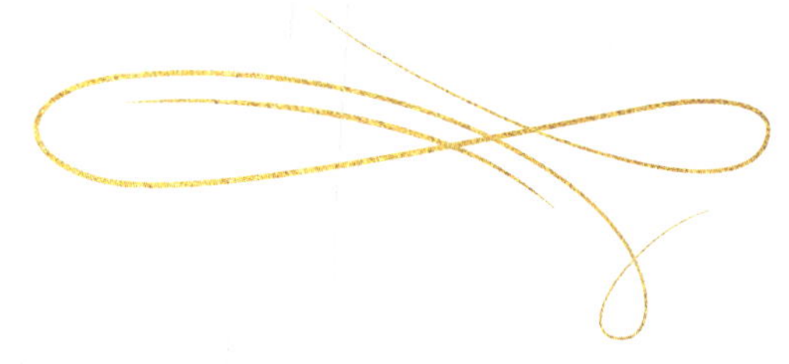

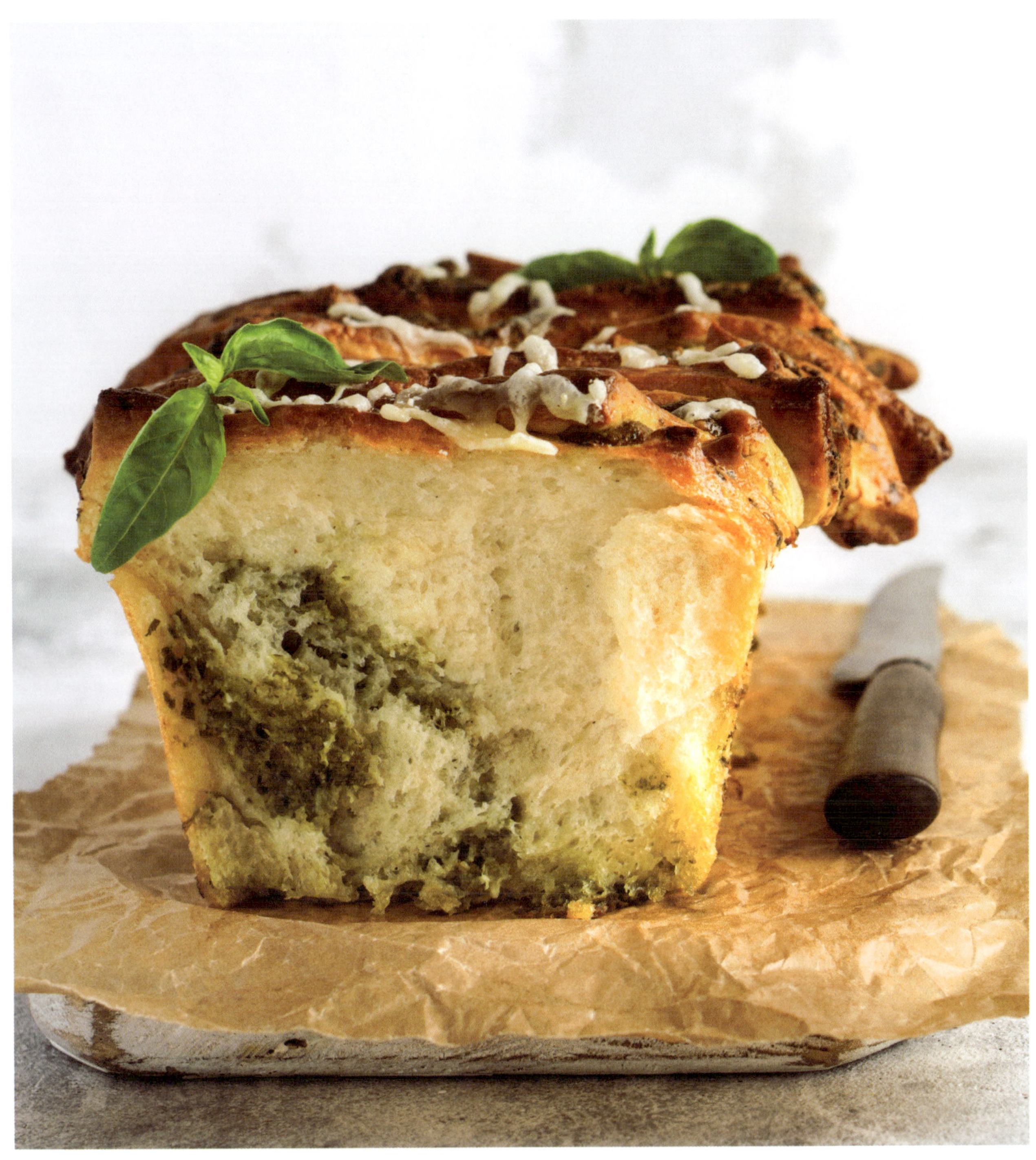

Pull-Apart Pesto Bread

SERVES 8

COOK TIME: HIGH 2 HRS 30 MINS

PULL-APART PESTO BREAD

3 cups (375g) plain flour

2 tsps baking powder

1 tsp salt

1 cup (250ml) buttermilk

1 egg, lightly whisked

115g butter, melted

⅓ cup (80g) pesto

2 tbsps olive oil

½ cup (60g) grated Cheddar cheese

½ cup (60g) grated mozzarella cheese

¼ cup (25g) grated Parmesan cheese

Fresh basil leaves to serve

Lightly grease the bowl of your slow cooker and line with greaseproof paper.

Whisk together the flour, baking powder and salt in a bowl. Make a well in the centre. Add the buttermilk, egg and melted butter. Mix with a flat-bladed knife until mixture comes together.

Turn the dough onto a lightly floured surface. Knead for 30 seconds or until smooth. Divide into eight pieces.

Place pesto and olive oil in a shallow bowl. Mix well.

Gently roll a piece of dough into a smooth ball and roll in the pesto mixture to coat. Transfer to prepared slow cooker. Repeat with remaining dough and pesto.

Cover and cook on high for 2 hours or until the bread is cooked through. Sprinkle with the cheeses, cover and cook for a further 30 minutes or until the cheese is bubbling.

Serve sprinkled with basil leaves.

Tomato and Rosemary Focaccia

SERVES 8-10
COOK TIME: LOW 30 MINS + HIGH 1-1¼ HRS
DAIRY FREE

7g sachet dried yeast
2 tsps caster sugar
1¼ cups (310ml) warm water
3 cups (375g) plain flour
Salt and pepper to taste
3½ tbsps olive oil
3 tsps chopped fresh rosemary leaves
1 tsp coarse salt
4-5 cherry tomatoes, finely chopped

Whisk yeast, sugar and ½ cup warm water in a jug. Set aside in a warm place for 15 minutes until bubbly.

Place flour in a large bowl. Season well with salt and pepper. Make a well in the centre. Add yeast mixture, 1 tablespoon oil and remaining warm water. Mix to form a sticky dough. Cover with plastic wrap. Set aside in a warm place for 15 minutes.

Grease bowl of slow cooker or line with greaseproof paper. Using lightly floured hands, transfer dough to slow cooker, spreading to almost cover base of cooker. Cover and cook on low for 30 minutes or until dough has doubled in size.

Using fingertips, press holes into the top of dough. Sprinkle with rosemary and drizzle with 2 tablespoons of remaining oil. Sprinkle with coarse salt. Cover and cook on high for 1 hour to 1 hour 15 minutes or until cooked and top is just firm to touch. Using two spatulas, carefully lift bread from slow cooker and transfer to a tray lined with greaseproof paper.

Preheat grill on high. Drizzle bread with remaining oil. Grill for 2-3 minutes or until top is golden, being careful not to burn paper.

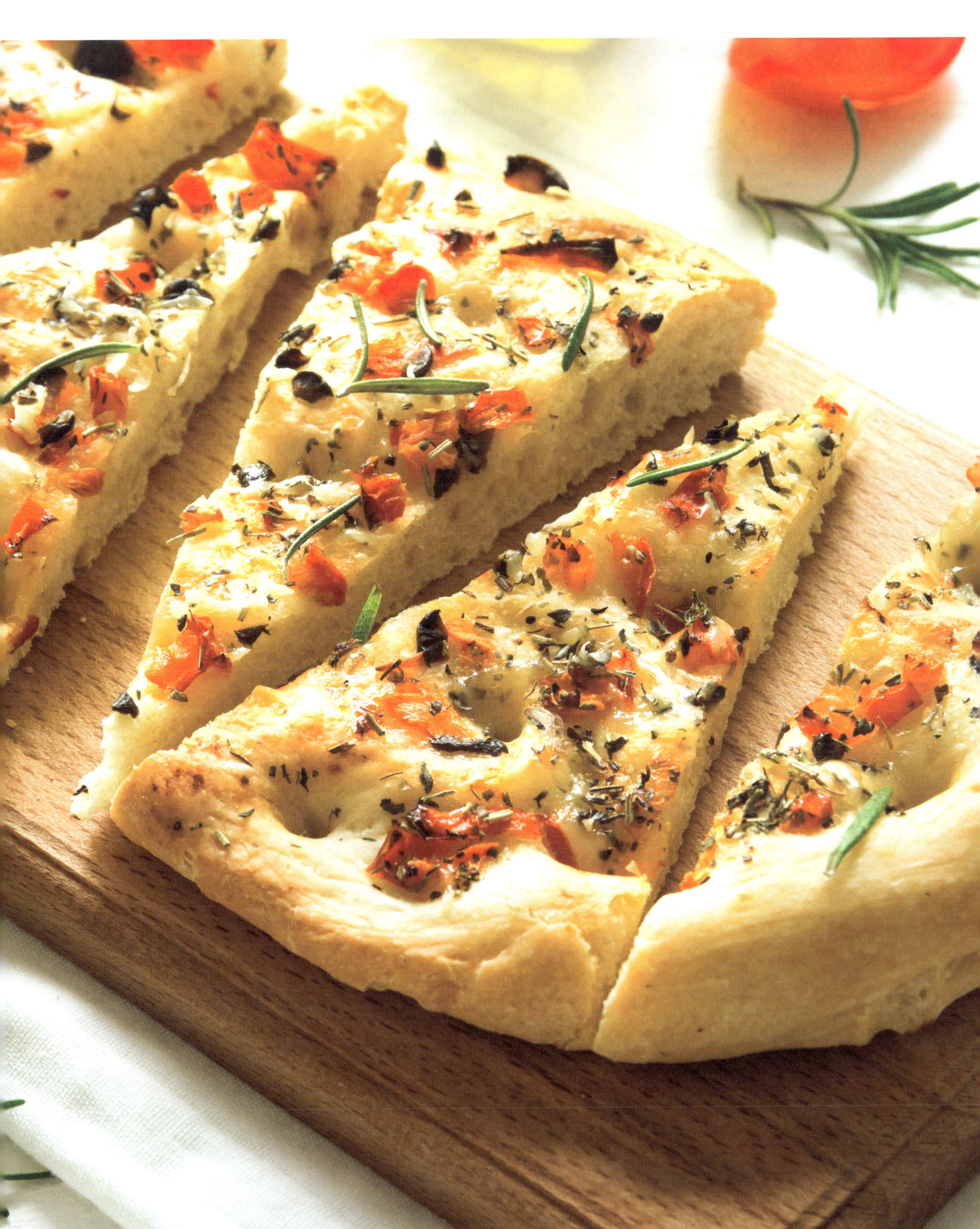

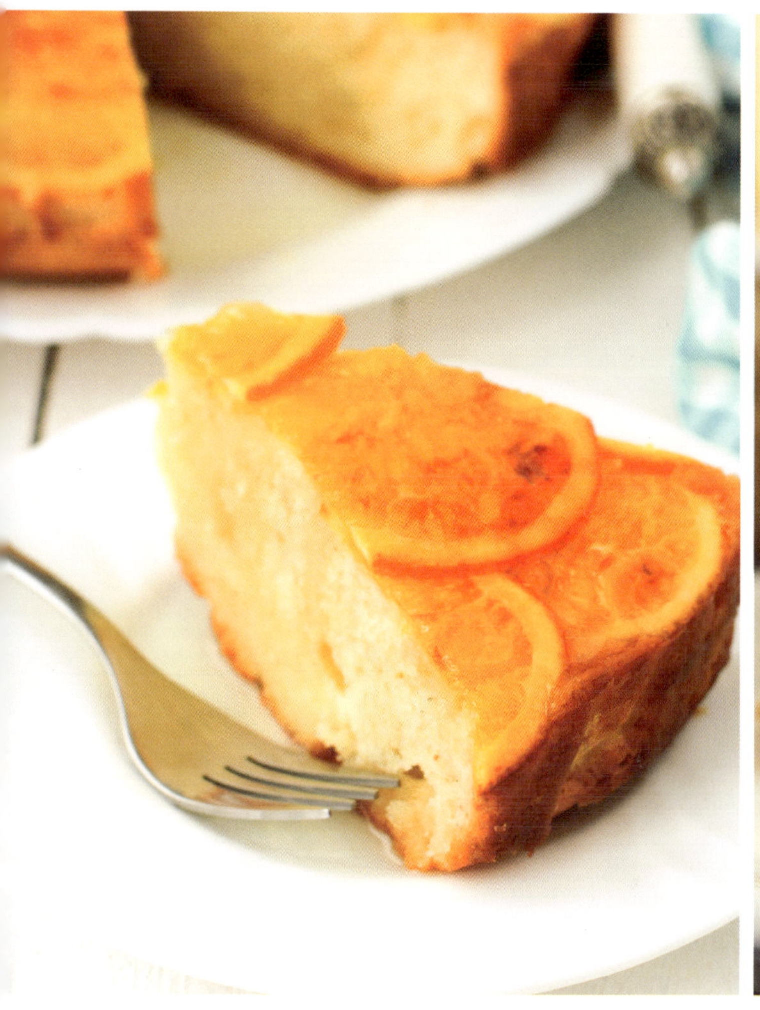

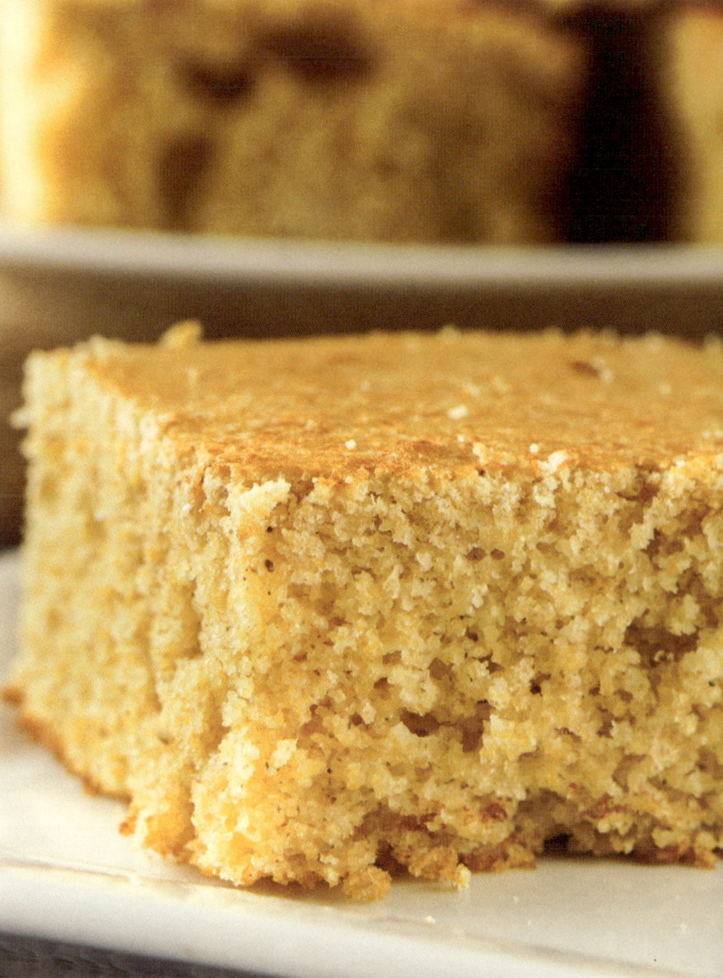

Gluten-Free Orange Upside-Down Cake

SERVES 8

COOK TIME: HIGH 2 HRS 30 MINS

DAIRY FREE

Cornbread

SERVES 8

COOK TIME: HIGH 2 HRS

GLUTEN-FREE ORANGE UPSIDE-DOWN CAKE

2 tbsps brown sugar
1 orange, thinly sliced
125g butter, softened
¾ cup (165g) caster sugar
2 eggs, lightly beaten
¾ cup (90g) gluten-free self-raising flour
¾ cup (90g) almond meal
¼ cup (60ml) freshly squeezed orange juice

Grease a deep, 20cm cake tin or loaf tin that will fit into your slow cooker. Line base and sides with baking paper, allowing a 2cm overhang.

Sprinkle brown sugar over base. Arrange orange slices over sugar.

Using an electric mixer, beat butter and caster sugar until light and fluffy. Add eggs, one at a time, beating until just combined. Stir in flour, almond meal and orange juice until just combined.

Carefully spoon mixture into cake or loaf tin. Smooth top with a rubber spatula.

Place cake tin into the slow cooker on top of two egg rings or an upturned saucer. Cover and cook on high for 2 hours 30 minutes or until an inserted skewer comes out clean.

Stand in tin for 5 minutes before inverting onto a plate. Serve warm.

CORNBREAD

2 tbsps butter
1 cup (125g) plain flour
1 cup (190g) polenta
1½ tbsps sugar
3 tsps baking powder
1 tsp salt
1 cup (250ml) buttermilk (or milk)
2 eggs

Place butter in the inset of a large slow cooker. Turn onto high and allow butter to melt.

Meanwhile, sift flour over a medium mixing bowl. Add polenta, sugar, baking powder and salt. Then add buttermilk and eggs and stir to combine.

Pour the cornbread batter into the slow cooker and smooth the surface evenly with a spatula or knife.

Cover and cook on high for 2 hours.

Almond Banana Loaf

SERVES 8

COOK TIME: HIGH 3 HRS 30 MINS

1 cup (125g) plain flour
1 tsp bicarbonate of soda
1 tsp salt
1 cup (120g) almond meal
½ cup (60g) almonds, roughly chopped (retain 1 tbsp to decorate)
125g butter, room temperature
1 cup (155g) brown sugar
2 eggs
1 tsp vanilla extract
3 large ripe bananas, mashed

Lightly grease the inset of a large slow cooker or grease a loaf tin.

Sift flour, bicarb and salt over a bowl. Add almond meal and almonds and stir to combine. Set aside.

Using a hand mixer or in the bowl of an electric mixer, beat butter and sugar until fluffy. Add eggs, one at a time, beating well after each addition. Stir in vanilla and the mashed bananas. Gradually add dry ingredients, stirring until the mixture is moist.

Pour batter into the slow cooker or the prepared tin. Smooth surface using a spatula and push retained almonds into the top. (If using a loaf tin, place a rack or scrunched-up foil on base of slow cooker before putting the tin into the cooker.)

Cover and cook on high for 2½ hours (if cooking in the inset itself) or 3½ hours if cooking in the loaf tin, until a skewer inserted in the centre comes out clean.

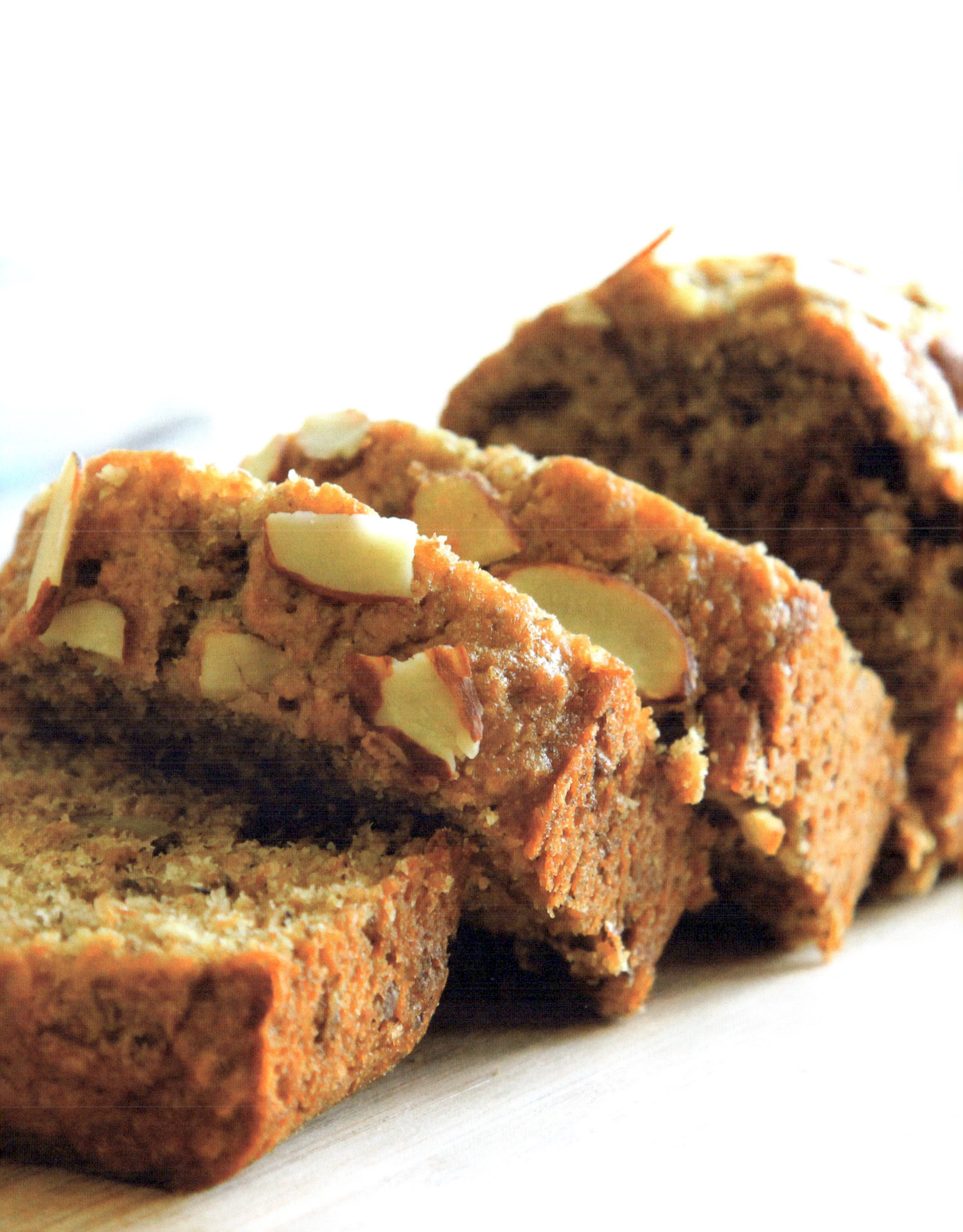

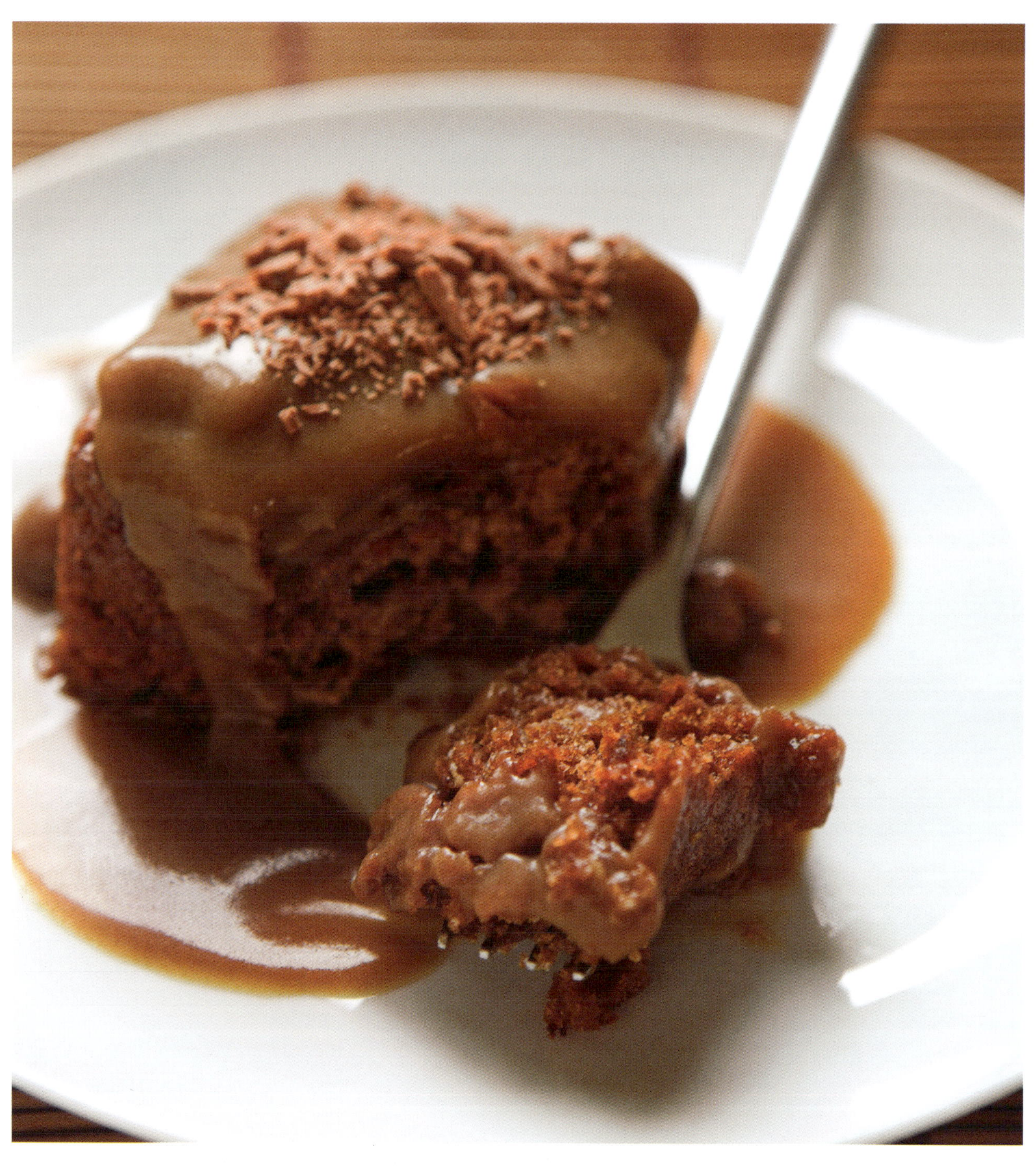

Sticky Toffee Pudding

SERVES 6

COOK TIME: LOW 3 HRS

STICKY TOFFEE PUDDING

2 cups (500ml) thickened cream
2 cups (310g) brown sugar
200g unsalted butter
¾ cup (185ml) water
1 cup (175g) pitted dates, finely chopped
1 tsp bicarbonate of soda
2 cups (250g) plain flour
½ cup (110g) caster sugar
1 tsp vanilla extract
2 eggs
¾ cup (185ml) milk
¾ cup (100g) milk chocolate, grated

In a saucepan, heat the cream, brown sugar and a third of the butter. Bring to the boil then reduce heat and simmer for 5 minutes. Set aside.

In a separate saucepan, add the water and the dates and bring to the boil. Add ¼ teaspoon of bicarb and stir through. Remove and allow to cool.

In a bowl combine the flour with the rest of the bicarb. In another bowl cream the remaining butter, caster sugar and vanilla with an electric mixer. Add the eggs, one at a time, and beat until smooth. Add the flour mixture to the butter mixture and add the milk gradually. Stir in the date mixture.

Spread the batter in the slow cooker and pour half of the cooled sauce over it. Place a tea towel over the top. Cover and cook on low for 3 hours. Drizzle on the rest of the sauce and sprinkle with grated chocolate just before serving.

Spinach and Feta Muffins

MAKES 12

COOK TIME: HIGH 1 HR

2¼ cups (280g) self-raising flour

Salt and pepper to taste

200g feta cheese, crumbled

1¼ cups (125g) finely grated Parmesan cheese

1 cup (250ml) milk

2 eggs

125g butter, melted and cooled

250g frozen spinach, thawed, moisture squeezed out and chopped

Preheat slow cooker on high for 20 minutes.

Sift flour into a bowl and season well with salt and freshly ground pepper. Stir in half each of the feta and Parmesan, then make a well in the centre. Whisk the milk and eggs together in a jug, then pour into the well. Add the melted butter. Use a spatula to gently fold together until just combined. Stir in the spinach.

Fill 12 silicone or paper cupcake cases three-quarters full. Mix together the remaining cheeses and sprinkle over each muffin.

Cover the slow cooker with a cotton tea towel, place lid on slow cooker and fold the tea towel back over the lid.

Cook for 1 hour on high or until an inserted skewer comes out clean.

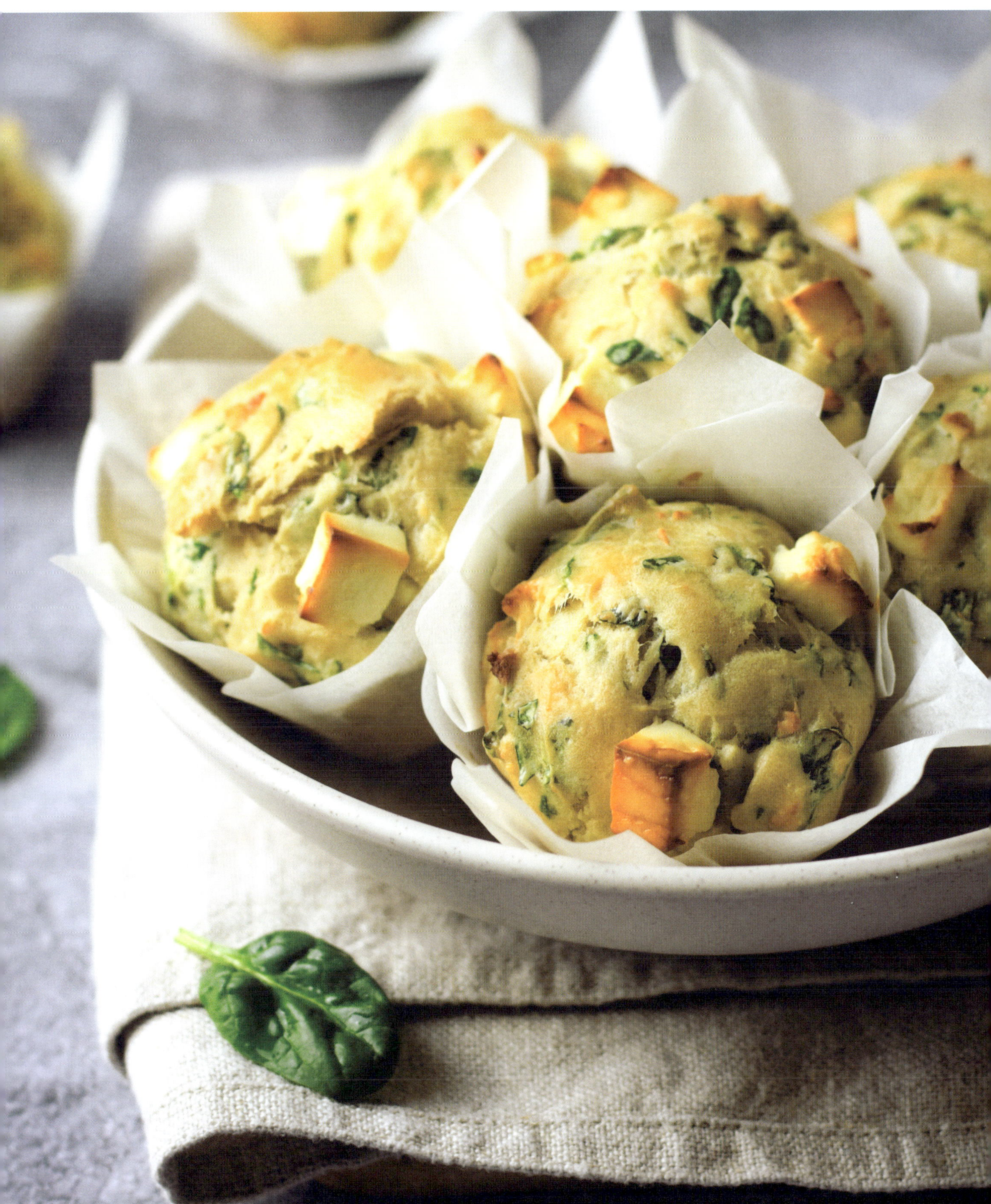

POTATO BUTTERMILK BREAD

2 potatoes, peeled and quartered
115g butter, room temperature
4 tsps active dry yeast
2 cups (500ml) buttermilk, room temperature
2 eggs, beaten
2 tbsps sugar
1½ tsps salt
1 tsp fennel seeds
6½ cups (800g) strong flour, sifted

Place potatoes in a saucepan and cover with water. Bring to the boil and cook for 10-12 minutes until fork tender. Drain and roughly mash with a fork.

Place potatoes and butter in the bowl of an electric mixer. Add yeast, buttermilk, eggs, sugar, salt and fennel seeds and beat slowly to combine.

Gradually add flour and stir until the dough is moist but not sticky.

Knead on low to medium speed using the dough attachment, or by hand, until the dough is smooth and elastic.

Grease a loaf tin with butter. Gently press the dough into the loaf tin and transfer tin to the slow cooker. (Place a rack or scrunched-up foil on base of slow cooker before putting the tin into the cooker.)

Turn the cooker onto high and cook for 1-3 hours. Check with an instant read thermometer after 1 hour, and keep checking every 30 minutes until cooked. When the thermometer reads 90°C, the bread is ready.

PUMPKIN CAKE

125g butter, softened
2 cups (310g) brown sugar, packed
3 eggs
2 tsps vanilla extract
2 cups (450g) pumpkin, cooked
1½ cups (185g) plain flour
1½ tsps baking powder
1½ tsps bicarbonate of soda
1 tsp cinnamon
¼ tsp nutmeg
¼ tsp ground ginger
Pinch of ground cloves
½ tsp salt

Take 2-3 sheets of heavy-duty aluminium foil, folded several times, and line the inside of a large slow cooker. Place a piece of baking paper inside the foil base.

Using an electric mixer, beat together butter and sugar until creamy. Beat in eggs one at a time until thoroughly combined. Add vanilla extract. Beat in pumpkin.

Fold in the flour, baking powder, bicarb, spices, and salt until a smooth batter forms.

Pour into prepared slow cooker. Cover and cook on high for 3 hours (check at 2 hours) or until a skewer inserted in the centre comes out clean.

Use the baking paper to lift cake from the slow cooker and allow to cool for 20 minutes before serving.

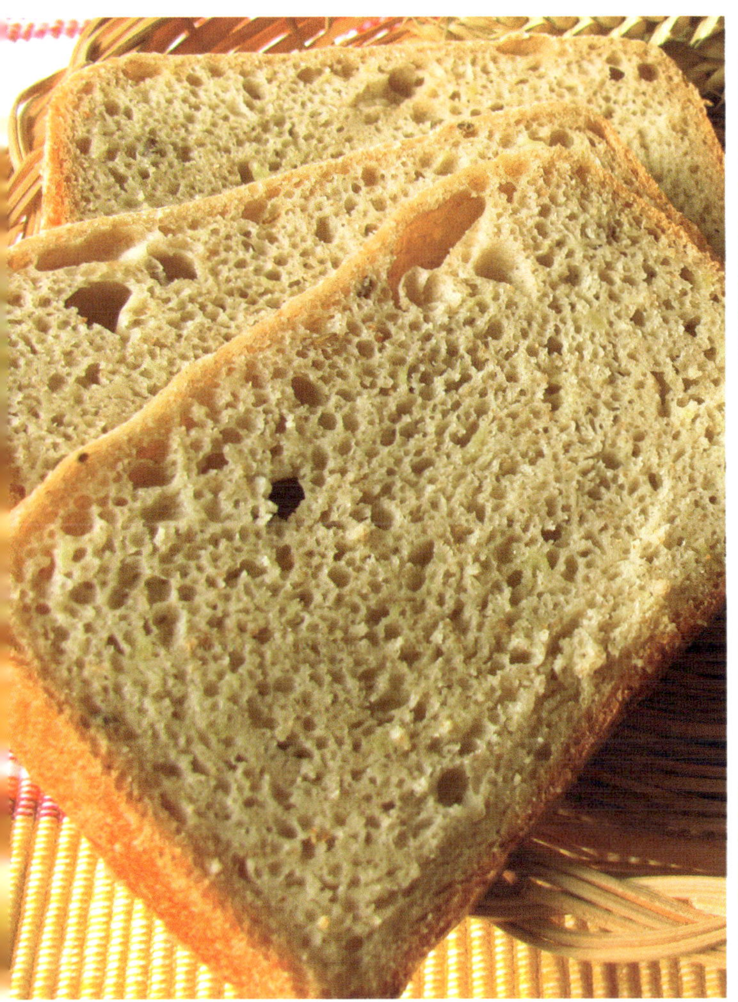

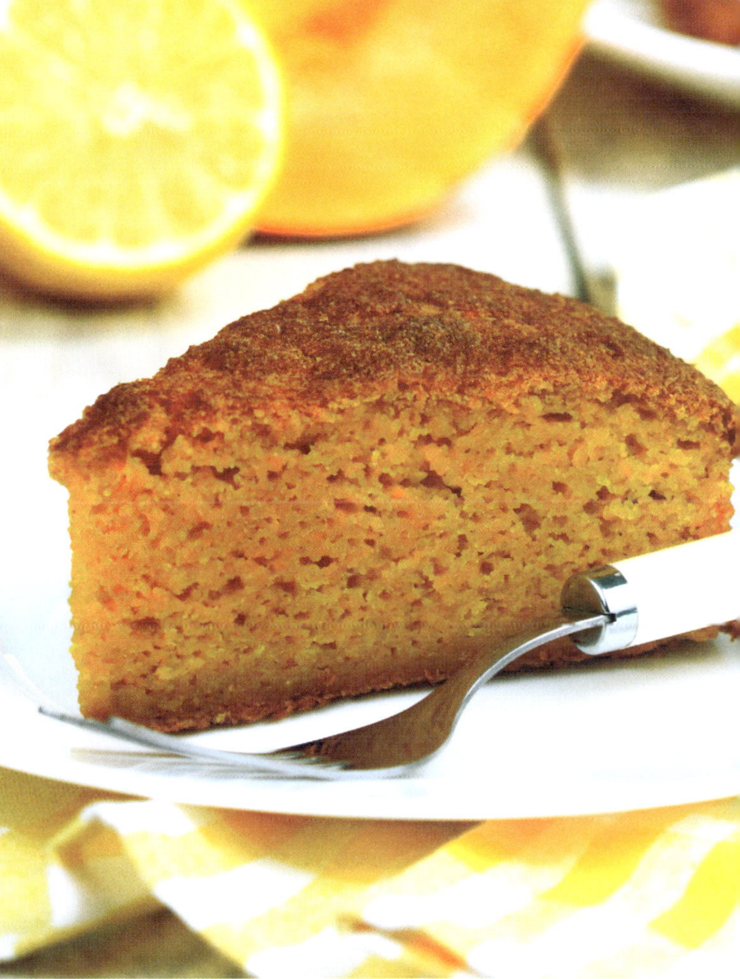

Potato Buttermilk Bread

SERVES 6

COOK TIME: HIGH 2 HRS

Pumpkin Cake

SERVES 10

COOK TIME: HIGH 3 HRS

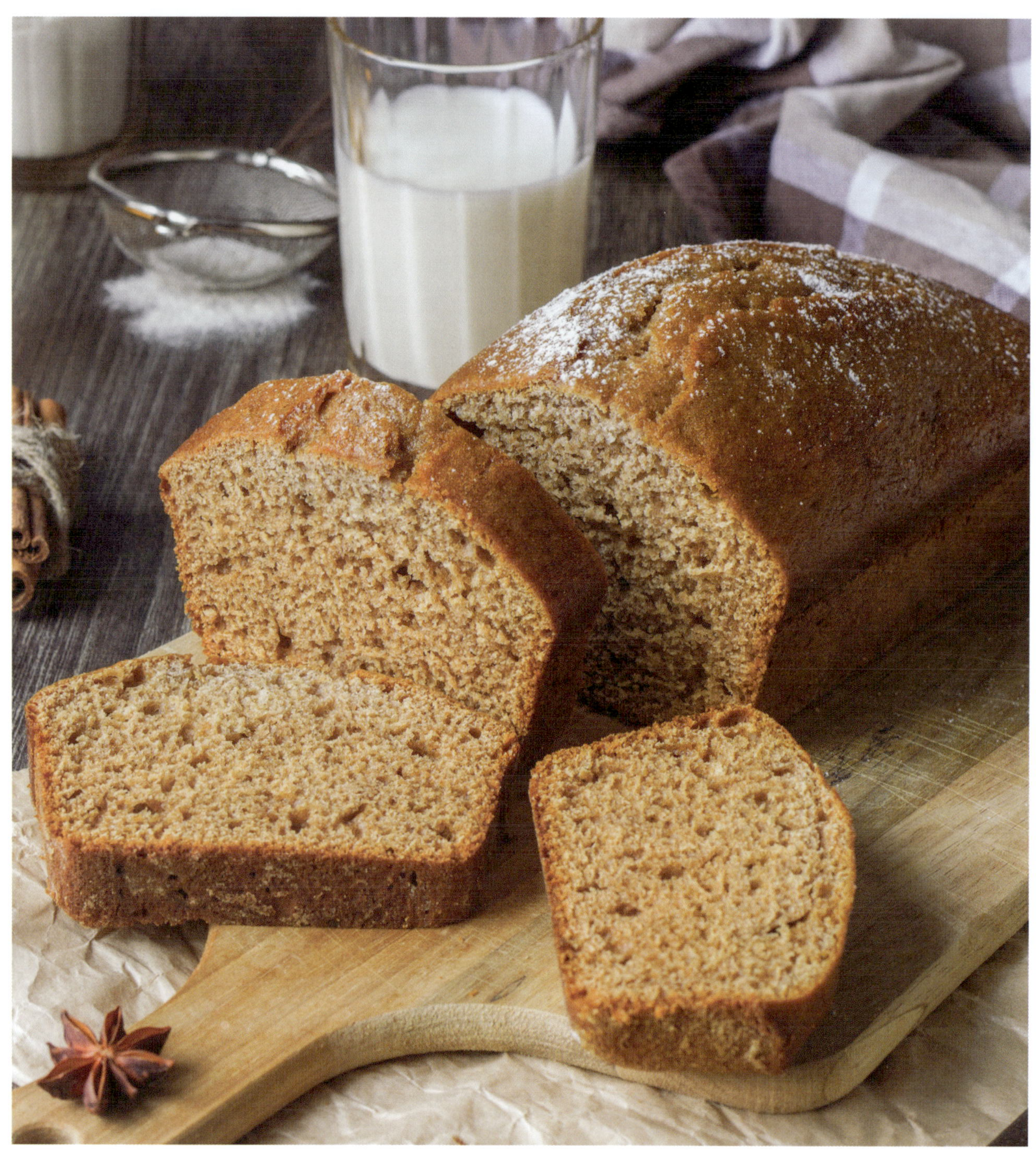

Spiced Honey Cake

SERVES 8

COOK TIME: HIGH 2 HRS 30 MINS

SPICED HONEY CAKE

4 cups (500g) plain flour
1⅔ cups (250g) brown sugar
2 tsps bicarbonate of soda
2 tbsps ground cinnamon
¼ tsp ground cloves
3 tsps ground cardamom
1 tsp ground star anise
¾ cup (200ml) milk
¾ cup (250g) honey
2 tbsps butter
2 tbsps icing sugar

Mix flour, sugar, bicarb, cinnamon, cloves, cardamom and star anise in a large bowl.

Place milk in a microwave-proof bowl with honey and warm through. Pour warm milk and honey into dry ingredients. Stir well to combine.

Grease a loaf tin with butter and line with greaseproof paper.

Pour the mixture into the tin.

In slow cooker bowl place two egg rings or an upturned saucer and about 3cm of water.

Place tin on egg rings in slow cooker bowl.

Cook on high for 2½ hours or until an inserted skewer comes out clean.

Dust with icing sugar to serve.

Tomato and Herb Bread

SERVES 10

COOK TIME: HIGH 2 HRS 30 MINS

1 cup (250ml) milk

1 tbsp white wine vinegar

2½ cups (310g) self-raising flour

2 tsps baking powder

½ cup (50g) grated Parmesan cheese

1½ cups (185g) grated mozzarella

1 cup (15g) fresh basil leaves, roughly chopped

2 cloves garlic, minced

Pinch of salt and pepper

1 cup (55g) sun-dried tomatoes, chopped

1 egg, beaten

Preheat the slow cooker on high for 20 minutes. Grease and line slow cooker with greaseproof paper or grease and line a loaf tin that fits inside your slow cooker. If using a loaf tin place in slow cooker on top of two egg rings or an upturned saucer.

In a small bowl add the milk and white wine vinegar and set aside for 5-10 minutes.

In a large bowl add flour, baking powder, cheeses, basil, garlic, salt and pepper, and sun-dried tomatoes. Stir to combine.

Pour prepared milk mixture into flour mixture and mix with a wooden spoon combine until a dough forms.

Mould into an oval shape and carefully place in your slow cooker or mould into a loaf shape and place in loaf tin in slow cooker.

Score the top of the loaf twice. Brush with beaten egg.

Cover the slow cooker with a tea towel, place lid on slow cooker and fold the tea towel back over the lid.

Cook on high for 2½ hours or until an inserted skewer comes out clean.

Remove and allow to cool slightly before slicing.

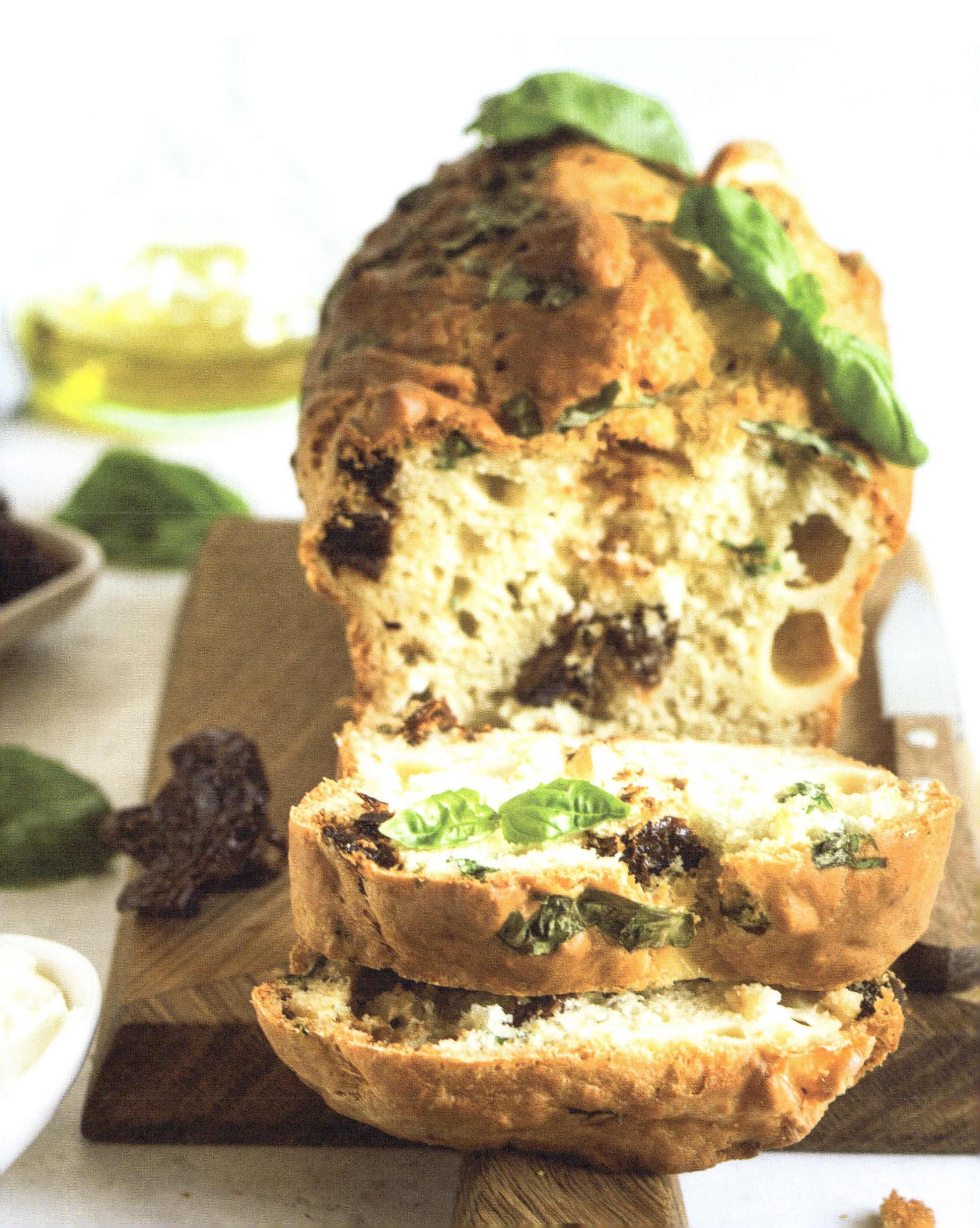

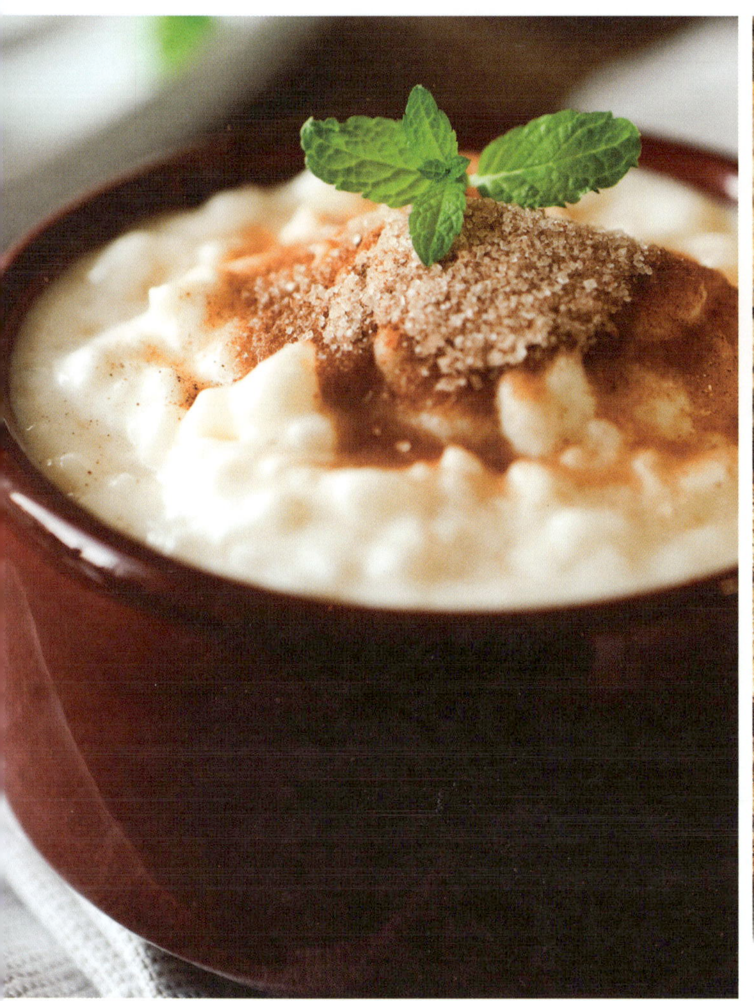

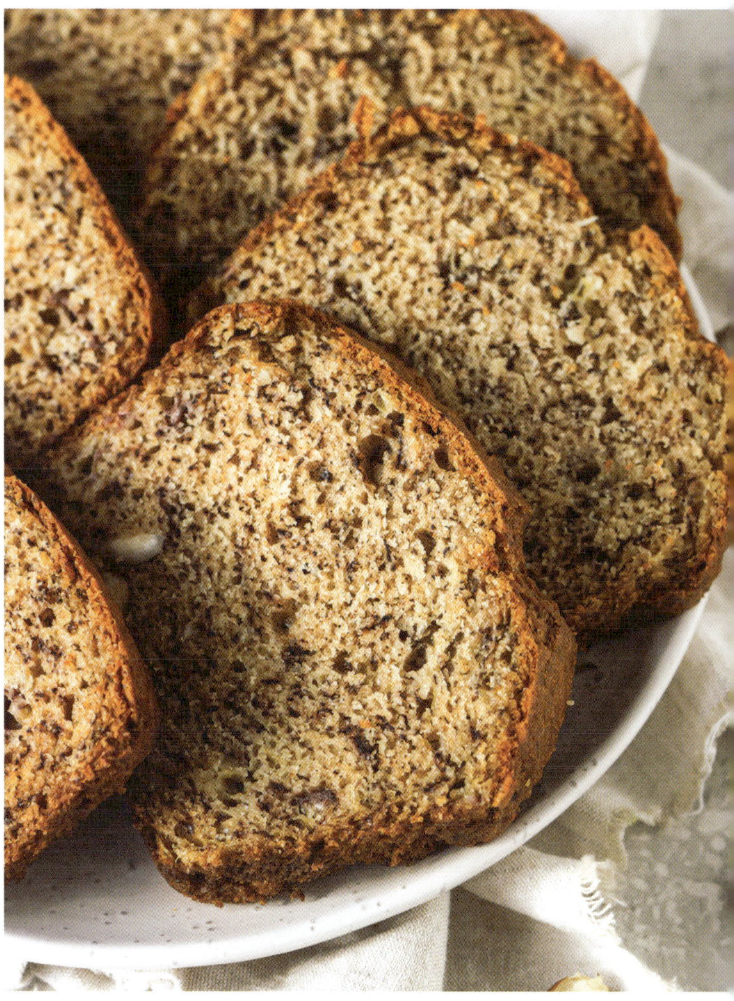

Creamy Rice Pudding with Cinnamon Sugar

SERVES 4

COOK TIME: LOW 6 HRS

GLUTEN FREE

Banana Bread

SERVES 10

COOK TIME: HIGH 2-3 HRS

CREAMY RICE PUDDING WITH CINNAMON SUGAR

1 cup (155g) Arborio rice
5 cups (1.25L) milk
¾ cup (165g) sugar
1 tsp vanilla extract
1 tsp ground cinnamon

Combine the rice, milk and ½ cup of sugar in the slow cooker and mix well. Add the vanilla extract and stir.

Cover and cook on low for 6 hours, stirring twice, until the rice is tender.

In a small bowl combine the rest of the sugar and cinnamon, and sprinkle over the cooked rice pudding.

BANANA BREAD

2 cups (250g) plain flour
1 tsp bicarbonate of soda
¼ tsp salt
½ cup (75g) chopped walnuts
115g butter, softened
1 cup (155g) sugar
2 large eggs
3 tbsps milk
1 tsp vanilla extract
4 small ripe bananas, mashed

Grease and flour the insert of the slow cooker or grease and line a loaf tin that fits into your slow cooker. If using a loaf tin place in slow cooker on top of two egg rings or an upturned saucer.

Preheat slow cooker on high for 20 minutes.

Mix flour, bicarb, salt and walnuts in a medium bowl.

In another bowl cream the butter and sugar together until light and fluffy. Add eggs one at a time. Add milk and vanilla and mix well. Stir in mashed banana.

Tip dry mixture into wet mixture and fold to combine.

Pour batter into slow cooker or loaf tin and cover with lid.

Cook for 2-3 hours on high or until an inserted skewer comes out clean. Allow to cool slightly before slicing.

Creme Caramel

SERVES 6
COOK TIME: LOW 3 HRS
GLUTEN FREE

2½ cups (600ml) milk
1 vanilla pod, split and seeded
¾ cup (160g) caster sugar
¼ cup (60ml) water
6 eggs (2 eggs, 4 egg yolks)

Pour the milk into a saucepan and add the split vanilla pod. Bring to a simmer over a medium heat, then leave to cool for 30 minutes. Remove the vanilla pod and discard.

In a separate pan add half of the sugar to the water and bring to the boil. Simmer for 15 minutes, until the sugar has dissolved and begun to caramelise. Distribute the sugar evenly between six ramekins.

In a mixing bowl whisk the rest of the sugar with the eggs and egg yolks. Once well combined, add the cooled vanilla milk, whisking continuously.

Divide the mixture between the ramekins and cover each with foil, securing with rubber bands. Place them in the slow cooker.

Fill the slow cooker with boiling water to halfway up the ramekins, and cook on low for 3 hours. Cool in the fridge before serving.

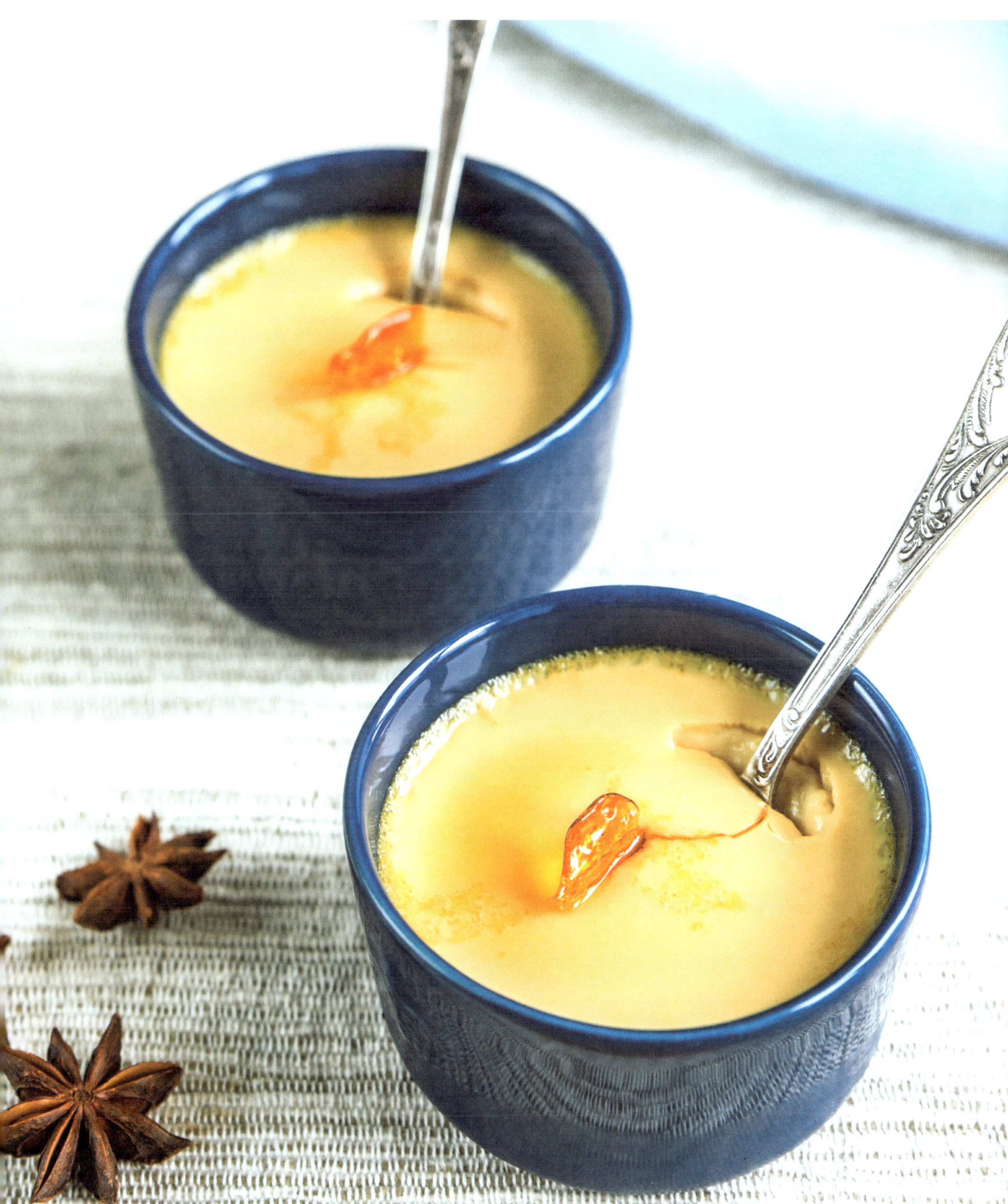

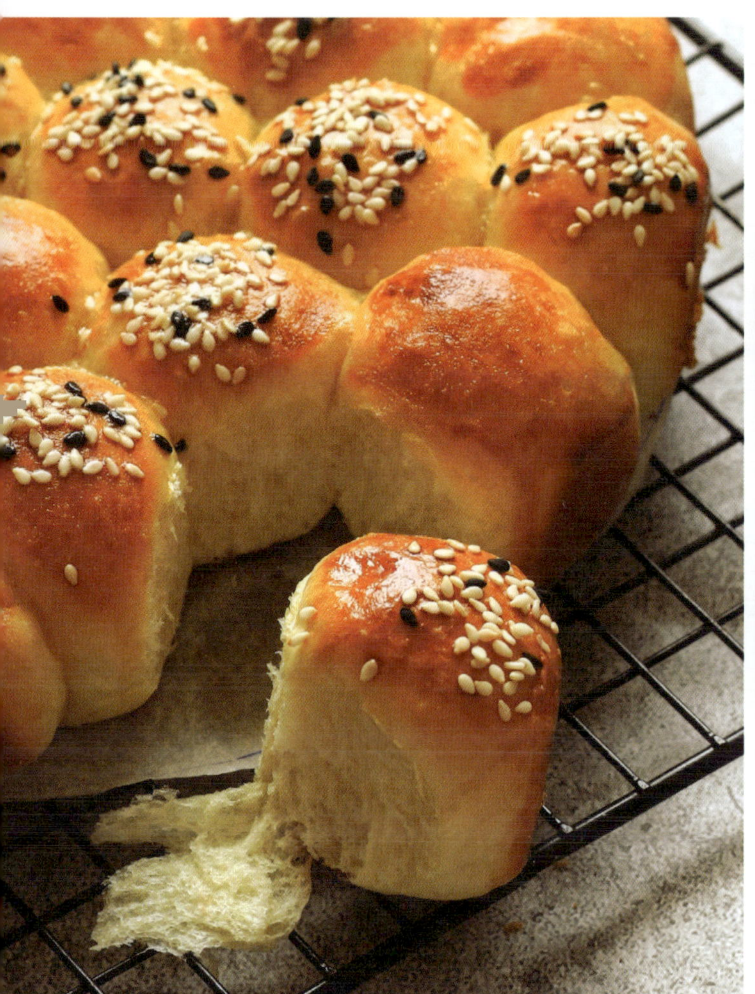

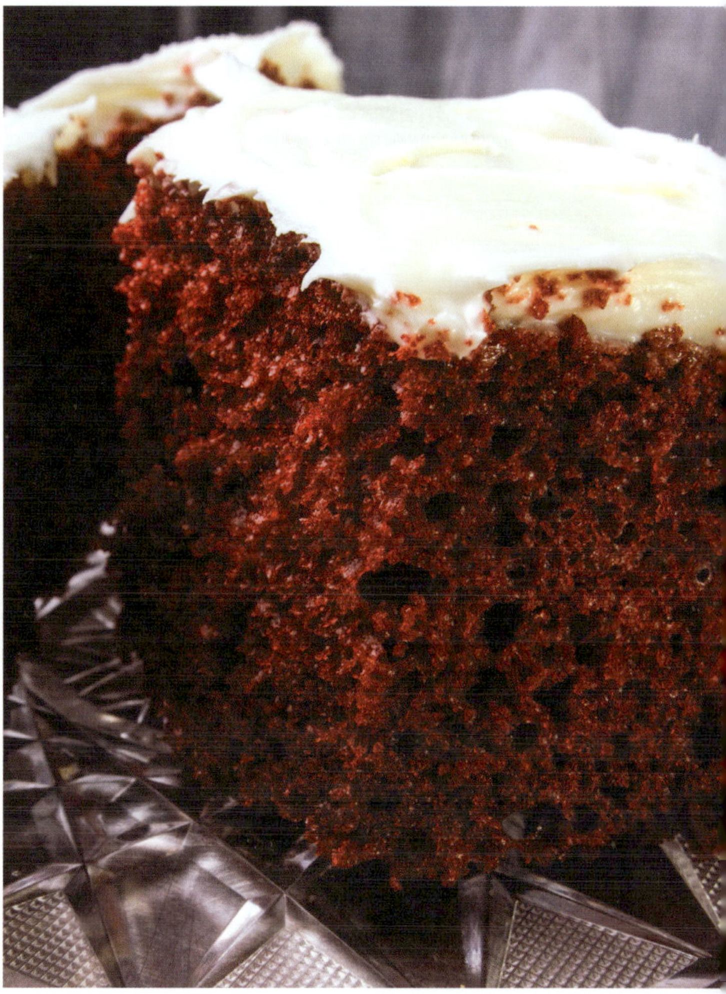

Milk Bread Rolls

SERVES 12

COOK TIME: 2 HRS 10 MINS

Red Velvet Cake

SERVES 8

COOK TIME: HIGH 3 HRS

MILK BREAD ROLLS

1 cup (250ml) warm milk
2¼ tsps (1 sachet) instant yeast
3 cups (375g) bread flour + more as needed
2 tbsps honey
2 tbsps sugar
2 tbsps butter, melted
2 tsps salt

TOPPING

1 tbsp butter, melted
2 tbsps black and white sesame seeds

Pour the warm milk into the bowl of a stand mixer, sprinkle in the yeast. Mix lightly, cover and set aside for 10 minutes until frothy.

Add the flour, honey, sugar, melted butter and salt. Using the dough hook, mix on medium speed for 5-6 minutes or until dough becomes soft and elastic and pulls away from the sides of the bowl.

Transfer the dough to a lightly floured work surface and cut into 12 equal pieces. Roll each piece into a ball.

Line slow cooker with greaseproof paper. Place dough balls in the lined slow cooker. Cover and cook on high for 90 minutes until the bottom of the bread is browned.

Remove from the slow cooker. Brush the tops with melted butter and sprinkle with sesame seeds.

Place under a hot grill for 1-2 minutes until the tops brown.

RED VELVET CAKE

2¼ cups (280g) plain flour
1 tsp bicarbonate of soda
1 tsp baking powder
1 tsp salt
2 tbsps cacao powder
200g butter
1¾ cups (385g) caster sugar
2 tsps vanilla extract
2 large eggs, room temperature
1 cup (250ml) buttermilk
1 tsp apple cider vinegar
½ cup (125ml) hot coffee
¼ cup (50ml) red food colouring

ICING

500g cream cheese
175g butter, room temperature
¼ tsp vanilla extract
4 cups (620g) icing sugar, sifted

In a large bowl sift together the flour, bicarb, baking powder, salt and cacao powder. In a separate mixing bowl cream together the butter and sugar until it resembles whipped cream. Add the vanilla and eggs and beat in gradually, one egg at a time.

Stir in the flour mix and when combined stir through the buttermilk and vinegar. Lastly stir in the coffee and add small amounts of red food colouring until you get a shade of red that you like.

Line the slow cooker with greased baking paper. Pour in the cake mix into the cooker. Place a clean tea towel over the top of the cooker and place the lid on top. Cook on high for 3 hours. Uncover and let cool in the cooker for 1 hour and then lift out onto a wire rack.

Whisk together the icing ingredients until light and fluffy and use to ice the cake once cool.

Pineapple Upside-Down Cake

SERVES 6

COOK TIME: LOW 2.5 HRS

¾ cup (120g, 4oz) brown sugar
3 tbsps butter, melted
½ tsp salt
Cooking spray
1 x 450g (1lb) can pineapple rings
¾ cup (165g, 6oz) sugar
1 egg plus 1 egg yolk
1 tsp vanilla extract
2 cups (250g, 8oz) plain flour
1 tsp bicarbonate of soda
¼ cup (60ml, 2fl oz)milk

In a bowl stir together the brown sugar, melted butter and half of the salt. Coat a cake tin that will fit your slow cooker with cooking spray, and spread the brown sugar mixture evenly in the bottom. Arrange the pineapple slices evenly over the sugar mixture.

In a large bowl beat the sugar, egg and egg yolk with an electric mixer until the mixture is thickened and smooth. Stir in the vanilla.

In a separate bowl, whisk together the flour, bicarb and the rest of the salt. Stir half of the flour mixture into the batter until almost incorporated. Add the milk and stir to combine. Add the rest of the flour mixture and stir until just combined. Spoon the batter over the pineapple in the tin spreading it to the edges. Place the cake tin into the slow cooker.

Place a tea towel over the slow cooker to absorb moisture and place the lid over the towel. Cook on low for 2 hours 30 minutes or until a skewer inserted in the middle comes out clean. Remove the slow cooker insert to a wire rack and allow the cake to cool for 20-30 minutes. Place a serving plate or large cutting board over the insert and carefully invert to release the cake.

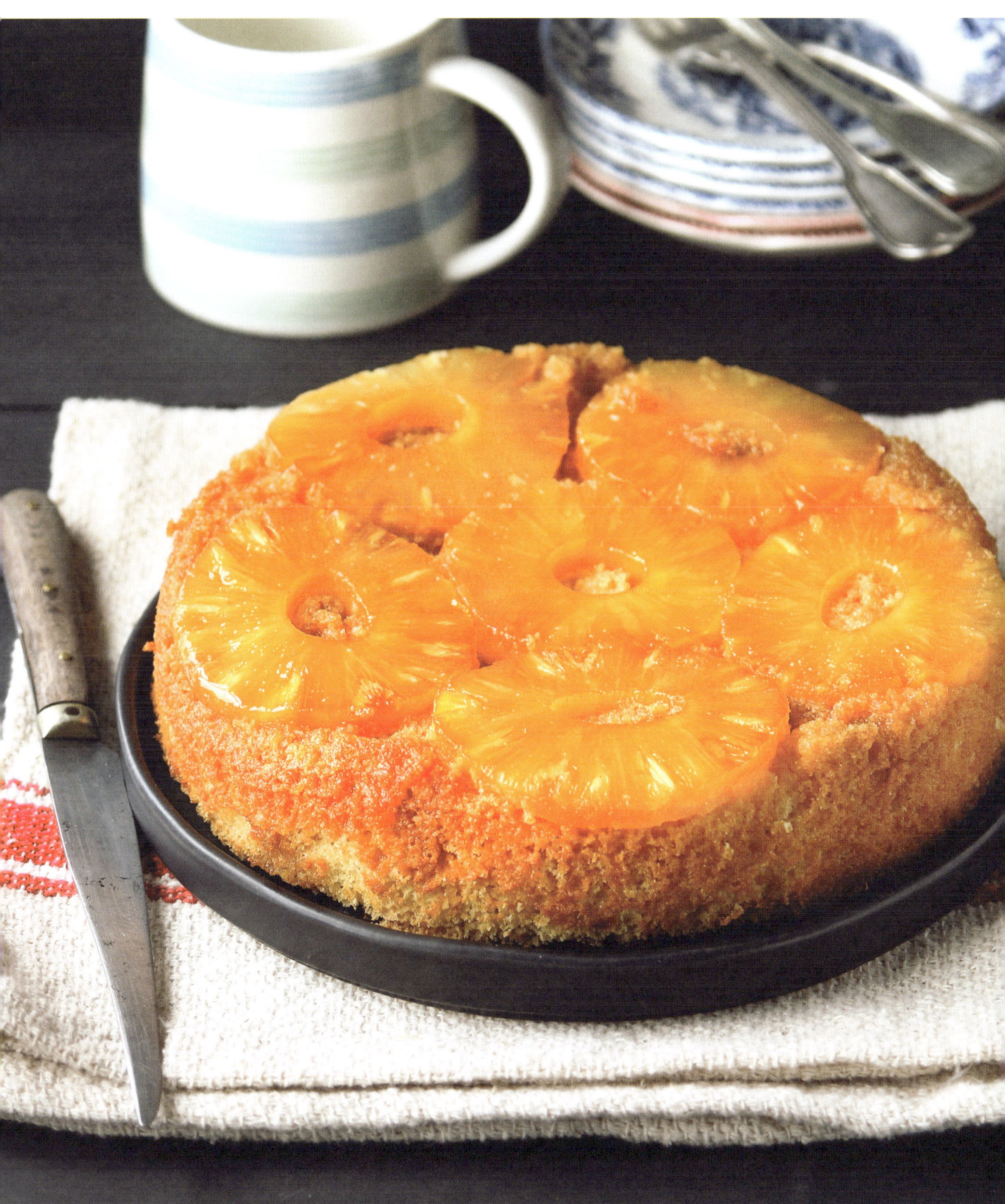

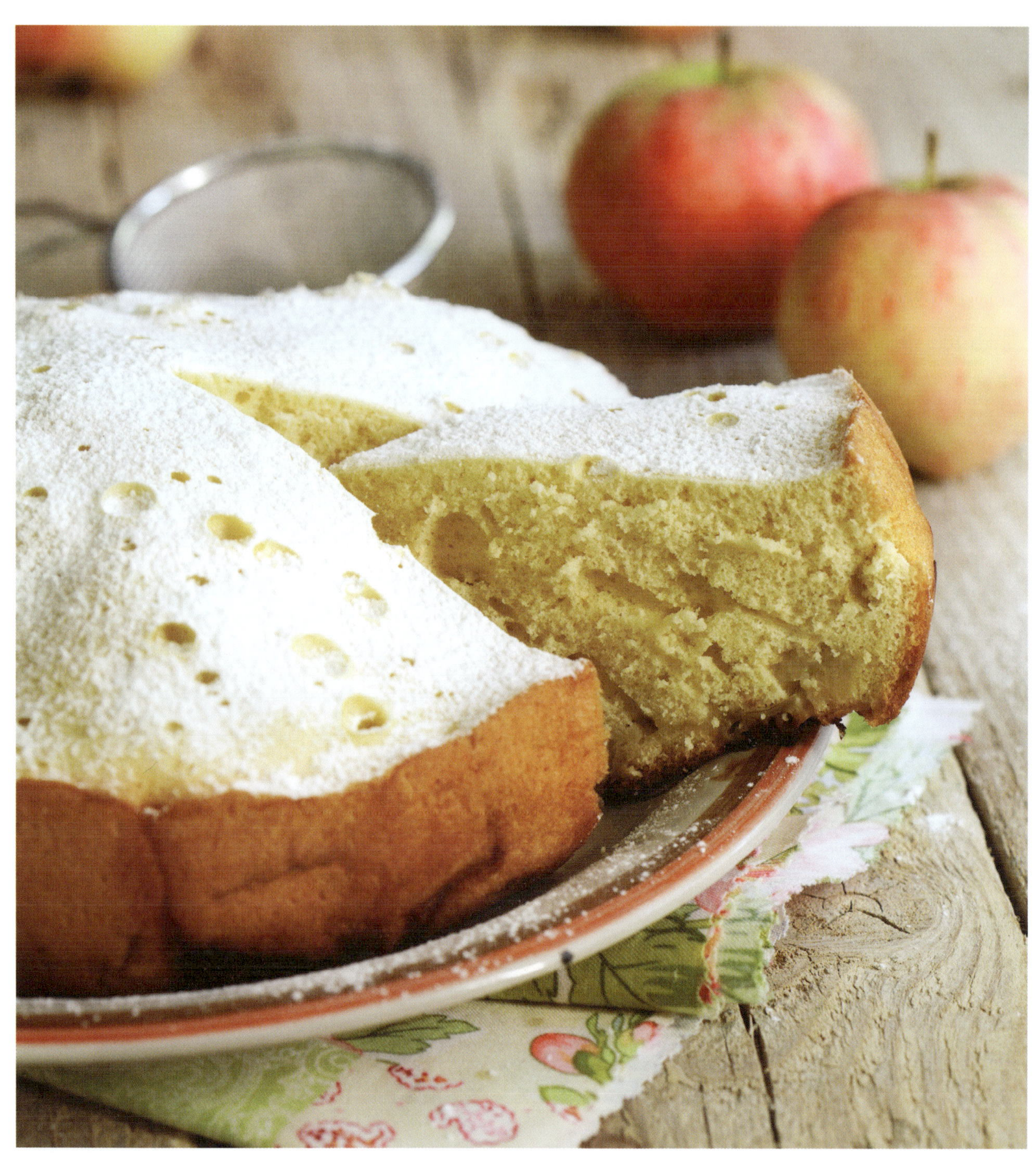

Apple Sponge Cake

SERVES 6

COOK TIME: HIGH 2 HRS

APPLE SPONGE CAKE

- 1 cup (220g) caster sugar
- ⅓ cup (40g) plain flour
- ⅓ cup (40g) self-raising flour
- ⅓ cup (50g) cornflour
- Pinch of salt
- 2 apples, peeled and grated
- 1 tbsp lemon zest
- 4 eggs, room temperature, separated
- 1 tbsp unsalted butter, melted
- ¼ cup (60ml) milk
- 2 tbsps icing sugar

Grease and line the insert of the slow cooker or grease and line a deep springform cake tin that fits into your slow cooker. If using a cake tin, place in slow cooker on top of two egg rings or an upturned saucer.

In a large mixing bowl, mix together sugar, flours and salt and make a well in the centre.

Drain and squeeze the grated apples to remove excess liquid.

Add the apple, zest, egg yolks, butter and milk and stir to combine thoroughly.

Beat the egg whites until stiff peaks form. Gently fold them into the apple mixture using a slotted spoon, keeping the batter as light as possible.

Pour into prepared cake tin in your slow cooker. Drape a tea towel over slow cooker then cover with lid and fold the tea towel back over the lid. Cook on high for 2 hours or until a skewer inserted into the middle comes out clean. It should be light and fluffy and golden.

Turn out onto a wire rack to cool, then dust with icing sugar to serve.

White Chocolate Chip Muffins

MAKES 20
COOK TIME: HIGH 40 MINS

2½ cups (310g) self-raising flour
½ tsp salt
1 tsp vanilla extract
⅔ cup (140g) caster sugar
2 eggs
1 cup (250ml) milk
50g butter, softened
1 cup (155g) white chocolate chips

Combine all ingredients in a large bowl. Mix well to combine.

Spoon into silicone cupcake cases or a lined muffin tray that will fit inside your slow cooker. Pour 1cm water into slow cooker bowl. Place a wire rack in the water and place cupcake moulds or muffin tray on top.

Drape a tea towel over the slow cooker and cover with the lid. Fold the tea towel back over the lid. Cook on high for 40 minutes or until an inserted skewer comes out clean.

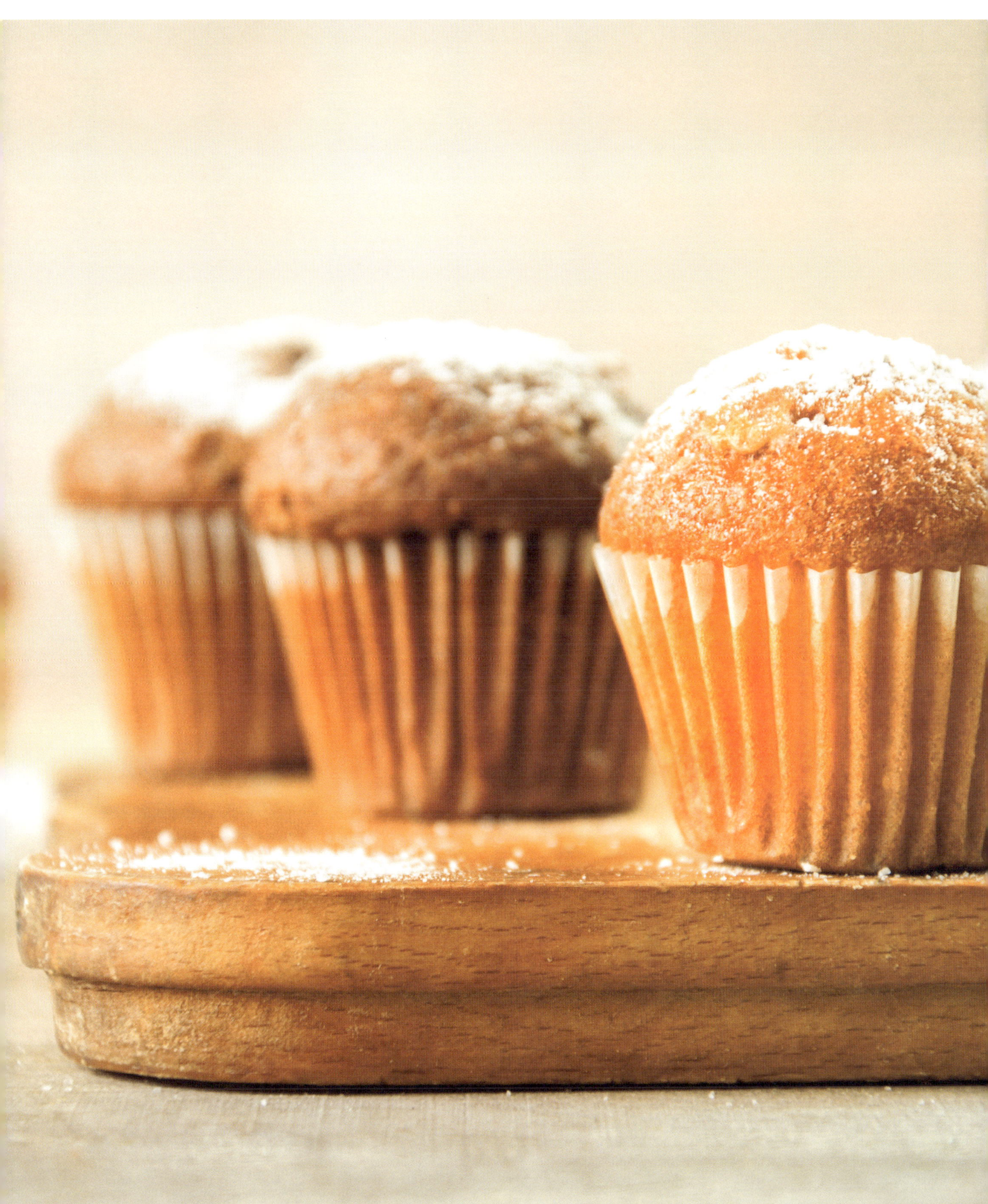

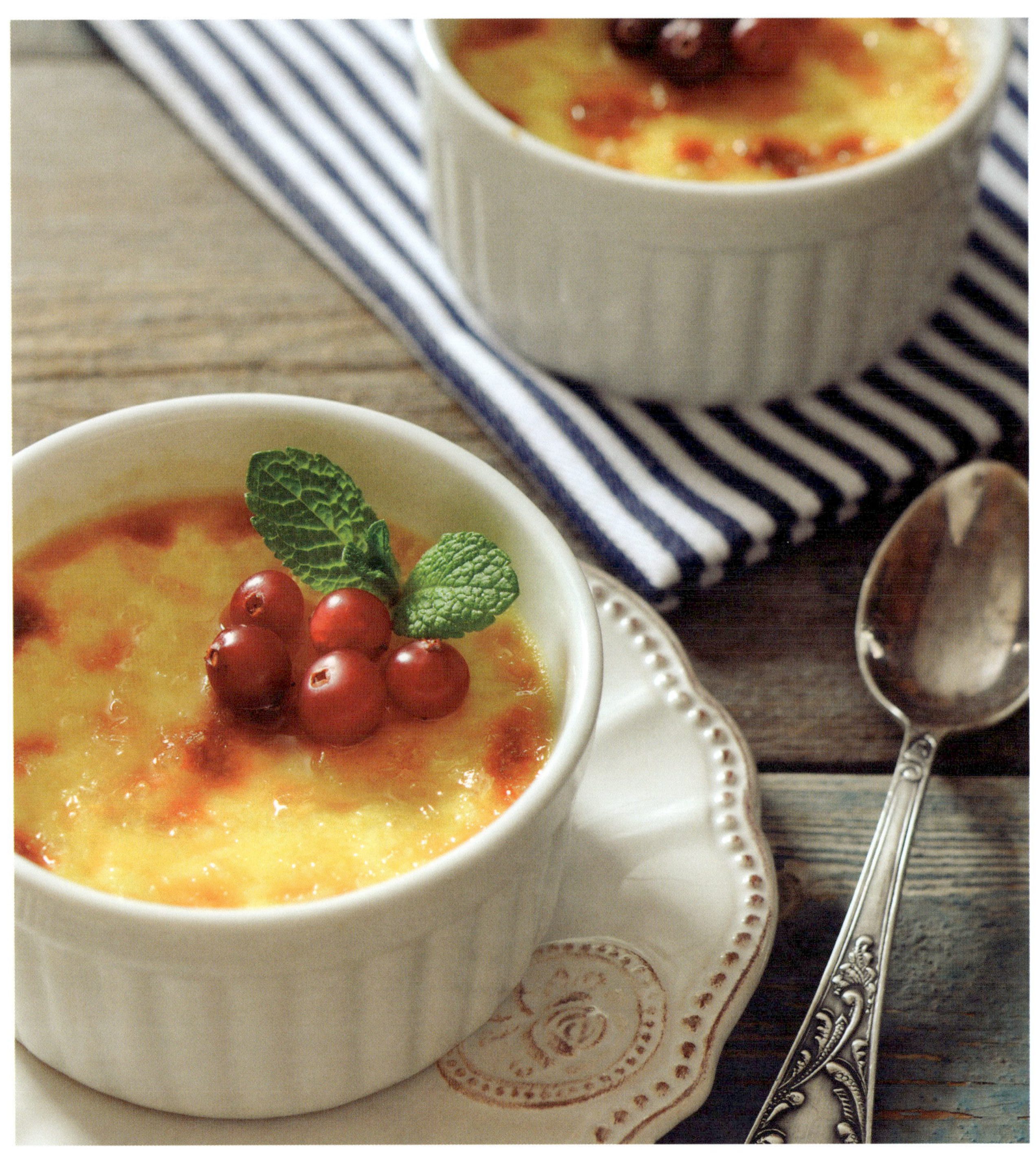

Creme Brulee

SERVES 4

COOK TIME: LOW 2 HRS

GLUTEN FREE

CREME BRULEE

4 large egg yolks

¼ cup (50g) caster sugar + extra for topping

¼ tsp salt

2 tsps vanilla extract

1⅔ cups (400ml) thickened cream

Fresh berries, to garnish

Mint leaves, to garnish

Whisk together the yolks, sugar, salt and vanilla. Gently whisk in the cream, then pour the mixture through a sieve into a measuring jug.

Pour the mixture into four ramekins and place them in the slow cooker. Fill the slow cooker with enough water to come halfway up the sides of the ramekins.

Cover the top of the slow cooker with a tea towel to absorb condensation then put the lid on and cook on low for 2 hours or until the mixture is set but jiggles slightly.

Remove the ramekins to a wire rack to cool. Place them in the fridge to chill for about 3 hours.

Sprinkle the extra caster sugar over each creme brulee, and brown the sugar with a culinary blowtorch (or place under a hot grill). Serve immediately, garnished with berries and mint.

Vanilla Cheesecake

SERVES 6
COOK TIME: HIGH 2 HRS

¾ cup (75g) sweet biscuits, crushed
¼ tsp ground nutmeg
2½ tbsps unsalted butter, melted
⅔ cup (140g) caster sugar
350g cream cheese
1 cup (240g) creme fraiche
1 tbsp plain flour
2 large eggs
1 tsp vanilla extract
1 tsp lime zest

In a large bowl mix the biscuits with the nutmeg, butter and 1 tablespoon of sugar. Press into the bottom of a cake tin that will fit your slow cooker.

Using an electric mixer, whisk the cream cheese, creme fraiche and flour for 1 minute. Add the rest of the sugar and beat for 2 minutes more. Add the eggs one at a time along with the vanilla and lime zest. Beat for another 30 seconds. Pour the mixture into the cake tin and smooth the top.

Place a tea towel at the bottom of the slow cooker and the cake tin on top. Pour enough water into the slow cooker so that it comes 2cm up the sides of the tin.

Place another tea towel over the top of the slow cooker, cover, and cook on high for 2 hours. Turn off the cooker and allow the cake to cool, without removing the lid, for another hour. Place the cake in the fridge to chill for at least 3 hours before serving.

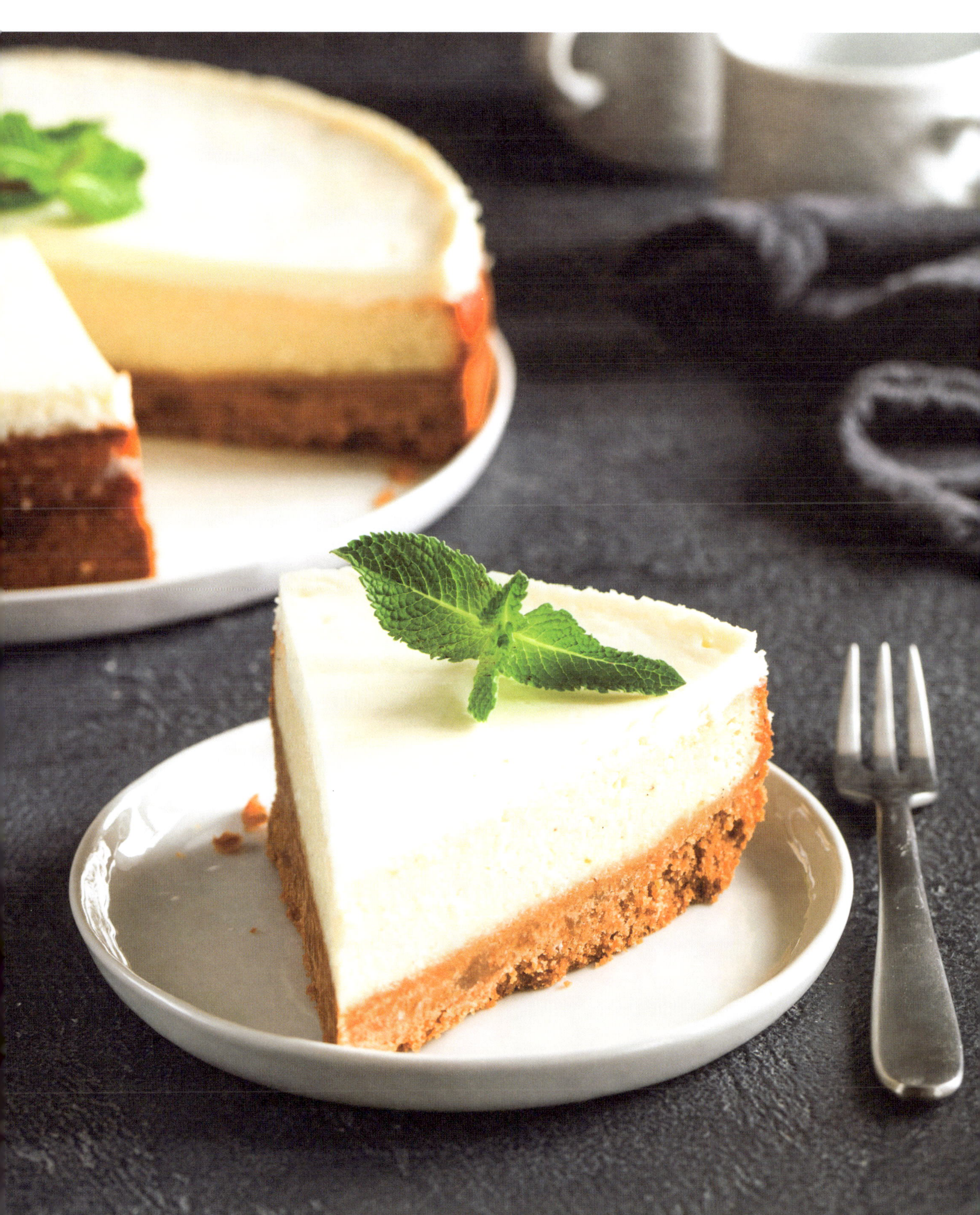

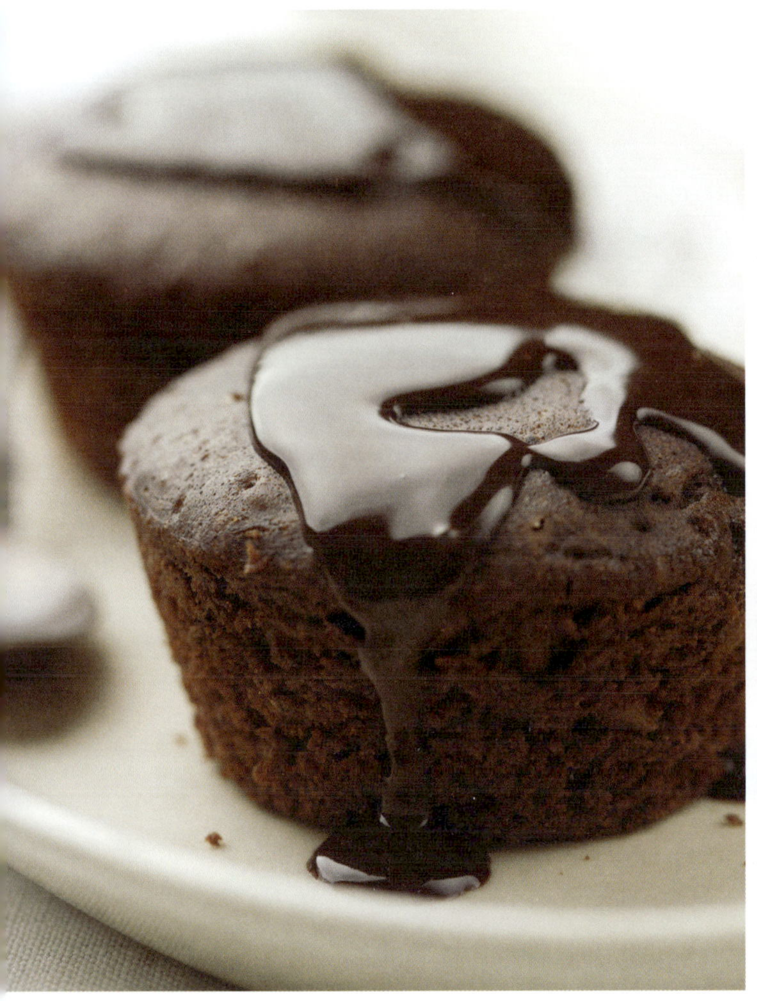

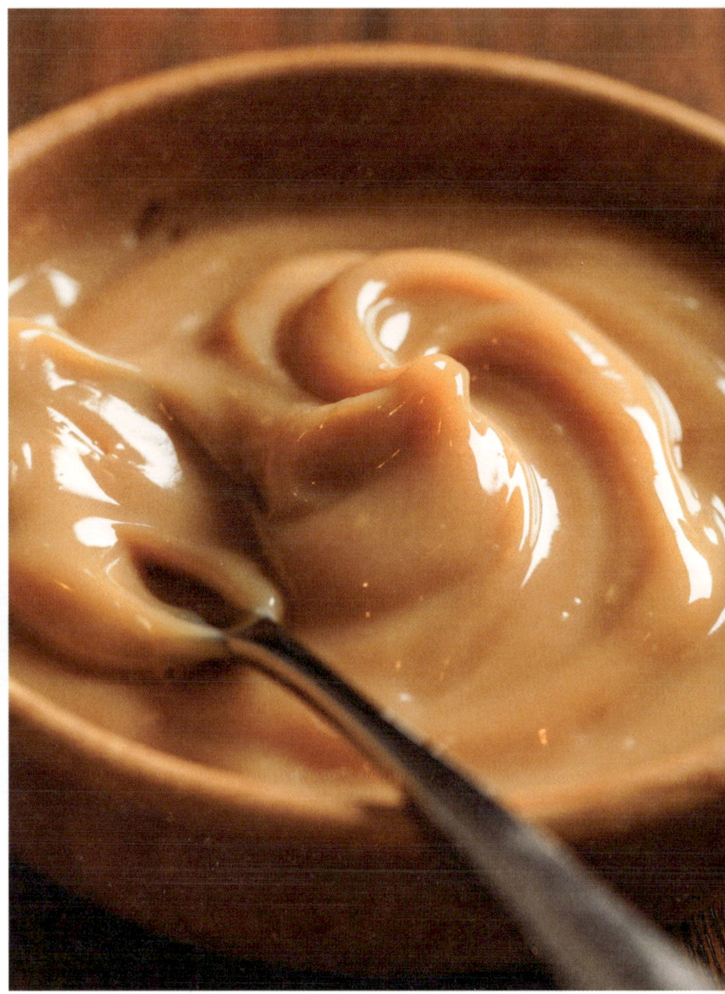

Mini Chocolate Muffins

MAKES 14

COOK TIME: HIGH 1 HR 45 MINS

Dulce de Leche

SERVES 4

COOK TIME: LOW 8 HRS

GLUTEN FREE

MINI CHOCOLATE MUFFINS

1 cup (125g) plain flour
2 tsps baking powder
5 tsps cocoa powder
½ cup (110g) caster sugar
⅓ cup (50g) + ½ cup (80g) dark chocolate chips
½ cup (125ml) milk
1 egg
1 tsp vanilla bean paste
2 tbsps olive oil or avocado oil + more for greasing

Place flour, baking powder, cocoa powder, sugar and ⅓ cup chocolate chips in a mixing bowl.

Place milk, egg, vanilla bean paste and oil in a separate jug and mix together.

Pour the wet ingredients into the dry ingredients and mix.

Brush 14 silicone mini muffin moulds with oil. Half fill each mould with muffin batter.

Place moulds in the slow cooker. Cover with a cotton tea towel, place lid on slow cooker and fold the tea towel back over the lid. Cook on high for 1 hour 45 minutes or until an inserted skewer comes out clean. Allow to cool then push out of muffin moulds.

Melt remaining chocolate chips in a bowl in the microwave, then drizzle over muffins.

DULCE DE LECHE

2 x 400g cans condensed milk

Place the two sealed cans of condensed milk in the slow cooker so they are standing upright. Fill the slow cooker with hot tap water, and cook on low for 8 hours.

Place the cans in cold water to cool before opening. Remove the dulce de leche from the cans and serve or store in jars.

Orange and Pistachio Cake

SERVES 8

COOK TIME: HIGH 1-2 HRS

4 eggs

⅓ cup (80g) caster sugar

4 tbsps honey

1½ cups (180g) plain flour

¾ cup (100g) pistachios, finely chopped

150g butter, melted

Juice and zest of 1 orange

SYRUP

3 tbsps honey

2 tbsps water

Juice of 1 large orange

TOPPING

¼ cup (30g) pistachios, roughly chopped

2 tbsps candied orange peel, sliced

1 tbsp honey

Grease and line slow cooker or use a slow-cooker liner and spray with cooking spray.

In a large bowl whisk together eggs, caster sugar and honey with an electric hand mixer for about 5 minutes until pale and thick.

Fold in the flour and chopped pistachios.

Stir in melted butter, orange juice and zest.

Pour mixture into the slow cooker. Cover and cook on high for 1-2 hours until an inserted skewer comes out clean.

Meanwhile make the syrup. Place honey, water and orange juice into a small pan over medium-low heat. Simmer for a few minutes until thick and syrupy.

When the cake is cooked, pour the syrup over the cake and allow it to absorb.

To serve, scatter with pistachios and candied peel and drizzle with honey.

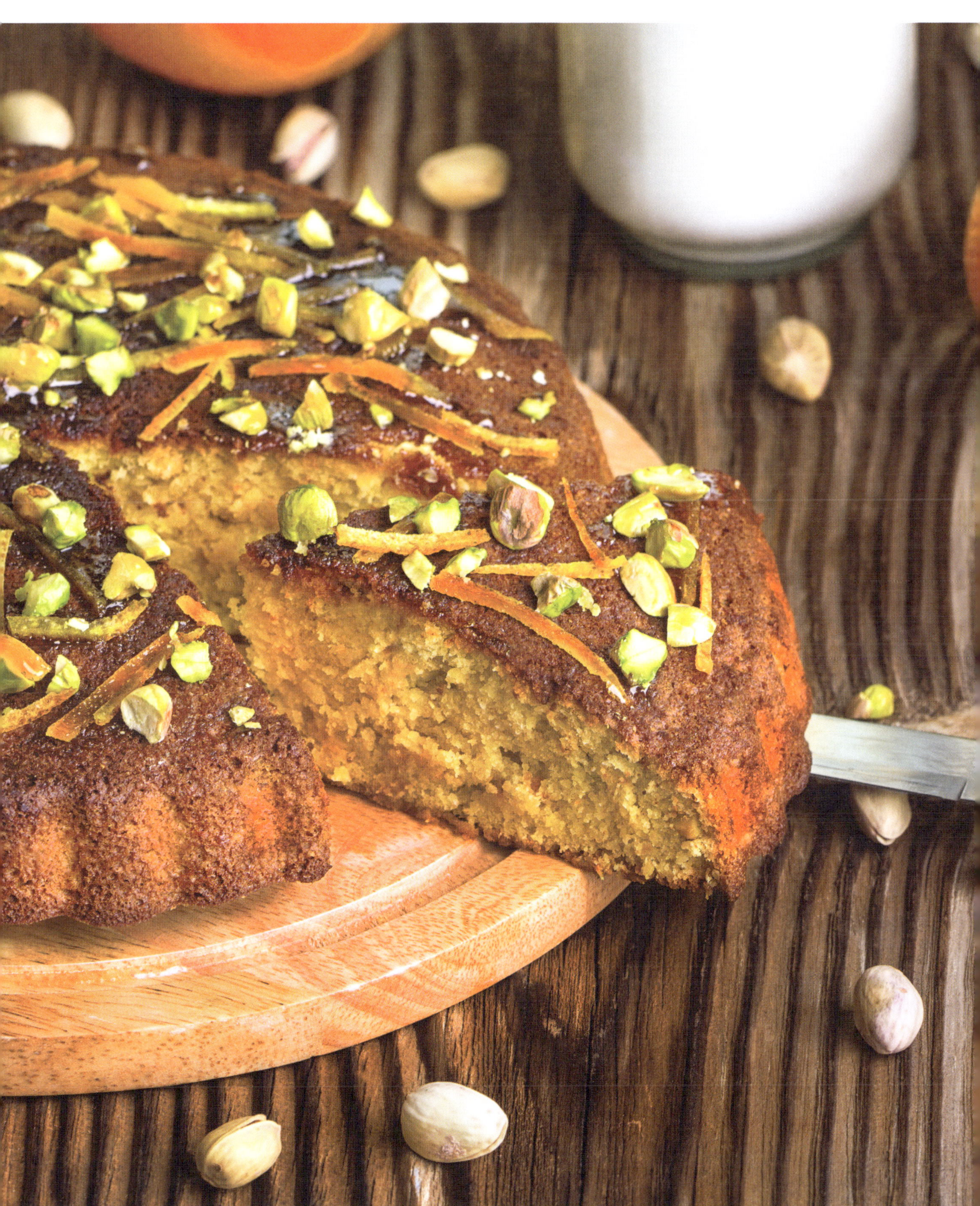

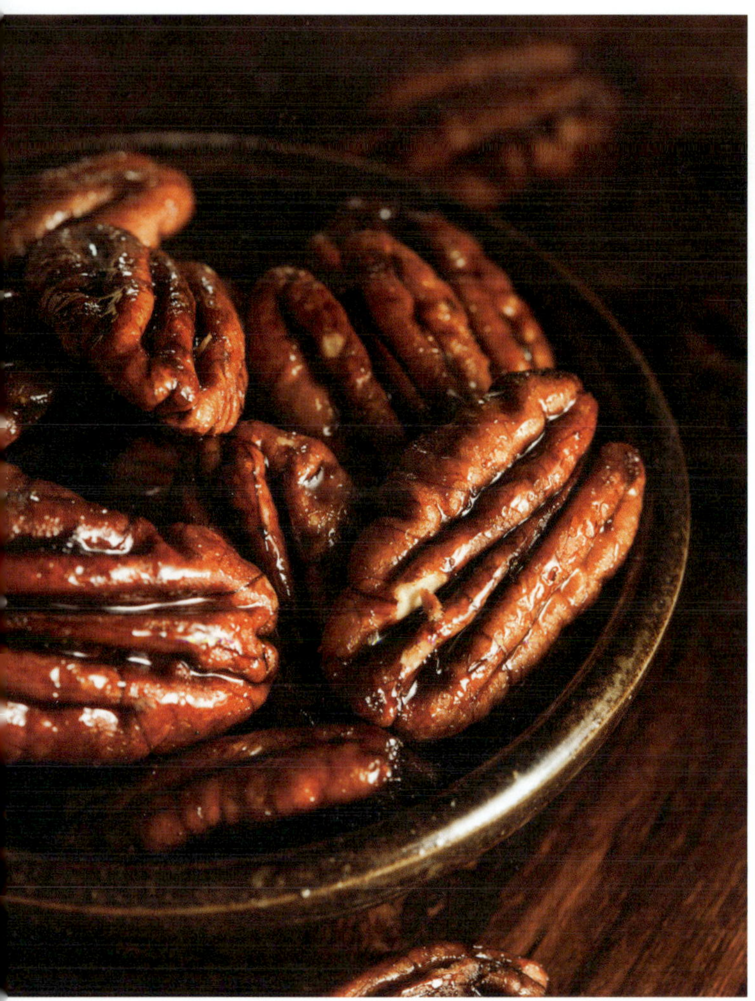

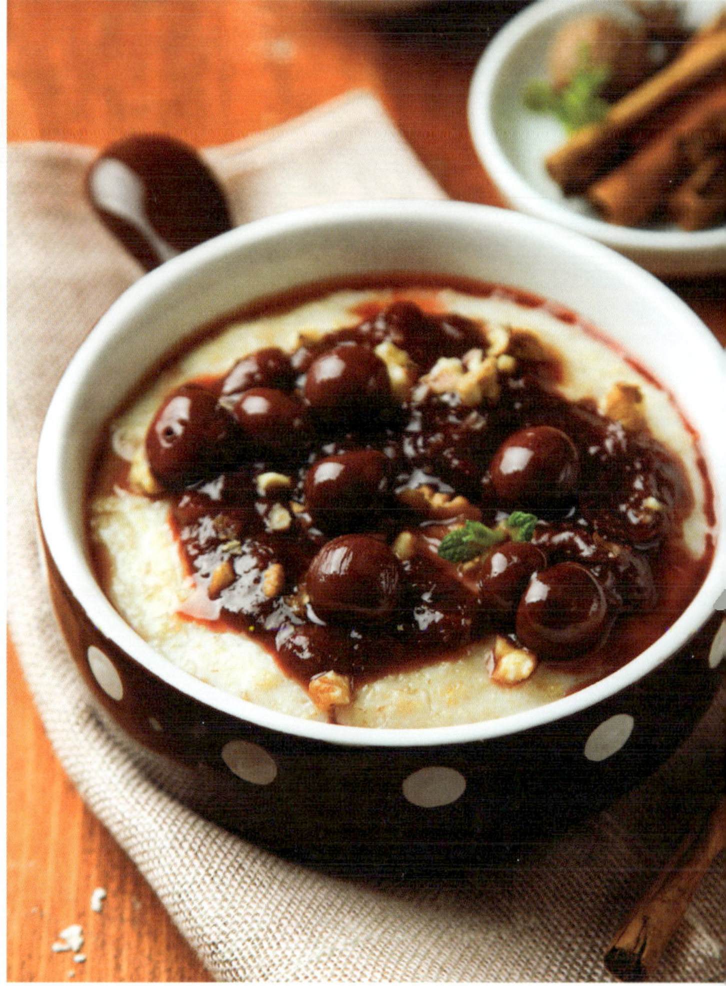

Candied Pecans

SERVES 4

COOK TIME: LOW 3 HRS

GLUTEN FREE • DAIRY FREE

Stewed Cherries

SERVES 4

COOK TIME: HIGH 3 HRS

GLUTEN FREE • DAIRY FREE

CANDIED PECANS

¾ cup (165g) caster sugar
½ cup (80g) light brown sugar
1½ tbsps cinnamon
1 egg white
2 tsps vanilla
5 cups (625g) pecans
¼ cup (60ml) water

Combine the sugar, brown sugar and cinnamon in a large mixing bowl. Set aside.

In a separate bowl whisk together egg white and vanilla until frothy.

Lightly grease the inset of the slow cooker. Place pecans inside and pour over the egg white mixture. Stir until nuts are evenly coated.

Sprinkle the cinnamon-sugar mix over the top and stir again to coat the nuts well.

Cover and cook on low for 3 hours. Stir every 20 minutes or so. Twenty minutes before cooking time is finished, add the water into the slow cooker and stir.

Remove from cooker and spread nuts out onto a baking tray to cool for 15 minutes before serving.

STEWED CHERRIES

600g cherries, pitted and halved
Juice of ½ lemon
1 cup (220g) caster sugar
1 tsp vanilla extract
½ cup (125ml) water
Rice pudding, to serve (optional, see recipe page 295)

Place the cherries, lemon juice, sugar and vanilla extract in the slow cooker and add the water.

Cook on high for 3 hours or until the cherries are softened and the water absorbed.

Serve with rice pudding, if desired.

Banana Choc Chip Loaf

SERVES 10

COOK TIME: HIGH 2-4 HRS

1¼ cups (275g) sugar
115g butter, softened
2 large eggs
3-4 ripe bananas, mashed
½ cup (125ml) milk
1 tsp vanilla extract
2½ cups (310g) plain flour
1 tsp bicarbonate of soda
½ tsp salt
1½ tsps cinnamon
½ cup (80g) dark chocolate chips

Preheat your slow cooker on high for 20 minutes. Grease and line a loaf tin that will fit inside your slow cooker. If your slow cooker is not big enough to hold a loaf tin, cook directly in your greased and lined slow cooker.

In a large mixing bowl, cream together the sugar and softened butter with an electric hand mixer. Add eggs one at a time and mix well to combine. Mix in the mashed bananas, milk and vanilla extract. Add flour, bicarb, salt and cinnamon. Stir with a wooden spoon to incorporate, making sure not to over mix, leaving the batter slightly lumpy. Stir in chocolate chips.

Pour batter into prepared loaf tin and place inside preheated slow cooker.

Cover the slow cooker with a cotton tea towel, place lid over slow cooker and fold the tea towel back over the lid. Cook on high for 2-4 hours until the bread is cooked through and a skewer inserted in the middle of the loaf comes out clean.

Remove the loaf tin from the slow cooker and allow the bread to cool for 10 minutes before removing bread from tin.

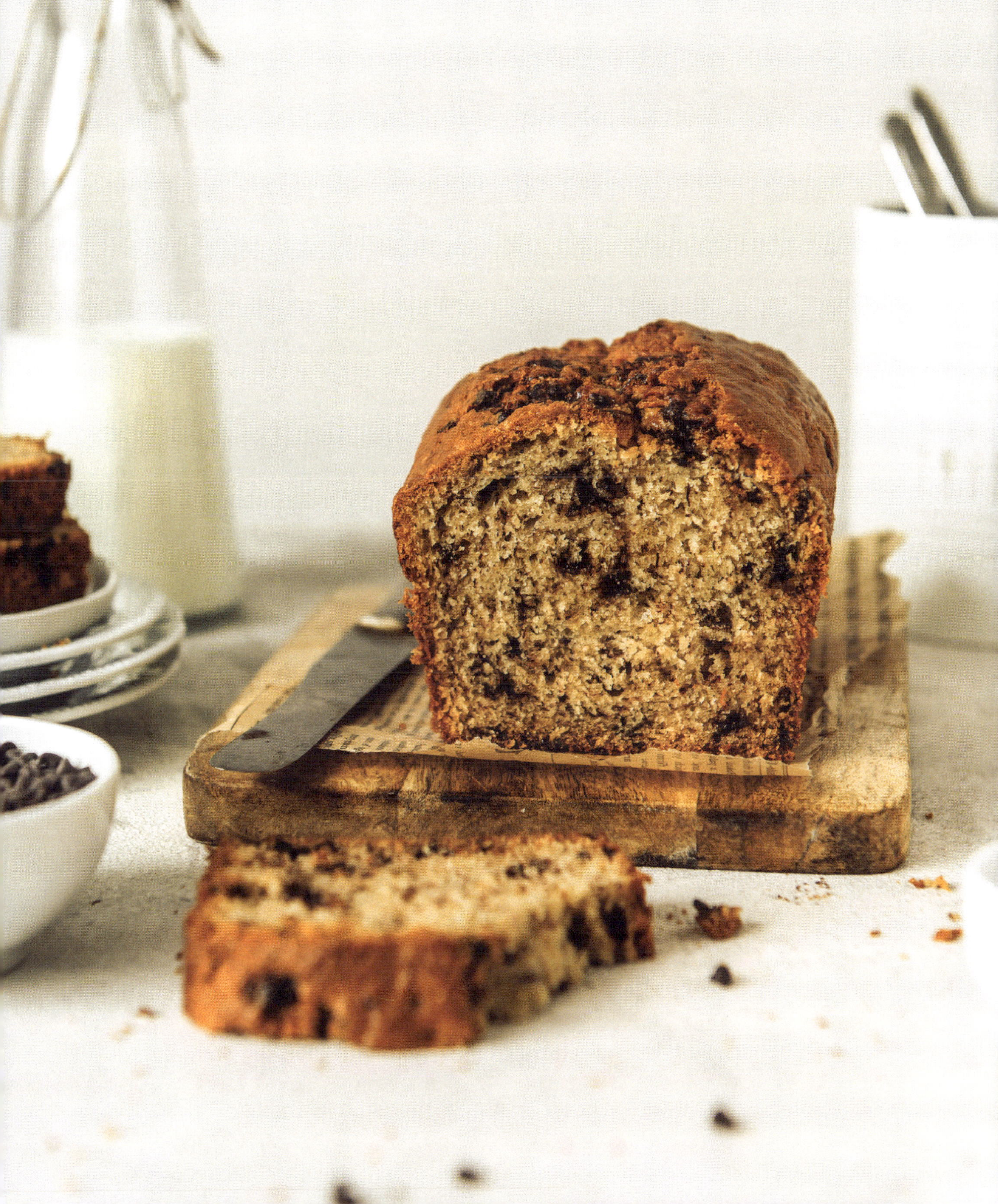

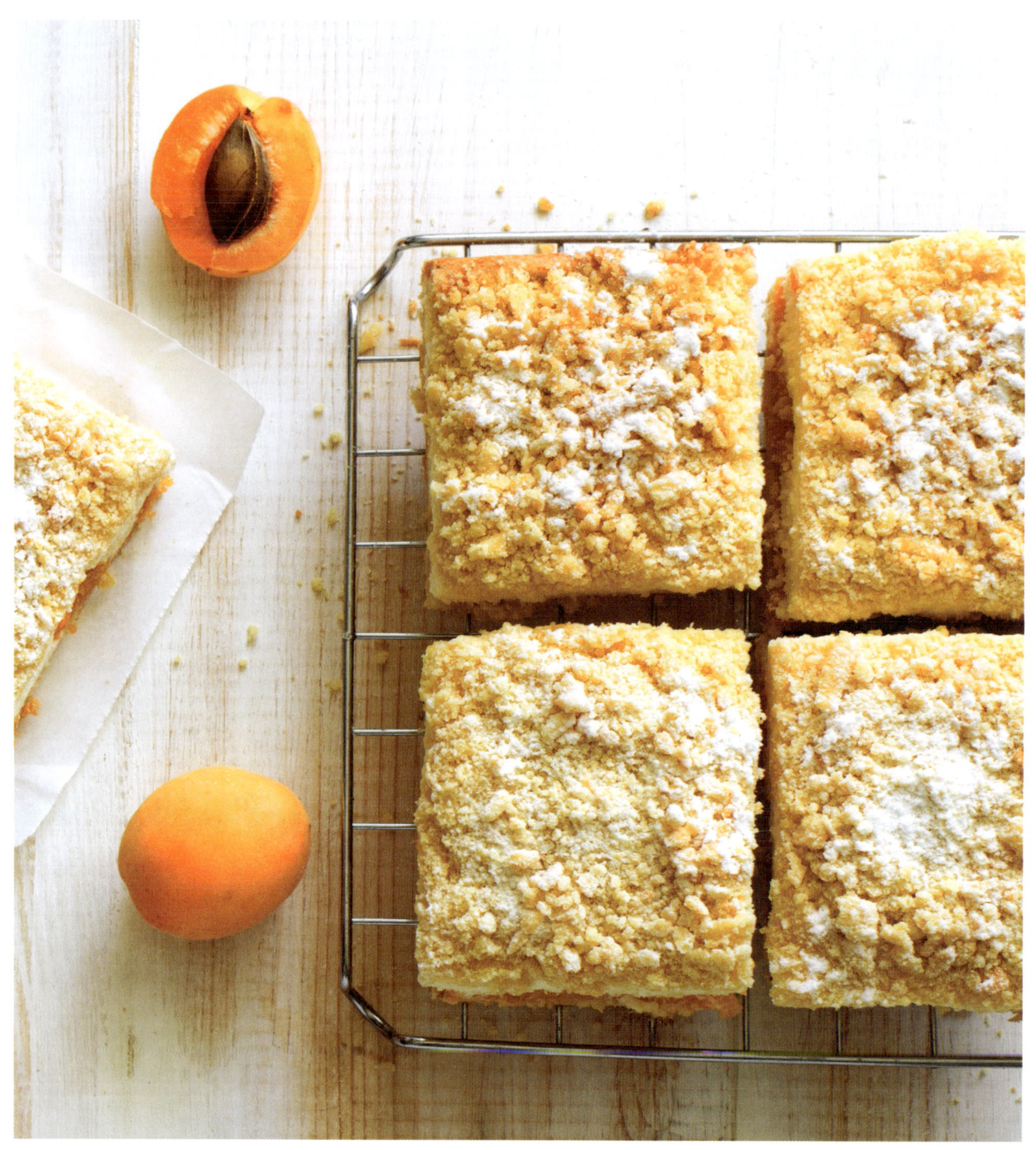

Apricot Crumble Slice

SERVES 16

COOK TIME: HIGH 2 HRS 30 MINS

APRICOT CRUMBLE SLICE

110g butter, room temperature, diced

1 cup (125g) plain flour

⅓ cup (60g) icing sugar

1-2 tbsps milk, as needed

⅔ cup (220g) apricot jam

CRUMBLE TOPPING

¾ cup (95g) plain flour

½ cup (100g) brown sugar

2 tbsps icing sugar + extra for dusting

110g butter, melted

Place a piece of greaseproof paper into your slow cooker, covering the base and coming halfway up the sides.

Place butter, flour and icing sugar into a food processor and pulse until the mixture forms a soft dough that just holds together. Add milk as needed if the dough is too dry.

Press into the base of slow cooker. Drape a tea towel over the slow cooker. Cover a with the lid, then fold the tea towel back over the lid. Cook on high for 30 minutes.

Remove the lid and spread the base with apricot jam.

To make the crumble topping combine the flour, brown sugar and icing sugar together in a bowl. Pour in the melted butter and mix until crumbly.

Pour the crumble over the base. Cover once more with tea towel and lid. Cook on high for 1½ -2 hours until golden brown and firm.

Allow to cool for 30 minutes before lifting the slice out of the slow cooker using the greaseproof paper. Allow to cool before dusting with icing sugar and serving.

SPICED RHUBARB

1 bunch rhubarb, chopped into 2cm pieces
2 green apples, peeled and chopped
2 tbsps brown sugar
1 vanilla bean
1 cinnamon stick
4 star anise
Small piece ginger, sliced
Juice of 1 orange

Place rhubarb and apple in the slow cooker. Sprinkle over sugar and stir to combine.

Cut vanilla bean down the centre and scrape out the seeds. Add seeds and bean to slow cooker.

Add cinnamon, star anise and ginger.

Squeeze orange juice over the other ingredients.

Cover and cook on high for 2 hours.

Serve with ice cream or over yoghurt or porridge.

BAKED APPLES

6 large apples
60g unsalted butter, softened
⅓ cup (50g) brown sugar
½ cup (60g) mixed nuts, chopped
½ cup (80g) mixed dried fruit
½ tsp ground cinnamon + extra to serve
½ tsp ground nutmeg
½ cup (125ml) water
1 tbsp honey

Cut a 2cm-deep lid horizontally off each of the apples and set aside.

Core the apples, trying to leave 1cm at the bottom to keep the filling inside.

In a bowl, combine butter, sugar, nuts, dried fruit, cinnamon and nutmeg. Spoon mixture into cored apples. Replace apple lids.

Place the apples into the slow cooker, sitting upright. Pour water into slow cooker around the base of the apples.

Cook on low for 3-4 hours or until tender.

Drizzle with honey and sprinkle with cinnamon to serve.

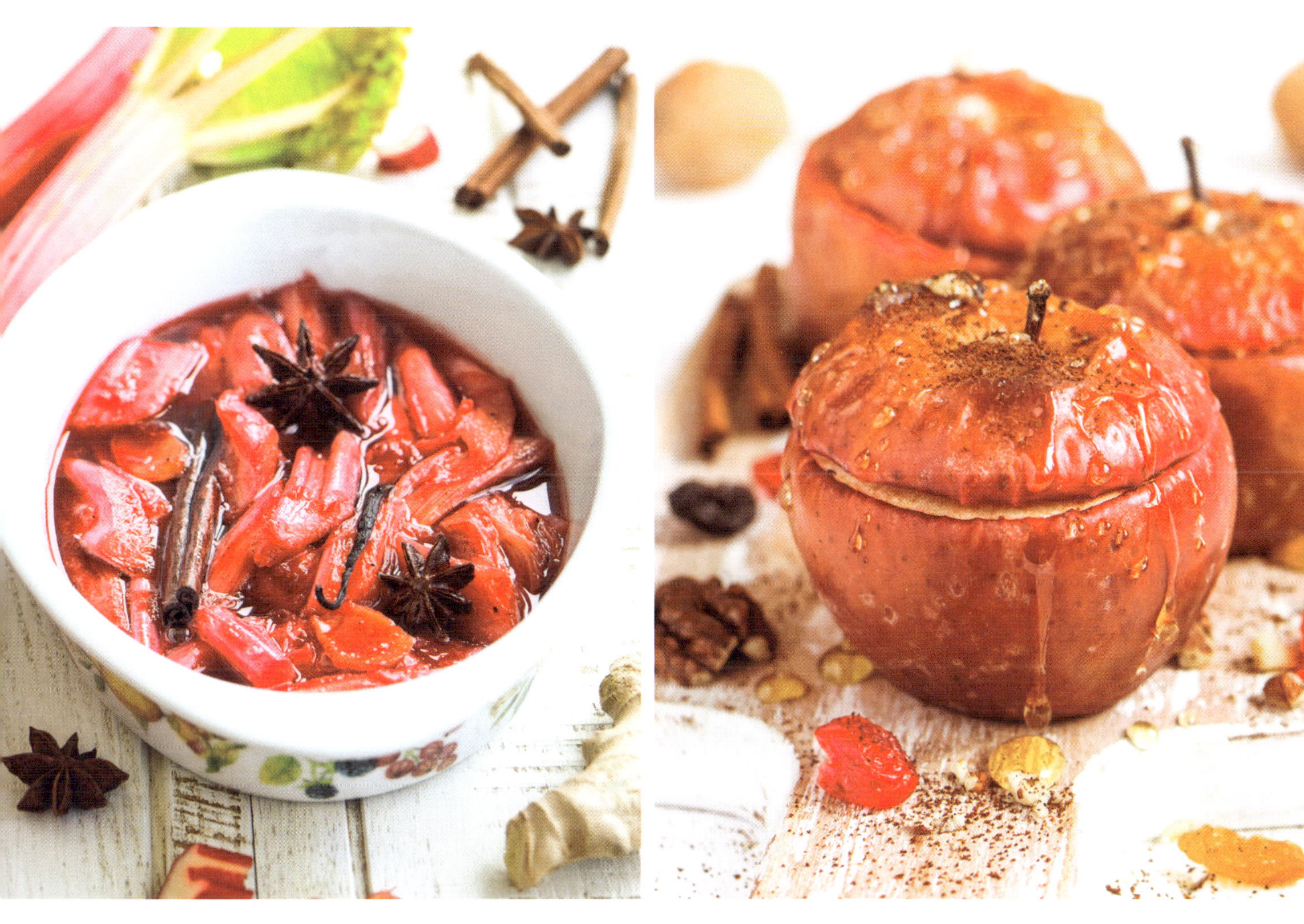

Spiced Rhubarb

SERVES 4-6

COOK TIME: HIGH 2 HRS

GLUTEN FREE • DAIRY FREE

Baked Apples

SERVES 6

COOK TIME: LOW 3-4 HRS

GLUTEN FREE

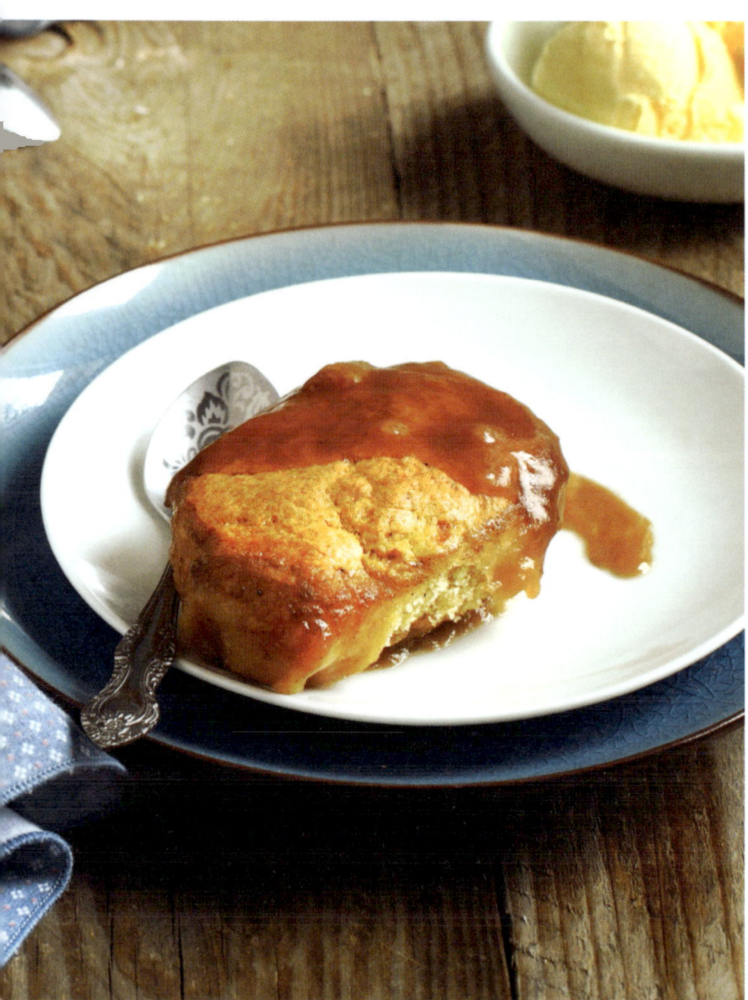

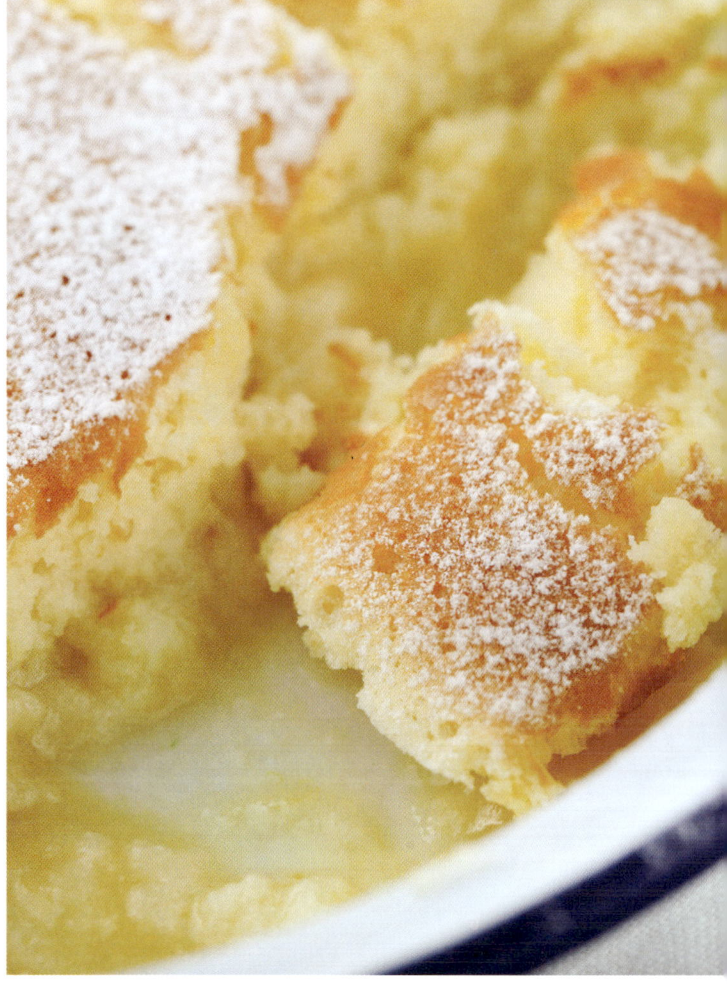

Caramel Dumplings

SERVES 6

COOK TIME: HIGH 1 HR 30 MINS

Lemon Delicious

SERVES 4

COOK TIME: LOW 4 HRS

CARAMEL DUMPLINGS

SAUCE

¾ cup (260g) golden syrup

½ cup (80g) brown sugar

50g butter, melted

2 cups (500ml) boiling water

DUMPLINGS

30g butter, softened

1½ cups (185g) self-raising flour

⅓ cup (80ml) milk

⅓ cup (115g) golden syrup

To make the sauce place golden syrup, brown sugar, butter and boiling water into slow cooker. Stir to combine.

To make the dumplings rub butter into the flour with your fingertips in a large bowl until it resembles breadcrumbs. Make a well in the centre and add the milk and golden syrup. Mix until well combined.

Roll the mixture into roughly 10 balls, then shape into logs. Carefully add the dumplings to the slow cooker, and lay on top of sauce.

Cover and cook on high for 1-1½ hours or until the dumplings are cooked through.

Spoon sauce over dumplings to serve.

LEMON DELICIOUS

150g unsalted butter, softened

1½ cups (330g) caster sugar

4 eggs, separated

¾ cup (90g) self-raising flour, sifted

1 tbsp lemon zest

⅓ cup (80ml) lemon juice

1½ cups (375ml) milk

Place butter and sugar in a large bowl. Use an electric hand mixer to beat together until light and fluffy.

Add egg yolks and whisk to combine.

Mix in the flour, lemon zest, lemon juice and milk.

In a separate bowl with a clean whisk, beat egg whites until soft peaks form. Gently fold into the cake mixture.

Lightly grease slow cooker, then pour in the cake batter.

Cover and cook on low for 4 hours until cooked through.

Moist Chocolate Cake

SERVES 12

COOK TIME: LOW 3 HRS

2 cups (310g) sugar
1¾ cups (215g) plain flour
¾ cup (90g) cocoa powder
1½ tsps baking powder
1½ tsps bicarbonate of soda
1 tsp salt
2 eggs
1 cup (250ml) milk
½ cup (125ml) vegetable oil
2 tsps vanilla extract
1 cup (250ml) boiling water
115g dark chocolate, chopped
½ cup (125ml) thickened cream
Grated chocolate and blueberries, to decorate

Grease and line the insert of the slow cooker or grease and line a deep springform cake tin that fits into your slow cooker. If using a cake tin, place in slow cooker on top of two egg rings or an upturned saucer.

In a large bowl, whisk together sugar, flour, cocoa, baking powder, bicarb and salt.

In a separate small bowl, mix together eggs, milk, oil and vanilla. Whisk in boiling water. Pour the wet ingredients into the dry and stir to combine.

Pour batter into the prepared slow cooker or cake tin. Drape a tea towel over slow cooker then cover with lid and fold the tea towel back over the lid

Cover and cook on low for 3 hours or until the cake starts to pull away from the sides of the slow cooker.

Turn off slow cooker and allow cake to rest for 30 minutes before turning on to a wire rack.

Meanwhile place chopped chocolate in a medium heatproof bowl. Heat the cream in a small saucepan over medium heat until gently simmering. Pour cream over chopped chocolate, then allow to sit for 2-3 minutes to gently soften the chocolate. With a metal spoon or small rubber spatula, slowly stir cream and chocolate until completely combined.

Allow to cool slightly then pour over cake. Top with grated chocolate and blueberries to serve.

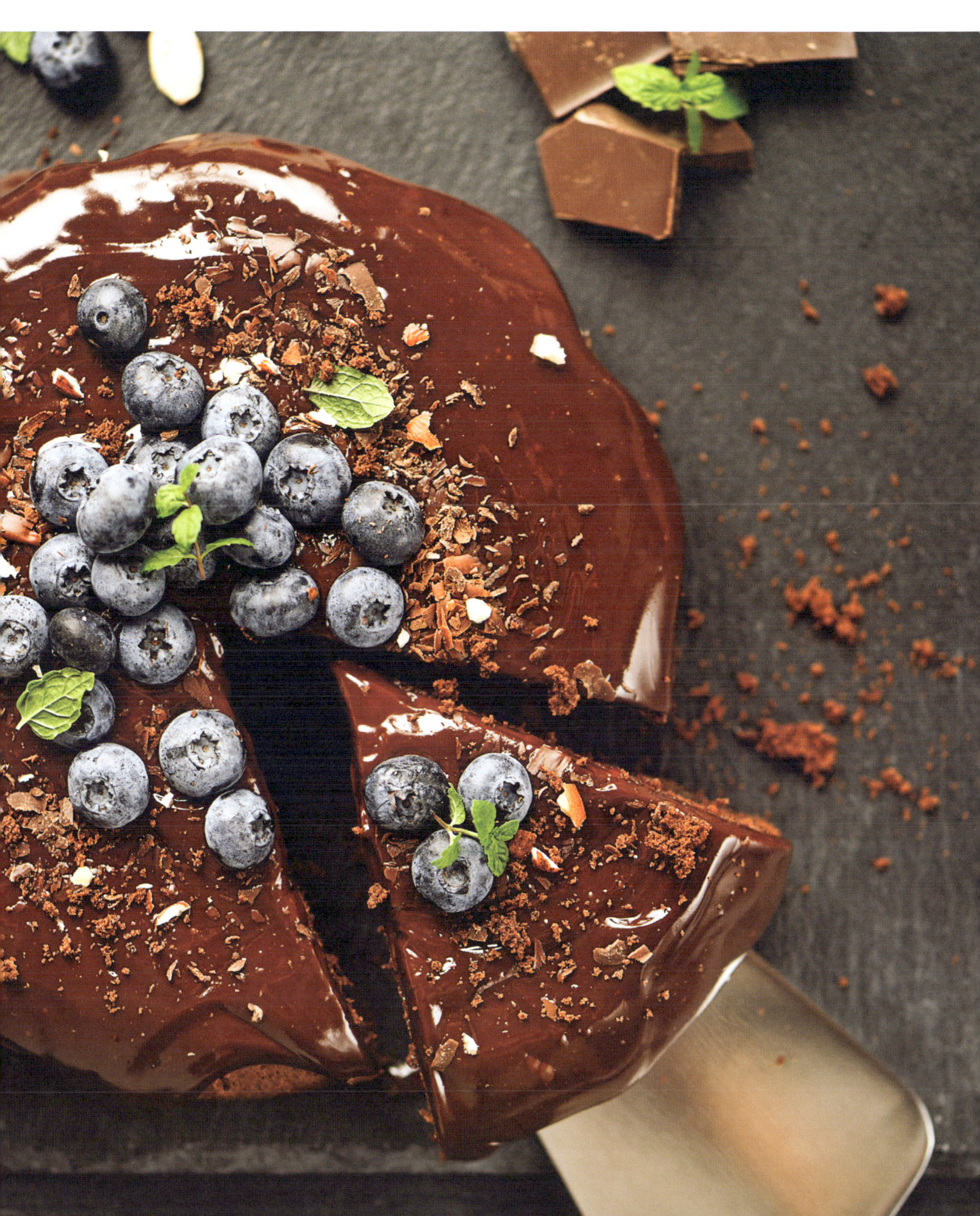

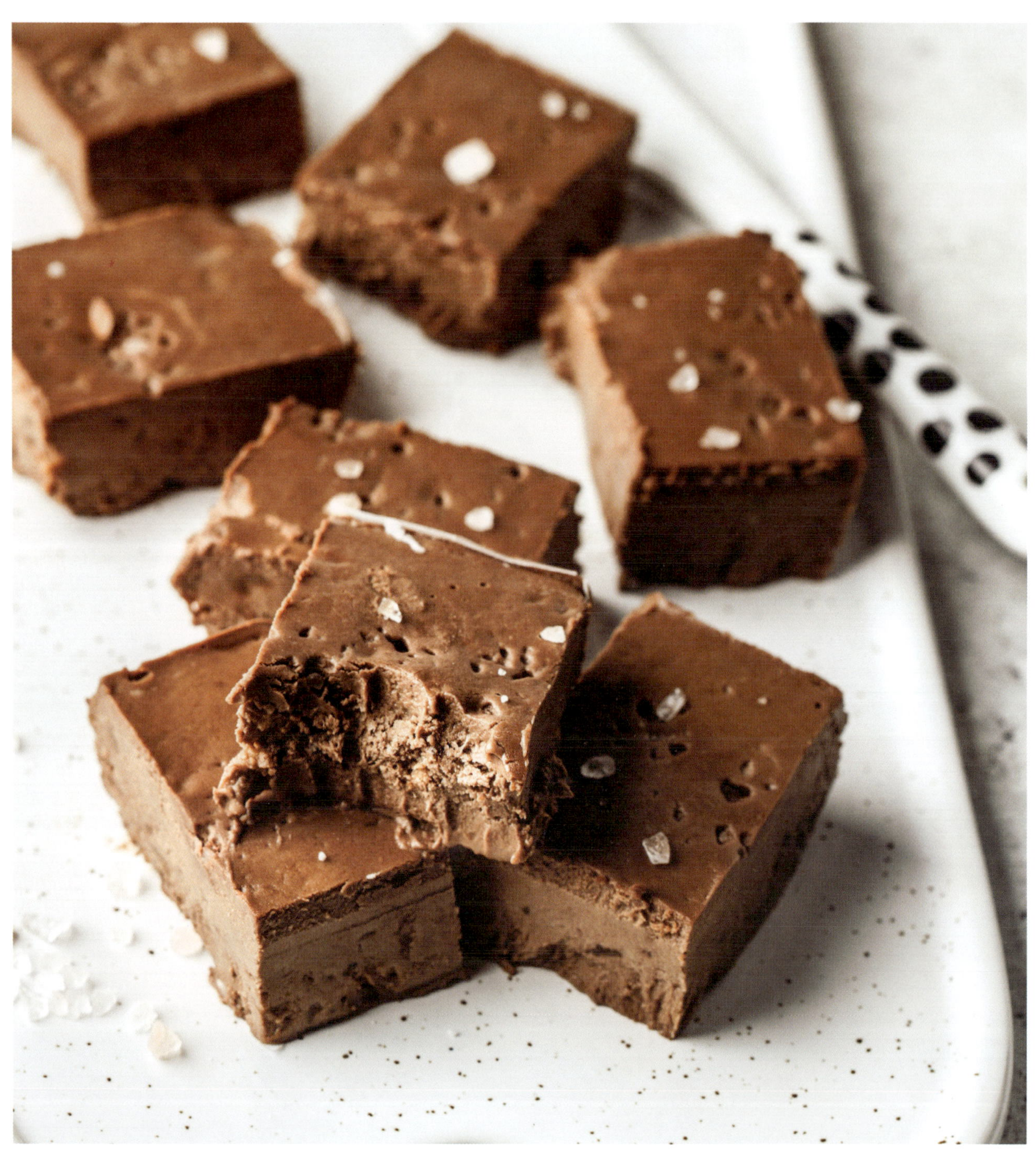

Chocolate Fudge

MAKES 20

COOK TIME: HIGH 30 MINS + LOW 2 HRS

GLUTEN FREE

CHOCOLATE FUDGE

500g dark chocolate (broken into pieces)
1 x 400g can condensed milk
1 tbsp butter
1 tbsp salt flakes

Line a 20cm square cake tin with greaseproof paper.

Place chocolate, condensed milk and butter in slow cooker.

Cook, uncovered, on high, stirring every few minutes, for 30 minutes or until chocolate is melted.

Turn down heat to low and cook for another 2 hours, stirring every 15-30 minutes.

Pour into the lined tin, allow to cool then place uncovered in the fridge for at least 2 hours to chill.

Cut into squares and sprinkle with salt flakes.

Rice Pudding with Peaches

SERVES 10

COOK TIME: LOW 7 HRS

GLUTEN FREE

PUDDING

8 cups (2L) full-cream milk

1 cup (155g) long-grain rice (such as jasmine or basmati)

¾ cup (165g) caster sugar

½ tsp salt

1 tsp vanilla extract

1 tbsp unsalted butter, melted

PEACHES IN SYRUP

120g butter

5 peaches, sliced

¼ cup (40g) brown sugar

1½ tsps ground cinnamon

1 cup (250ml) orange juice

To cook the rice, place all the rice pudding ingredients in the slow cooker and stir to combine.

Cover and cook on low for 7 hours.

Half an hour before the rice pudding is ready, prepare the peaches.

In a large frying pan, heat the butter over medium heat until the butter begins to foam.

Place the peach slices in the butter and sprinkle over the brown sugar and cinnamon.

Cook them for 4 minutes on each side until golden.

Remove the peaches and add the orange juice to the pan. Stir through. Simmer for 5 minutes until reduced and thickened then remove from heat.

Ladle a dessertspoon of the sauce into the bottom of each serving glass or bowl. Almost fill with rice pudding, then place four peach slices on top and drizzle over a tablespoon of the sauce.

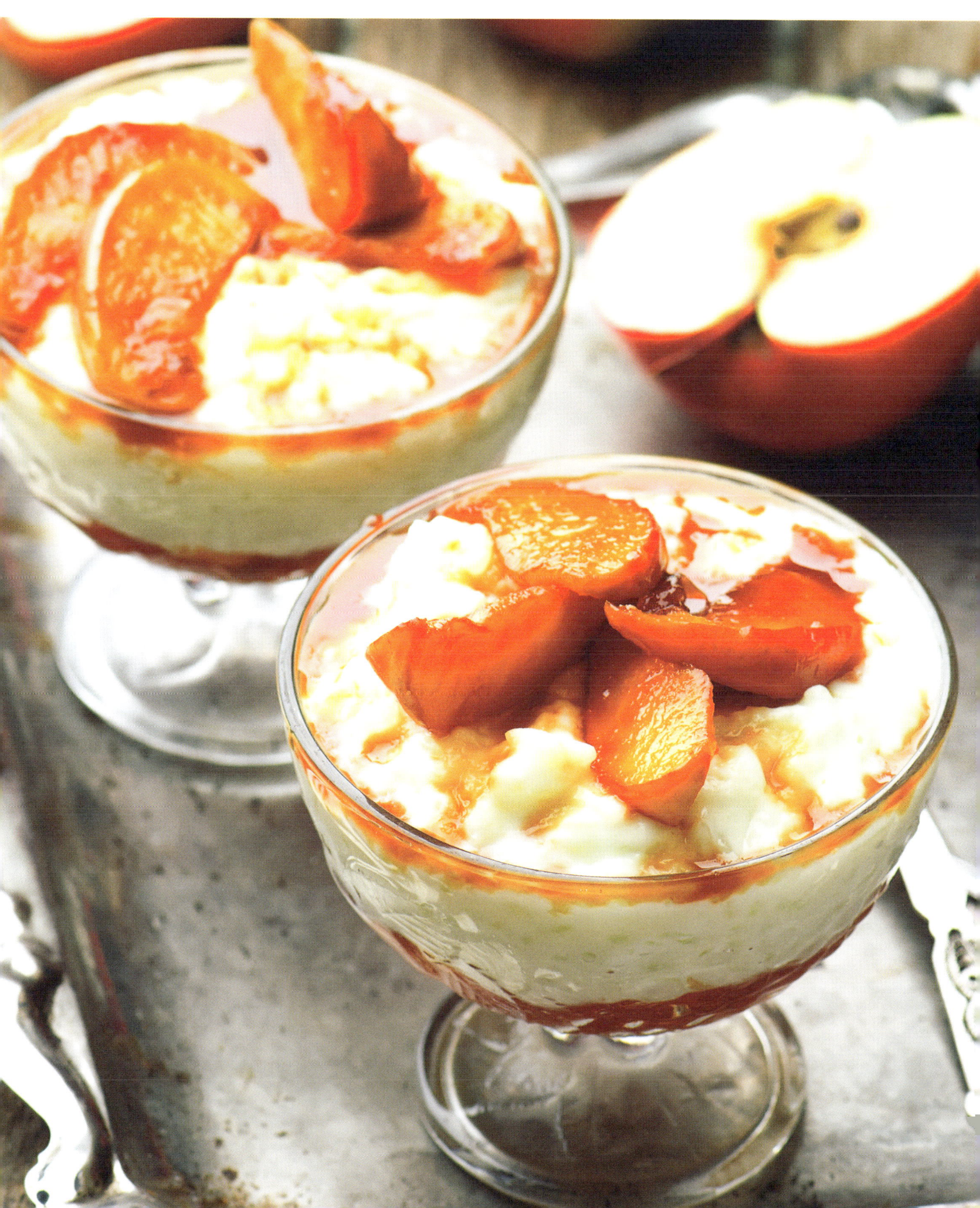

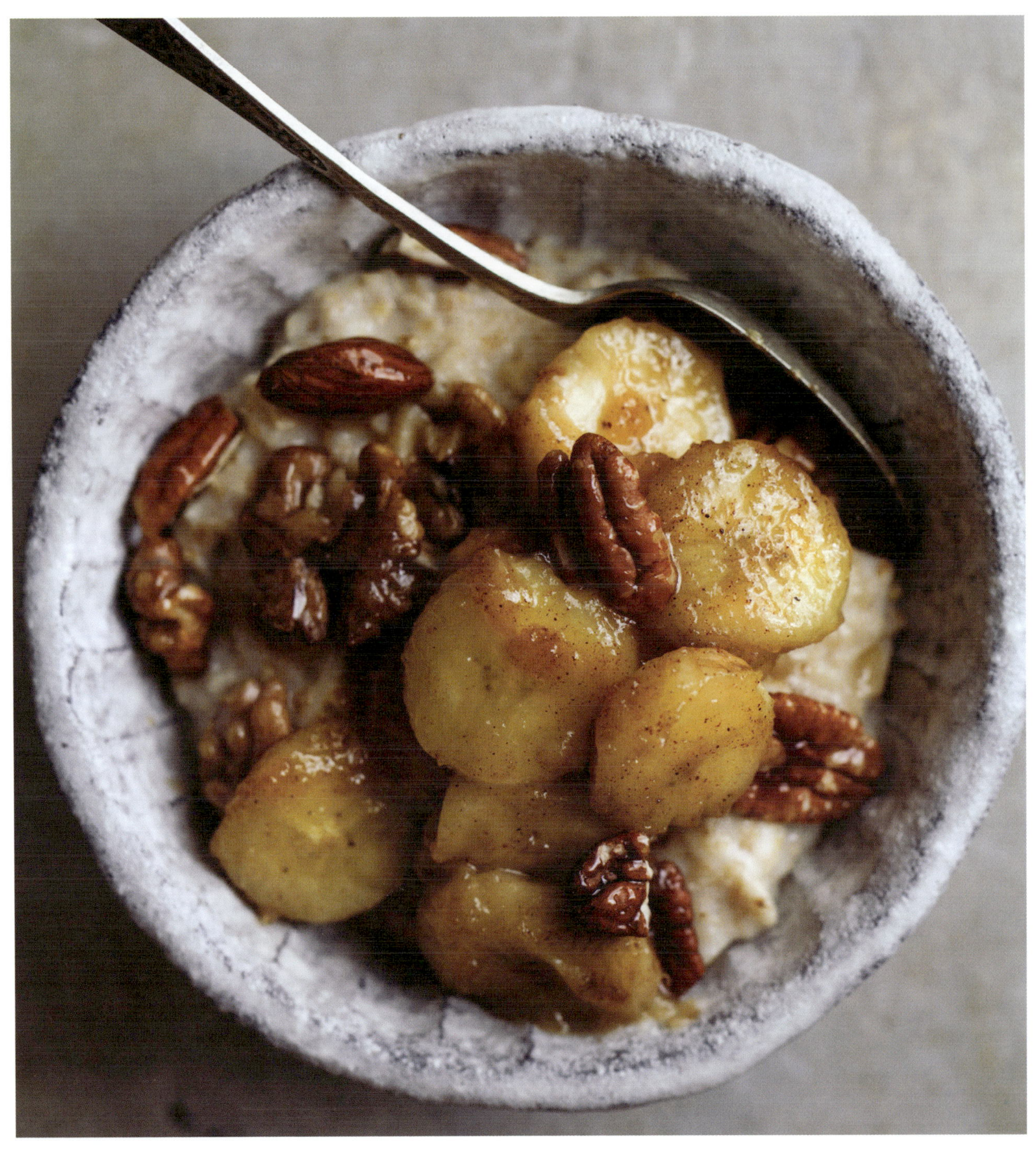

Caramelised Banana and Nuts

SERVES 4

COOK TIME: LOW 2 HRS

GLUTEN FREE

CARAMELISED BANANA AND NUTS

4 large bananas, peeled and roughly chopped
1 cup (155g) brown sugar
60g butter, melted
¼ cup (60ml) rum (optional)
1 tsp vanilla extract
½ tsp ground cinnamon
⅓ cup (40g) walnuts, roughly chopped
⅓ cup (40g) almonds
Rice pudding, to serve (optional, see recipe page 295)

Layer the banana pieces at the bottom of the slow cooker. In a large bowl combine the sugar, butter, rum (if using) vanilla and cinnamon. Pour over the bananas in the slow cooker, cover and cook on low for 1 hour 30 minutes or until heated through.

Add the walnuts and almonds, stir, and cook for another 30 minutes.

Serve with rice pudding.

Cheesecake with Caramel Sauce

SERVES 20

COOK TIME: LOW 5-7 HRS

12 digestive biscuits

6 tbsps melted butter + more for greasing

700g cream cheese

1¼ cups (275g) sugar

1½ cups (375ml) sour cream

5 large eggs

3 tbsps plain flour

1 tbsp vanilla extract

½ tsp salt

CARAMEL SAUCE

¼ cup (40g) dark brown sugar

1 tbsp butter

1 tbsp cream

Fold two pieces of greaseproof paper into long, 5cm-wide strips. Fold and place into slow cooker, to go down sides, across the bottom and up the sides again (these will be tabs to lift out the cheesecake when it is complete).

Grease and line slow cooker with greaseproof paper.

Place biscuits in a food processor and pulse into crumbs. Pour in butter and pulse to combine. Pour mixture into slow cooker and press evenly over the bottom.

Combine cream cheese and sugar in food processor; pulse until smooth. Add sour cream, eggs, flour, vanilla and salt. Puree until extremely smooth.

Pour filling over crust. Cover and cook on low for 5-7 hours, until an inserted skewer comes out clean.

Remove lid and transfer slow cooker insert to the fridge and chill for 3 hours.

Meanwhile heat sugar in pan over low heat, stirring regularly, for about 15 minutes. When the sugar is melted add butter and stir to combine. Then add cream and whisk well. Remove from heat and set aside to cool.

Carefully lift the entire cheesecake out of the insert by the paper tabs. Peel the paper back and drizzle with caramel sauce.

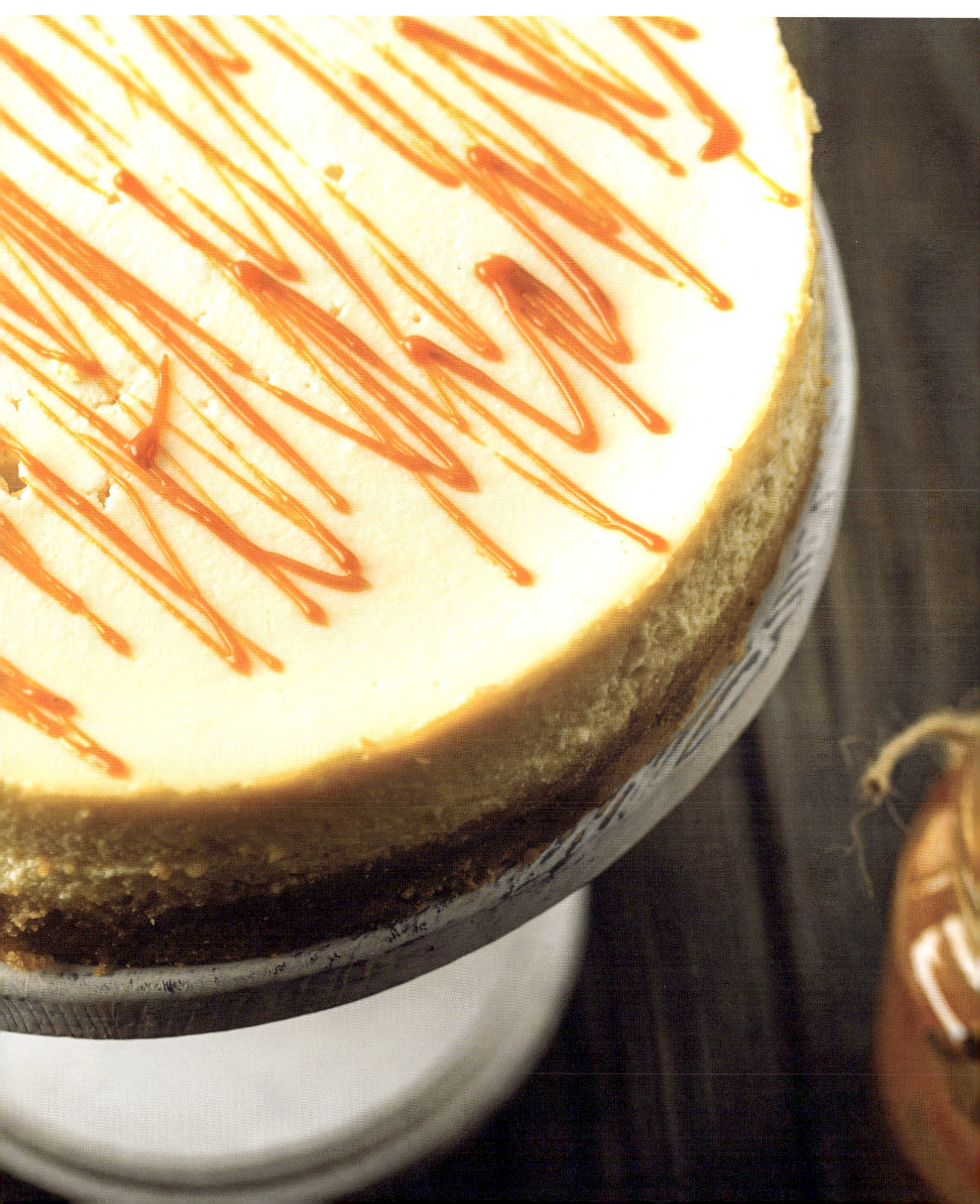

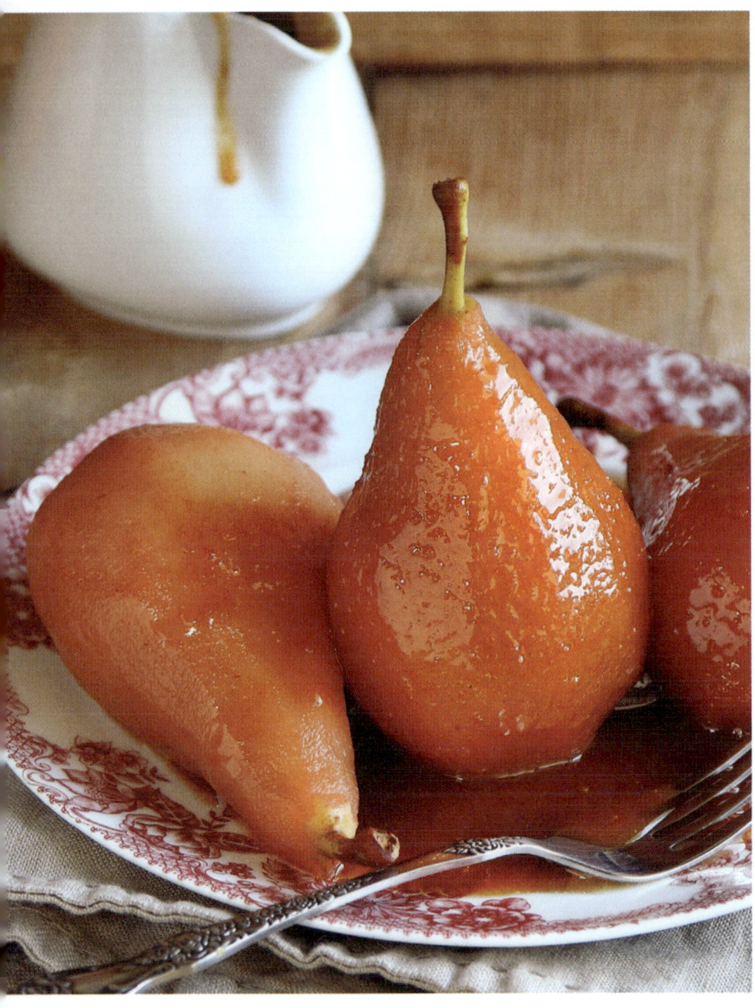

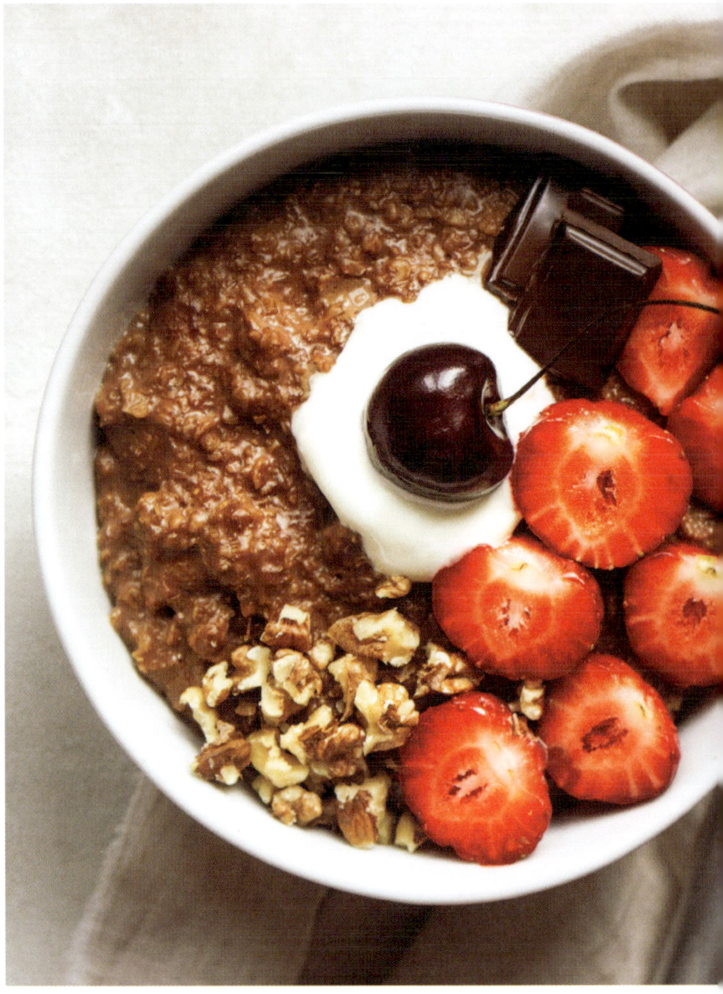

Poached Pears

SERVES 6

COOK TIME: HIGH 3 HRS

GLUTEN FREE

Chocolate Porridge

SERVES 4

COOK TIME: LOW 6 HRS

POACHED PEARS

6 firm Beurre Bosc pears

½ cup (80g) packed light brown sugar

⅓ cup (115g) honey

2 tbsps Cointreau

1 tbsp unsalted butter, melted

2 tsps finely grated orange zest

¼ tsp ground cardamom

1 tbsp arrowroot flour

3 tbsps orange juice

Peel the pears and leave stems intact, then sit them upright in the bottom of the slow cooker.

Mix together the rest of the ingredients except the arrowroot and orange juice.

Pour the mixture over the pears.

Cook, covered, on high heat for 2 hours 45 minutes until the pears are tender. Remove the pears and place in pre-warmed individual dessert bowls.

Keep the slow cooker on high heat. Mix together the arrowroot and orange juice and pour into the remaining liquid in the slow cooker. Stir for 15 minutes or until the sauce has thickened to desired consistency.

Spoon the sauce over the pears and serve them warm.

CHOCOLATE PORRIDGE

Butter for greasing

2 cups (180g) steel-cut oats

4 cups (1L) milk

1 cup (250ml) water

¼ cup (30g) cocoa powder

2 tbsps maple syrup

2 tsps vanilla extract

Pinch of salt

⅓ cup (80ml) thickened cream

Optional toppings: dark chocolate squares, cherries, strawberry halves, chopped walnuts

Grease slow cooker with butter.

Pour oats, milk, water, cocoa powder, maple syrup, vanilla and salt into a bowl. Mix well then pour into slow cooker.

Cook on low for 6 hours.

Serve into bowls and spoon over a dollop of cream. Finish with your choice of toppings.

Coconut and Cream Cake

SERVES 6

COOK TIME: HIGH 1 HR 30 MINS

1 cup (220g) caster sugar
½ cup (125ml) coconut oil
250g unsalted butter
3 large eggs
2 cups (250g) plain flour
1 tsp bicarbonate of soda
½ cup (125ml) coconut milk
220g cream cheese
3 cups (465g) icing sugar
½ tsp salt
1 tsp vanilla extract
Fresh raspberries, to garnish

In a bowl beat the caster sugar, coconut oil and half of the butter until fully combined. Mix in the eggs one at a time, continuing to beat, followed by the flour, bicarb and coconut milk.

Lightly grease the slow cooker and pour the batter in. Place a tea towel over the top to absorb condensation. Cover and cook on high for 90 minutes or until a toothpick comes out clean. Allow the cake to stand for 15 minutes in the slow cooker before removing.

For the frosting, beat the cream cheese and the rest of the butter in a large bowl using an electric mixer, until light and fluffy. Gradually beat in the icing sugar until well combined, followed by the salt and vanilla extract. Spread the topping on the cooled cake.

Garnish with the raspberries.

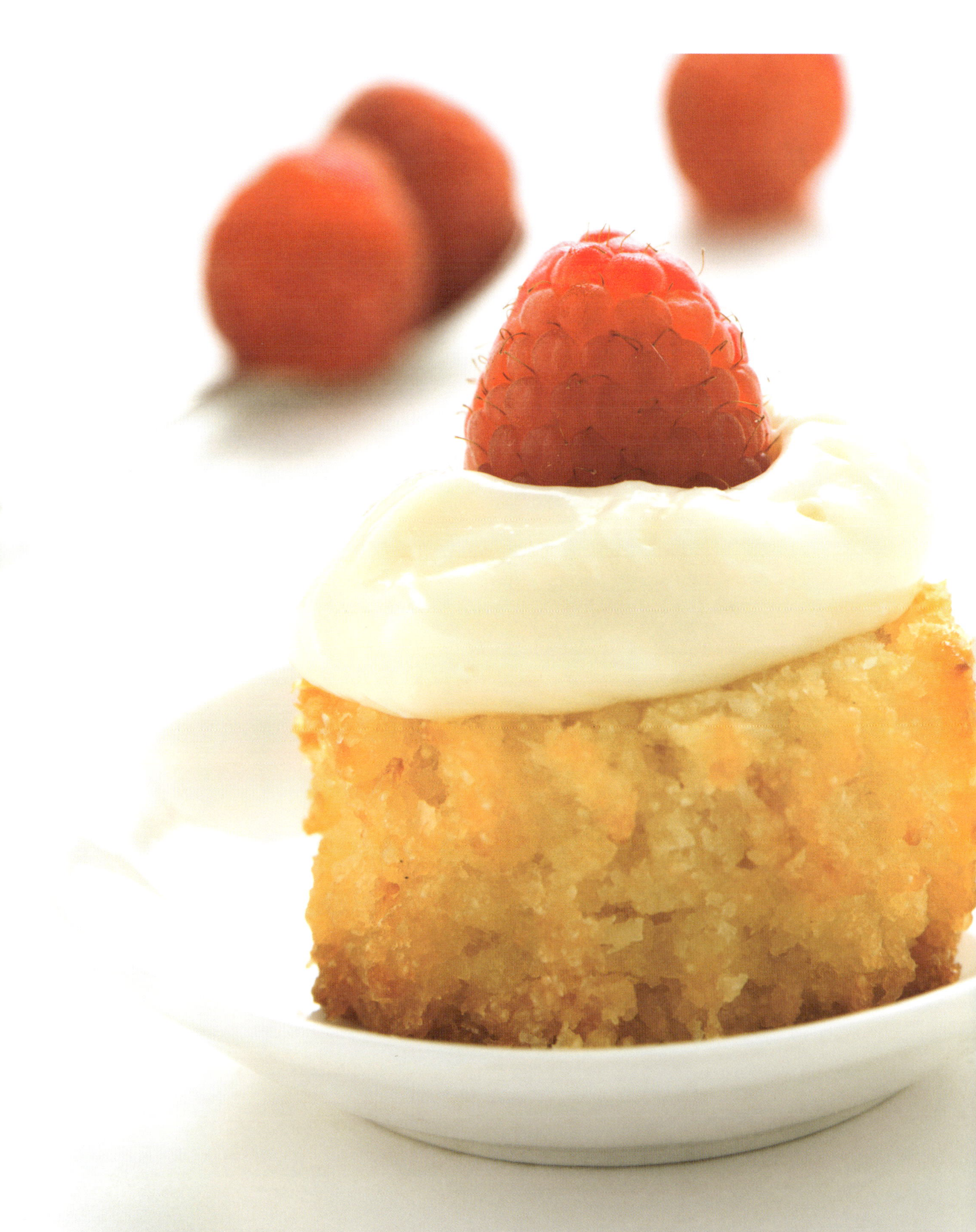

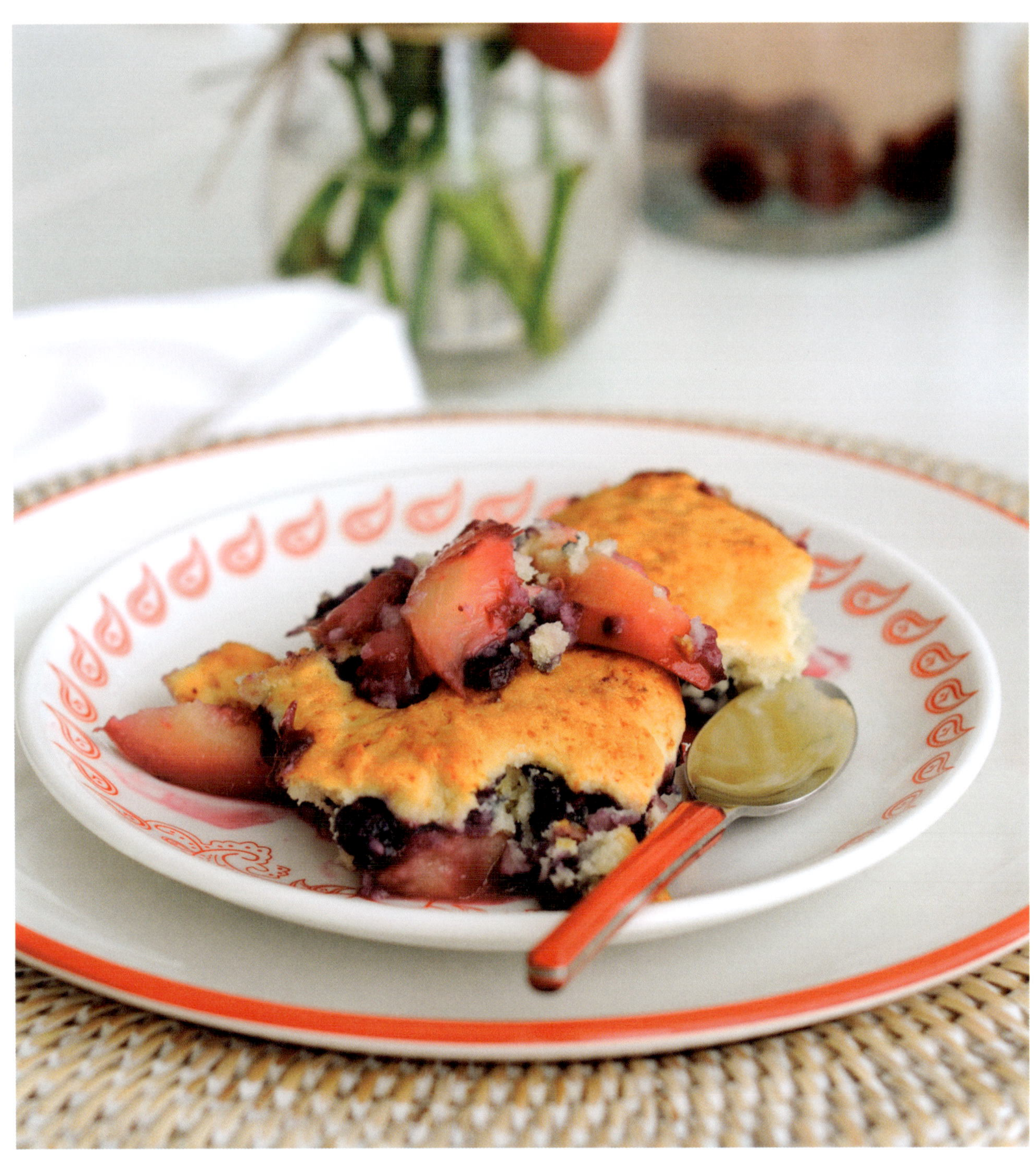

Pear and Berry Cobbler

SERVES 4

COOK TIME: HIGH 3 HRS

PEAR AND BERRY COBBLER

4 pears, peeled, cored and cut into wedges
2 cups (300g) mixed berries, frozen or fresh
⅓ cup (70g) caster sugar + 1 tbsp extra
¼ cup (30g) plain flour
1 tsp vanilla extract
1½ cups (185g) self-raising flour
120g butter
¾ cup (185ml) buttermilk

Place the pears, berries, ⅓ cup of sugar, plain flour and vanilla extract in the slow cooker and stir to combine. Stand for 10 minutes or until the berries start to release their juices.

Meanwhile, combine the self-raising flour and extra sugar in a large bowl. Add the butter and use your fingers rub the butter through the flour mixture until it resembles fine breadcrumbs.

Make a hole in the centre of the mixture and pour in the buttermilk. Stir until a soft, sticky dough is formed.

Spoon the mixture into the slow cooker with the pear and berries. Cover and cook on high for 3 hours or until the dough mixture is cooked through and the fruit is tender.

Molten Chocolate Puddings

SERVES 4-6

COOK TIME: HIGH 3 HRS

- 90g unsalted butter, softened + more for greasing
- 1½ cups (185g) self-raising flour
- 1 cup (220g) caster sugar
- ½ tsp vanilla bean paste
- 4 tbsps cacao powder
- 1 large egg, room temperature, lightly beaten
- ¾ cup (185ml) full-cream milk
- 1 cup (155g) brown sugar
- 2½ cups (625ml) boiling water
- 1½ tbsps icing sugar

Preheat the slow cooker for 20 minutes on high.

Use butter to grease six small ramekins or four large ramekins, depending on what your slow cooker can hold.

Sift the flour into a large mixing bowl, then whisk in caster sugar, butter, vanilla paste, 2 tablespoons cacao powder, egg and milk. Mix everything well then divide the batter between the ramekins.

Sprinkle the brown sugar and remaining 2 tablespoons cacao powder over the top of the puddings.

Line the bottom of the slow cooker with a folded piece of foil to create a level surface. Place the ramekins on top of the foil. Then gently pour the boiling water over the top of each. Pour extra water into the bottom of the slow cooker to come halfway up the sides of the ramekins.

Cook on high for 3 hours.

Remove the ramekins and dust the tops with icing sugar.

Serve warm.

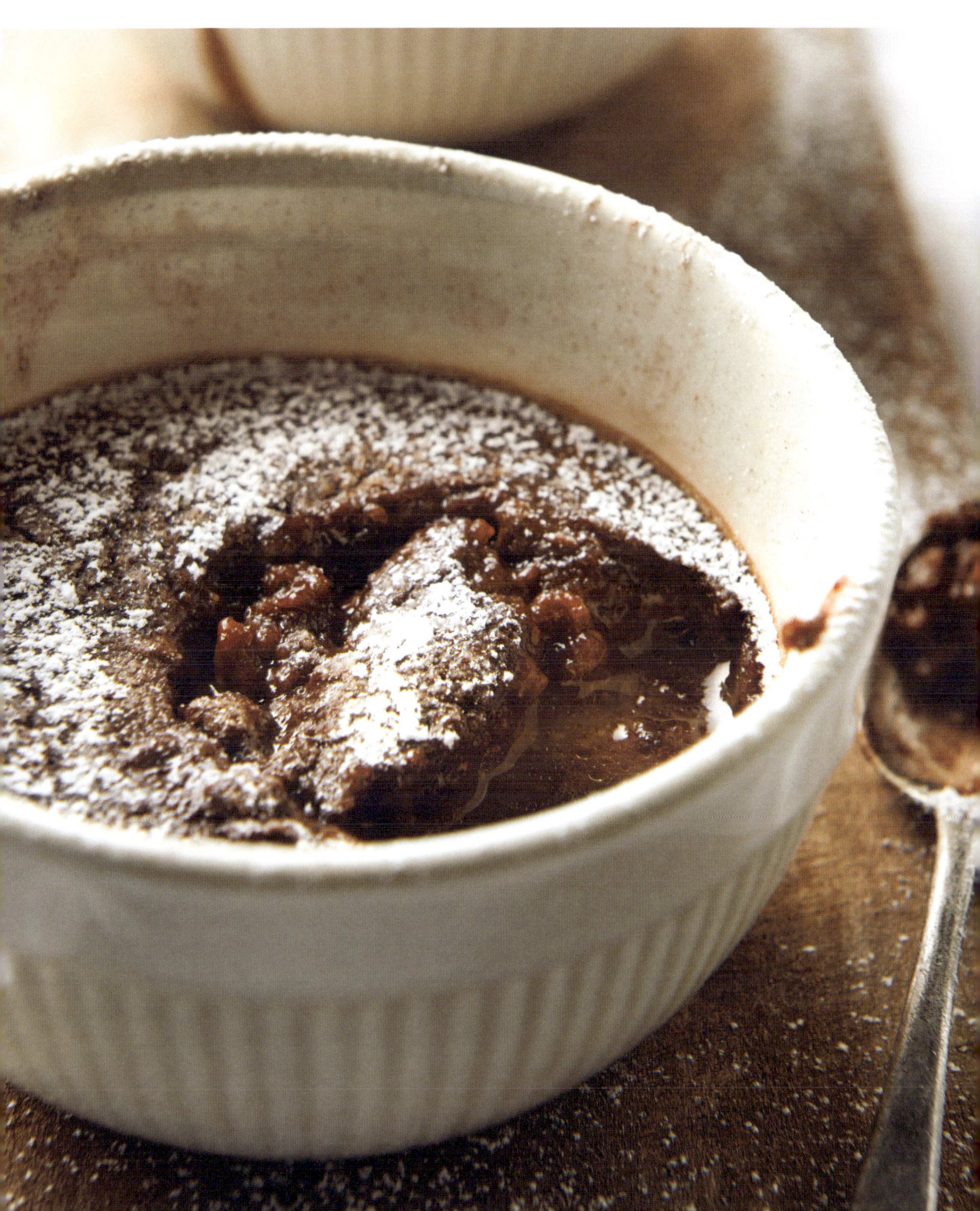

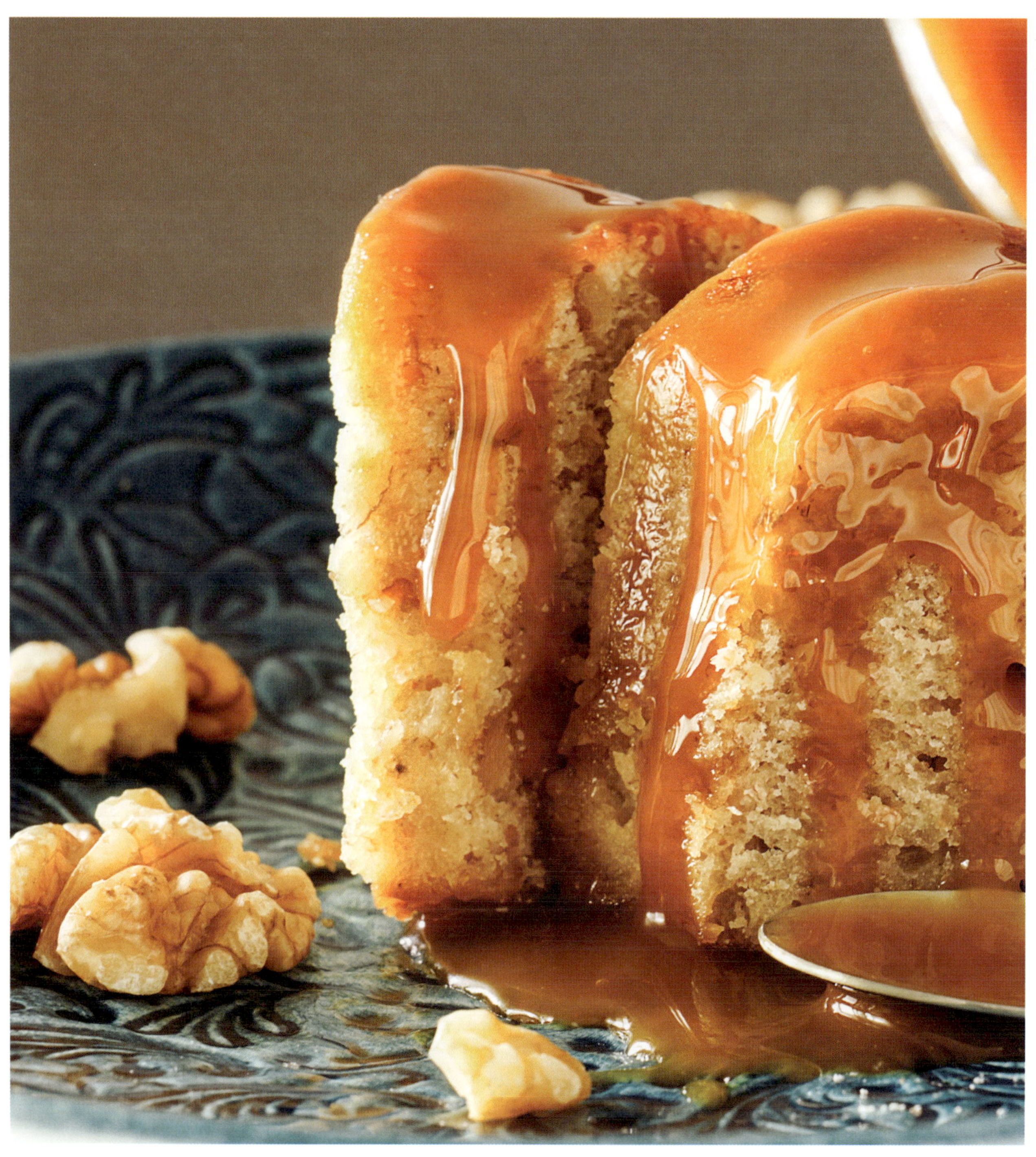

Banana Cake with Caramel Sauce

SERVES 8

COOK TIME: HIGH 1½-2 HRS

BANANA CAKE WITH CARAMEL SAUCE

Butter or cooking spray for greasing

2 large eggs

½ cup (125ml) olive oil or melted coconut oil

¾ cup (120g) light brown sugar

2 tsps vanilla extract

½ cup (30g) chopped walnuts

3 large ripe bananas, mashed

2 cups (250g) plain flour

1 tsp baking powder

½ tsp bicarbonate of soda

¼ tsp salt

1 tsp cinnamon

SAUCE

½ cup (80g) light brown sugar, packed

1½ cups (375ml) boiling water

2 tbsps butter, melted

Grease the inside of slow cooker or use a slow-cooker liner and spray with cooking spray.

In a large bowl mix together eggs, oil, sugar and vanilla. Whisk to combine. Add walnuts and banana and stir through. Add flour, baking powder, bicarb, salt and cinnamon. Mix well.

Pour mixture into slow cooker, spread out evenly with a spatula.

In another bowl add sugar, boiling water and butter. Whisk to combine. Pour over batter in slow cooker. It will turn into caramel sauce as it cooks.

Cover and cook on high for 1½-2 hours, or until the edges are set and golden brown and an inserted skewer comes out clean.

Index

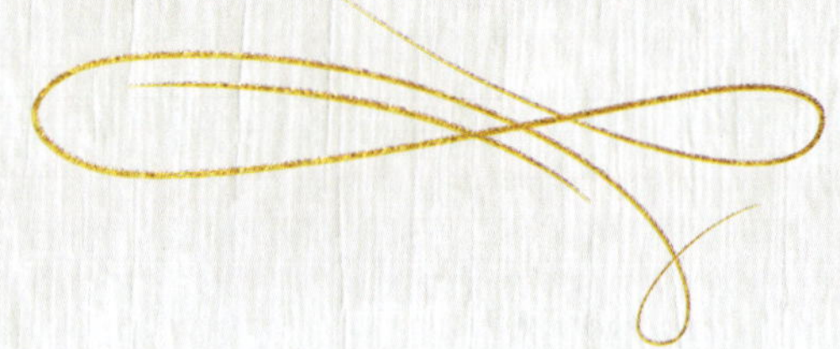

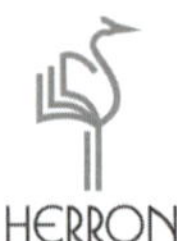

HERRON

First Published in 2024 by Herron Book Distributors Pty Ltd
14 Manton St
Morningside
QLD 4170
www.herronbooks.com

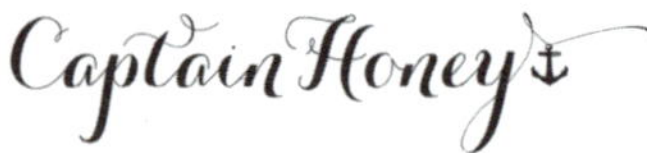

Custom book production by Captain Honey Pty Ltd
12 Station St
Bangalow
NSW 2479
www.captainhoney.com.au

Recipes in this book were previously published in: *Slow Cooker Kitchen* (2017)
6 Ingredients: Slow Cooker (2017), Slow Cooker (*Appliance Series* – 2021),
Best Ever: Slow Cooker Cookbook (2023)

Cataloguing-in-Publication. A catalogue record for this book is available from the National Library of Australia

ISBN 978-1-922944-68-9

Cover image and pg 6, 14-15, 91 © Nadine Greeff - Stocksy.com
Image pg 9 © Helen Rushbrook - Stocksy.com
All other images used under license from Shutterstock.com

Printed and bound in China

5 4 3 2 1 24 25 26 27 28

NOTES FOR THE READER

All reasonable efforts have been made to ensure the accuracy of the content in this book. Information in this book is not intended as a substitute for medical advice. The author and publisher cannot and do not accept any legal duty of care or responsibility in relation to the content in this book, and disclaim any liabilities relating to its use.

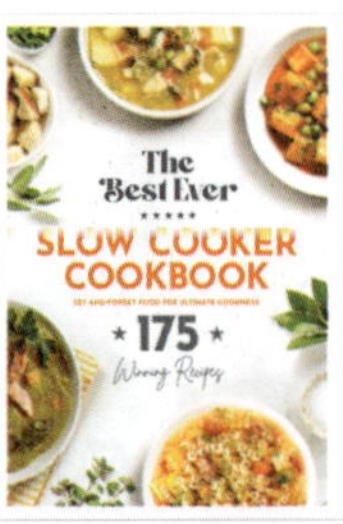

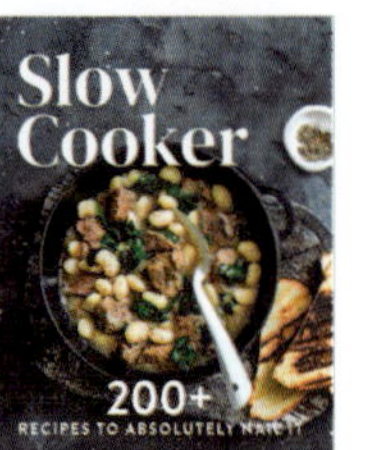

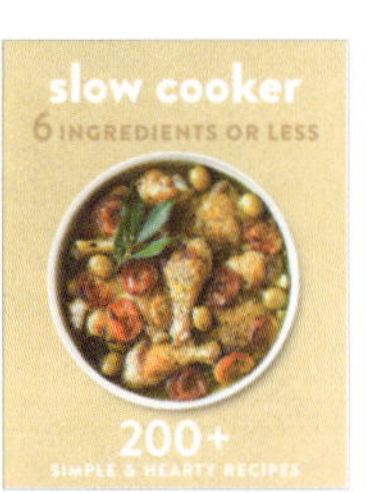

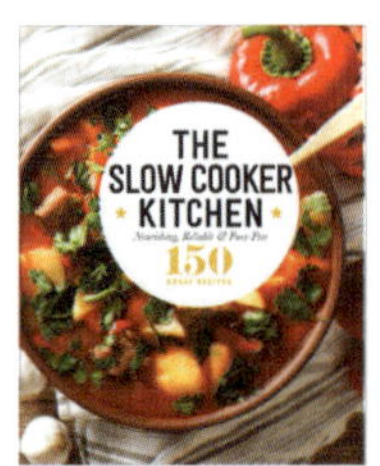

NOTE ABOUT REVIEWS

Thanks to the many customers who sent in complimentary comments about our slow cooker cookbooks, or left great reviews on the websites of our key retailers like Kmart.

With thanks, we feature a few of these reviews on the back cover of this book. We appreciate your support and are excited that you loved the recipes.